# The Health of the People

## The African Regional Health Report

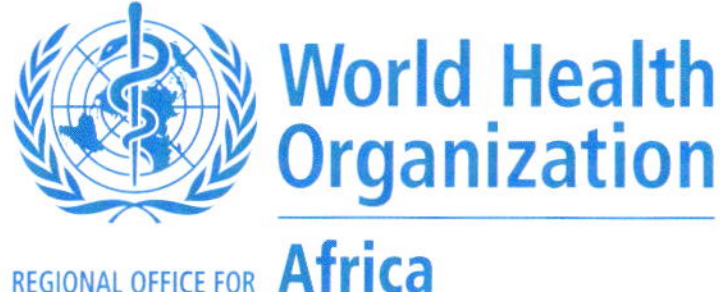

**WHO Library Cataloguing-in-Publication Data**

World Health Organization. Regional Office for Africa.
 The health of the people : the African regional health report.

 1.Public health  2.Development  3.Delivery of health care
 4.Health status  5.Africa  I.Title.

 ISBN 92 9023 103 3                    (NLM classification: WA 541 HA1)




This report has been prepared by a core team from the African Regional Office of the World Health Organization (WHO) under the general guidance of Dr. Luis G. Sambo and Dr. Paul-Samson Lusamba. The core team was coordinated by Drs. Derege Kebede, Amidou Baba-Moussa, and Doyin Oluwole; and included Drs. Rufaro Chatora, Alimata J. Diarra-Nama, Antoine Kabore, Chris Mwikisa, and James Mwanzia. The following have also contributed to the report:  Drs. Djamila Cabral, Colette Dehlot, Abayneh Desta, Antonio Filipe Jr, Joses Muthuri Kirigia, Allel Louazani, Magda Robalo, Moeti Matshidiso, Patience Mensah, Fidelis Morfaw, Seipati Mothebesoane-Anoh, Tigest Ketsela, Benjamin Nganda, Dosithée Ngo Bebe, Louis H. Ouedraogo, Martins Ovberedjo, Thebe A. Pule, Edoh Soumbey-Alley, Thomas Sukwa, Prosper Tumusiime and Rui Gama Vaz. The assistance of the following staff from WHO's African Regional Office is gratefully acknowledged: Thérèse Agossou, Sam Ajibola, Doris Durao, Wenceslas H. Kouvividila, Jennifer Nyoni, Jean Y. Ramde, and, Khoko Soumahoro.

This report was edited and produced by the team from the Bulletin of the World Health Organization: Saba Amdeselassie, Diane d'Arcis, Fiona Fleck, Laragh Gollogly, Sophie Guetaneh Aguettant, Gael Kernen, Hooman Momen, Brenda Morris, Ian G. Neil, Kaylene Selleck, Ramesh Shademani.

The following journalists contributed material to this report: Mawusi Afele (Ghana), Arthur Asiimwe (Rwanda), Judith Basutuma (Burundi), Lauren Beukes (South Africa), Richard Brass (United Kingdom), Pam Chepki (United Republic of Tanzania), Phil Dickie (Switzerland), Anil Gundooa (Mauritius), Karen Iley (Angola), Pushpa Jamieson (Malawi), Douglas Kimani (Kenya), Pelekelo Liswaniso (Zambia), Peter Masebu (Senegal), Rodrick Mukumbira (Botswana), Helen Nyambura (United Republic of Tanzania), Paul Okunlola (Nigeria), Abiodun Raufu (Nigeria), Tsitsi Singizi (Zimbabwe), Sarah Venis (Ethiopia), Charles Wendo (Uganda), Jacqui Wise (South Africa).

The assistance of the following WHO staff is gratefully acknowledged: Samira Aboubaker, James Bartram, Robert Beaglehole Michel Beusenberg Zoe Brillantes, Jose Carlos Martines, Carlos Corvalan, Timothy Evans, Michelle Funk, Maria Guraiib, Mie Inoue, Doris Ma Fat, Elizabeth Mason, Colin Mathers, Zoe Matthews, Jane McElligott, Chandika Indikadahena, Quazi Monirul Islam, Federico Montero, Tunga Namjilsuren, Ariel Pablos-Mendez, Gilles Poumerol, Thomson Prentice, Shekhar Saxena, Kenji Shibuya, Laura Sminkey, Nadia Soleman, Tessa Tan-Torres, Michel Thieren, Phyllida Travis, Colin Tutuitonga, Nathalie Van de Maele, Mark van Ommeren, Jelka Zupan.

The assistance of Don de Savigny and Kamran Abbasi is also gratefully acknowledged.


Printed in  Switzerland

**More information about this publication can be obtained from:**
WHO – Regional Office for Africa
Brazzaville / Republic of Congo

# Contents

# Boxes



# Figures

## *Tables*

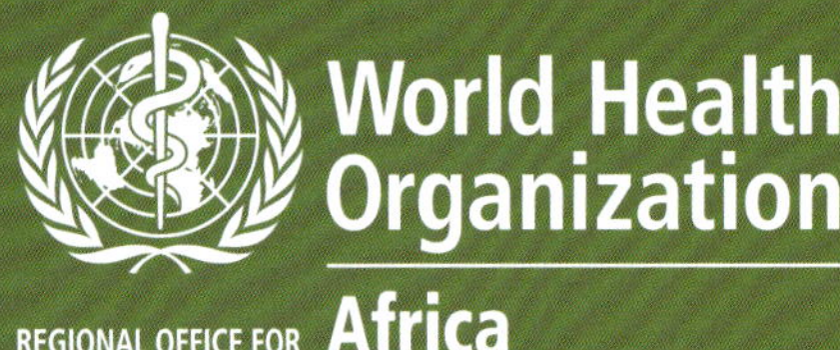


Dr Luis Gomes Sambo
Regional Director
WHO – Regional Office for Africa

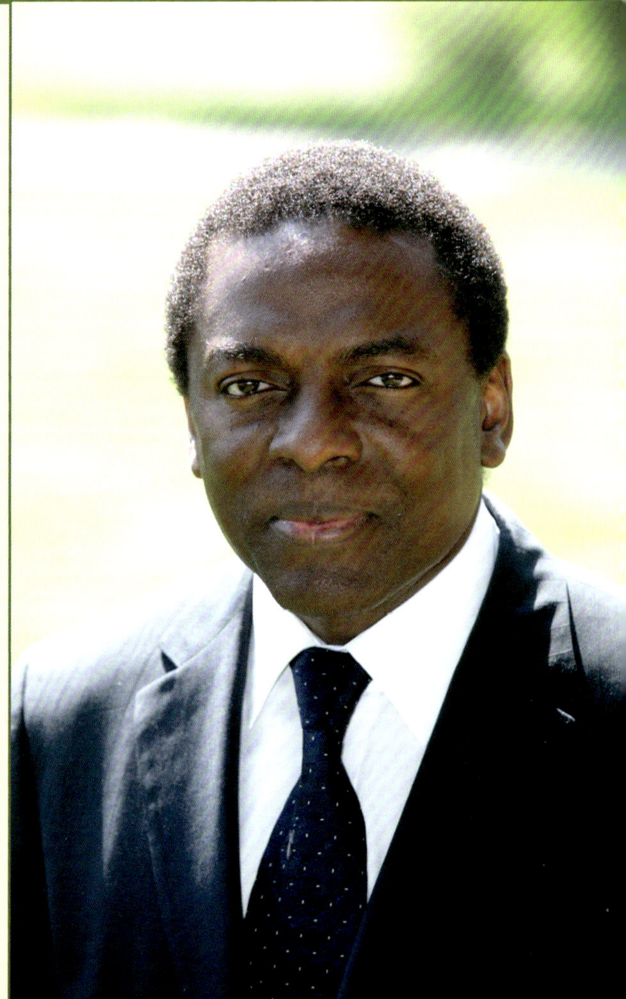

*Much can be done to prevent disease and disability through the promotion of healthy lifestyles and health education. ... We know which treatment, diagnostic and preventive methods are needed and what works in Africa. We also have the institutions. This report shows clearly that health systems are the key to providing a range of essential health care. African governments and their partners need to invest more funds to strengthen the continent's fragile health systems.*

# Message from the Regional Director

Every year millions of Africans are dying needlessly of diseases that are preventable and treatable. *The Health of the People: the African Regional Health Report* provides vital reading for those who want to understand why and what can be done about it.

The vast majority of people living in Africa have yet to benefit from advances in medical research and public health. The result is an immense burden of death and disease that is devastating for African societies. This report looks at: HIV/AIDS, tuberculosis and malaria, and the pregnancy-related conditions that kill mothers and babies. It also highlights the lesser known problems of chronic diseases, such as diabetes and hypertension, and other noncommunicable conditions, such as mental illness and injuries.

The challenges are many, including: weak and fragmented health systems; inadequate resources for scaling up proven interventions; limited access to the health services and technologies that are available; poor management of human resources for health; recurrent natural and man-made disasters and emergencies; and extreme poverty.

And yet these pages do not merely recount tales of misery, indeed, they describe in detail some of Africa's public health success stories that may serve as a models for others in the continent. Much can be done to prevent disease and disability through the promotion of healthy lifestyles and health education. ... And when people become sick with malaria or suffer with other health problems, the solutions are within our grasp. ... We know which treatment, diagnostic and preventive methods are needed and what works in Africa. We also have the institutions. WHO is working tirelessly with WHO's 46 Member States in the African Region to help build and reinforce health systems that are central to improving the health of the people across the Region.

This report shows clearly that health systems are the key to providing a range of essential health care. African governments and their partners need to invest more funds to strengthen the continent's fragile health systems.

The challenge for African governments and their partners is to coordinate the provision of health care more effectively than ever before, and to ensure that all funds are used in an accountable manner to the benefit of the African people. On behalf of the African Regional Office of WHO, I would like to express our gratitude to the 46 Member States and our partners in the Region for their commitment to improving the health of their people.

Dr Luis Gomes Sambo
Regional Director
WHO – Regional Office for Africa

*This report is an excellent review of the public health situation across the WHO African Region, that includes 46 African countries that are all Member States of the African Union. ... The African Union Commission fully supports the central message of this report: that African governments and their partners need to do more to build and reinforce health systems to deliver essential health-care interventions to people living on this continent.*

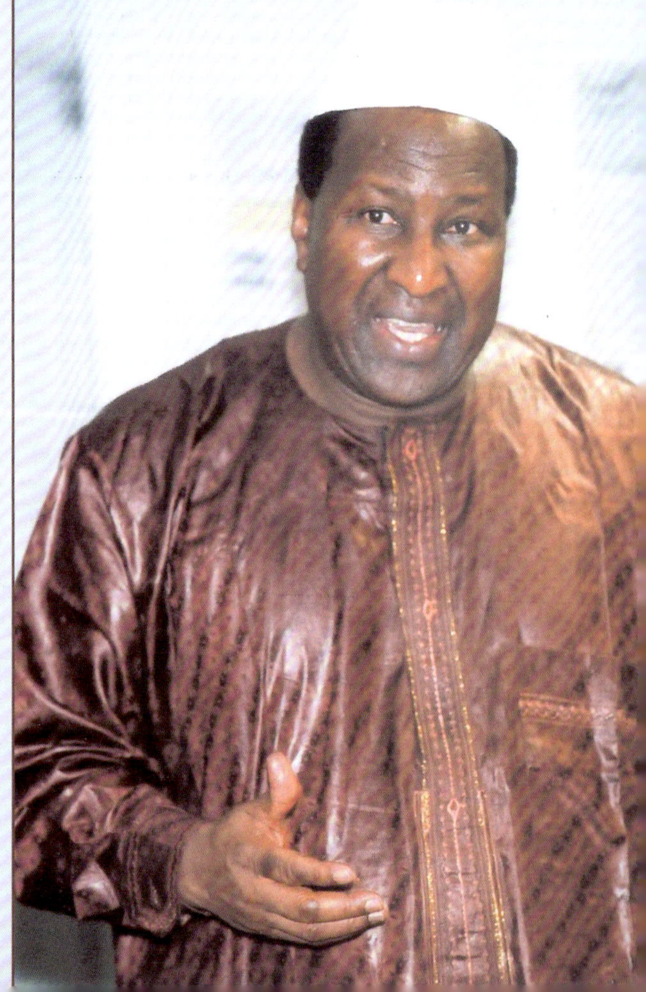

# *Foreword*

# Chairperson of the African Union Commission

Public health in Africa has come under the international spotlight in recent years. The sheer enormity of the disease burden in African countries and the often inadequate response has prompted many regional and international initiatives. More funds than ever before have been pledged for health in Africa, yet many problems prevail.

This report is an excellent review of the public health situation across the WHO African Region, that includes 46 African countries that are all Member States of the African Union. *The health of the people: the African regional health report* provides vital insight into why Africa has such a heavy burden of premature death and disease, but also a valuable overview of the interventions that work and need to be extended to everyone who needs them.

The African Union Commission has been working closely with WHO's African Regional Office in several public health areas. In May 2006, the African Union Commission, in collaboration with United Nations agencies and other development partners held a Special Summit on HIV/AIDS, tuberculosis and malaria in Abuja, Nigeria, to look at progress so far and the way forward to achieve universal access to treatment for these diseases by 2010.

In collaboration with WHO and other United Nations' agencies, the African Union launched a campaign this year to prevent HIV/AIDS in Africa. We want to promote widespread awareness of HIV and how it is caused through media campaigns and public health education. We want more Africans to embrace HIV counselling and testing and we want governments to ensure that HIV prevention services are available — along with antiretroviral therapy — for everyone who needs them.

Violence is a major public health problem in Africa. The African Union's 53 Member States declared 2005 the African Year of Prevention of Violence, and the African Union and WHO are working closely on violence prevention in Africa. The African Union supports key health partnerships and initiatives, including the STOP–TB partnership and the Road Map on the Reduction of Maternal and Newborn Morbidity and Mortality in Africa.

Much progress has been made in the fight against polio by the Global Polio Eradication Initiative, but more efforts by African governments and their partners are needed to ensure that new outbreaks are quickly brought under control and that high immunity levels are maintained in all populations through vaccination. The African Union has been working closely with WHO and other partners on a preparedness and response plan to reduce the risk of bird flu and human pandemic influenza.

The African Union Commission fully supports the central message of this report: that African governments and their partners need to do more to build and reinforce health systems to deliver essential health-care interventions to people living on this continent.

H.E. Prof. Alpha Omar Konaré,
Chairperson of the African Union Commission

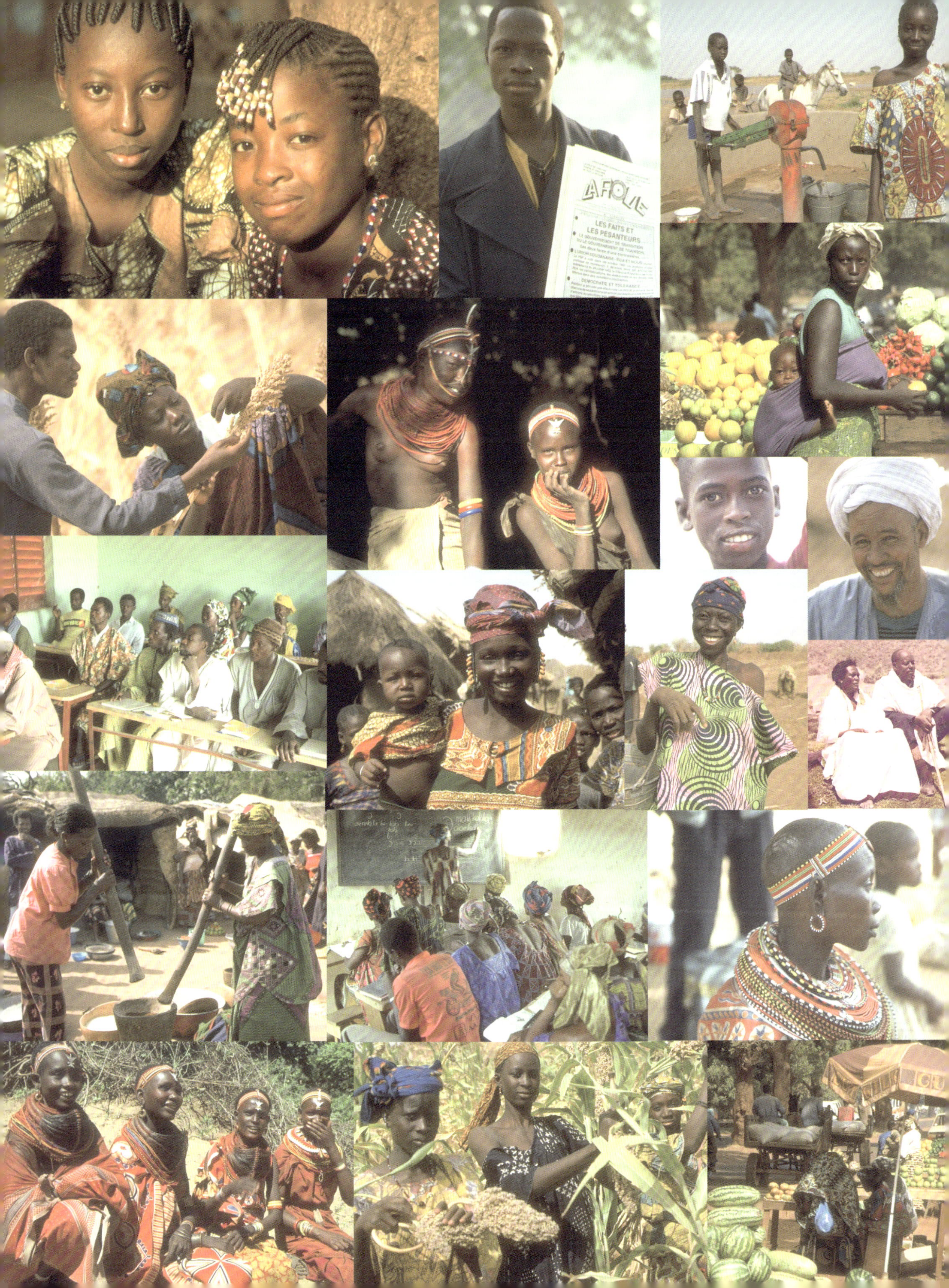

# *Executive summary*

## *The health of the people*

This report comes at a crucial time, when much attention is being devoted to Africa and when African countries are finding their own voice and their own solutions to their problems. *The health of the people: the African regional health report* provides an overview of the public health situation across the 46 Member States of the African Region of the World Health Organization. This report charts progress made to date in fighting disease and promoting health in the African Region. It reviews the success stories and looks at areas where more efforts are needed to improve people's health.

The central message of the report is clear: African countries will not develop economically and socially without substantial improvements in the health of their people. The health-care interventions — treatments, diagnostic and preventive methods — that are needed in this Region are known. The challenge for African countries and their partners is to deliver these to the people who need them, and the best way to do this is to establish well-functioning health systems.

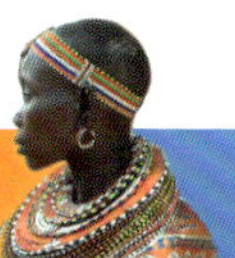

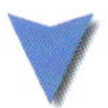

## Chapter 1: *Health and development in Africa*

Economic development is impossible without major investments to apply tried-and-tested health-care interventions that work. This chapter shows how much the severe burden of disease hampers social progress and economic development in many African countries. Ill-health pushes people into the poverty trap. Poverty is a major factor determining ill-health, as well as being both a cause and an outcome of ill-health. Several studies have sought to quantify the macroeconomic impact of the disease burden (see Table a).

Governments in the African Region and their development partners need to invest more in health care. Recent rapid economic growth in some African countries provides an opportunity to do this. Their partners need to increase donor funds to scale up tried-and-tested public health interventions. A paradigm shift is needed: African countries and their partners need to address the underlying factors that determine ill-health. Investing in health, therefore, means investing in water, sanitation, environment, education, women's empowerment, governance and other related sectors.

WHO's African Region lags behind other regions of the world in terms of human development. This limited development is largely attributable to the Region's immense burden of infectious diseases, particularly that of HIV/AIDS, tuberculosis and malaria. This chapter describes the macroeconomic impact of the Region's heavy burden of infectious diseases as well as of unhealthy environments; maternal, newborn and child death and disease; and the growing burden of noncommunicable diseases.

There are positive indications that things are changing as Member States of the Region and their partners continue to demonstrate the will to address poverty and development by bringing health issues to the forefront. This is demonstrated by regional initiatives, such as the New Partnership for Africa's Development (NEPAD) and efforts by the G8 and global financial institutions to cancel debt and encourage least-developed countries to channel

Table a
Burden of disease in the African Region 2002

| Burden of disease in DALYs* by cause and mortality stratum in the African Region | | |
|---|---|---|
| | | Mortality stratum |
| | High child, high adult (000) | High child, very high adult (000) |
| 1   AIDS | 14 620 | 49 343 |
| 2   Malaria | 20 070 | 20 785 |
| 3   Respiratory infections | 18 976 | 16 619 |
| 4   Perinatal conditions | 10 869 | 10 485 |
| 5   Diarrhoea | 11 548 | 11 689 |
| 6   **Top five subtotal (1 – 5)** | **76 083** | **108 921** |
| 7   Other communicable diseases | 39 234 | 41 484 |
| 8   Communicable diseases (6 and 7) | 115 317 | 150 405 |
| 9   Noncommunicable diseases | 30 124 | 34 727 |
| 10   Injuries | 14 974 | 15 829 |
| Total   **Total (8 – 10)** | **160 415** | **200 961** |

The Member States of the Region have been divided into mortality strata on the basis of their levels of mortality in children under five years of age and in males aged 15–59 years as described on pp. 156–7 of the 2004 *World health report*.

*   See glossary for explanation.

Source: *The world health report 2004*. Geneva. World Health Organization; 2004.

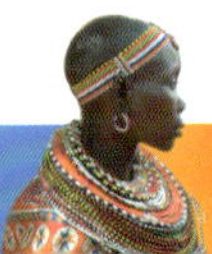

the resulting savings into health and related sectors. Chapter 1 reviews these and other current initiatives to combat high mortality and morbidity in Africa, including regional efforts, such as the Abuja Declaration and international efforts, including the United Kingdom's Commission for Africa and the UN Millennium Development Goals (MDGs). More needs to be done to encourage African nations to honour the pledge they made in Abuja to allocate 15% of their national budgets to health. Similarly, developed countries should honour the pledge they made to committing 0.7% of their gross domestic product (GDP) to development assistance.

The challenges for public health in the African Region are enormous. But with true commitment and resolve by governments in the Region and their development partners, these challenges can be overcome, helping countries in the Region to move closer to achieving the MDGs.

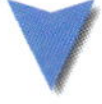

## Chapter 2: *Maternal, newborn and child health*

This chapter describes Africa's "silent epidemic", the tragedy that millions of mothers, newborn babies and children die every year from preventable, treatable causes. It summarizes the trends of death and disease among mothers during pregnancy and childbirth, and of their children in the African Region. Progress in this area of health was made in the 1970s and 1980s, as African states established health-care systems providing antenatal and emergency obstetric care. Improved child survival became a global phenomenon during those years, largely due to immunization and the success of oral rehydration therapy for diarrhoeal diseases. But since the early 1990s, little or no progress has been made in maternal, newborn and child health in many parts of the Region largely due to the HIV/AIDS epidemic and armed conflicts. In some parts of the Region, progress in maternal, newborn and child health has been reversed.

Major global efforts to address the situation have so far produced limited results. Few countries in the Region are likely to achieve MDG 4 on child health and MDG 5 on maternal health (see Fig. a and Fig. b). The obstacles and challenges are many: conflict and emergencies, HIV/AIDS, inadequate resource allocation and weak health systems. Renewed efforts are now under way to make motherhood safer; prevent mother-to-child transmission of HIV; provide family planning services; and manage childhood illness.

This chapter looks at some success stories, for example, in the countries and districts that have improved maternal, newborn and child health in the Region. It reviews the tried-and-tested interventions, such as skilled birth attendance, immunization and family planning, that need to be scaled up and replicated throughout the Region. Furthermore, women need to receive better education to improve their economic and social status and, in turn, their own health and that of

**Fig, a**

Under-5 mortality (deaths per 1000 live births) in the African Region



Based on data from: *The world health report, 2005.* Geneva: World Health Organization; 2005.

**Fig. b**

Maternal mortality (deaths per 100 000 live births) in the African Region



Based on data from: *The world health report, 2005.* Geneva: World Health Organization; 2005.

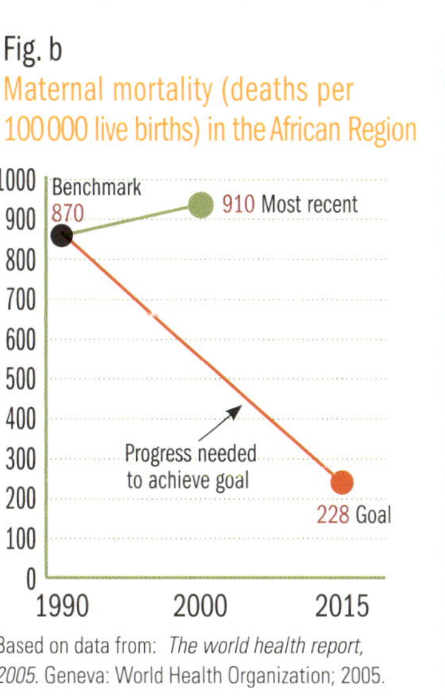

their families. Governments in the Region have committed themselves to improving the health of mothers, newborn babies and children. Now they need to act by allocating more funds to this vital, but neglected area of public health.

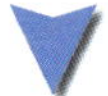

## Chapter 3: *Infectious diseases in Africa*

Infectious diseases are a major obstacle to human development in the African Region. This chapter recalls that people in Africa suffer from a vast range of preventable and treatable infectious diseases. It reviews the challenges for infectious disease control in the Region and shows how factors, such as climate, geography and parasites, make this task especially difficult.

Chapter 3 charts the Region's successes in controlling certain infectious diseases, such as river blindness and leprosy, as well as vaccine-preventable diseases, such as polio. It looks at the diseases in the Region that are prone to epidemics, such as cholera, meningitis, Lassa fever and yellow fever, and the neglected diseases, such as Buruli ulcer and sleeping sickness.

The chapter also takes a detailed look at three diseases of major public health concern: HIV/AIDS, tuberculosis and malaria, which kill more than three million people in the Region every year. HIV/AIDS prevalence is particularly high in southern African countries (see Fig. c). This high prevalence increases the occurrence of other infectious diseases, particularly tuberculosis. However, the shortage of health workers is hampering efforts to provide health care for this and other problems.

Chapter 3 describes the devastating effect of these three infectious diseases on society — hardship, impoverishment, countless lives lost and reduced productivity — and how governments are forced to divert scarce resources to tackle these diseases, spinning countries on an inescapable cycle of poverty and ill-health. But it also charts the progress made in the Region in rolling out antiretroviral treatment for HIV/AIDS in recent years.

It outlines some of the solutions that work in the Region. Tried-and-tested public health interventions — for example the provision

### Fig. c

HIV prevalence among 15–24-year-olds in selected sub-Saharan African countries, 2001–03

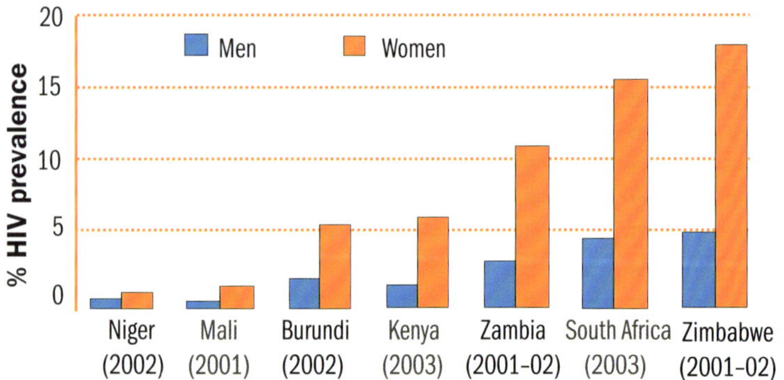


Sources: Burundi (Enquête Nationale de Séroprévalence de l'infection par le VIH au Burundi. Bujumbura, Décembre 2002). Kenya (Kenya Demographic and Health Survey 2003). Mali (Enquête Démographique et de Santé. Mali 2001). Niger (Enquête Nationale de Séroprévalence de l'infection par le VIH dans la population générale agée de 15 à 49 ans au Niger (2002)). South Africa (Pettifor AE, Rees HV, Steffenson A, Hlongwa-Madikizela L, MacPhal C, Vermaak K, Kleinschmidt I: HIV and sexual behaviour among young South Africans: a national survey of 15-24 year olds. Johannesburg: Reproductive Health Research Unit, University of Witwatersrand, 2004). Zambia (Zambia Demographic and Health Survey 2001-2002). Zimbabwe (The Zimbabwe Young Adult Survey 2001-2002) .

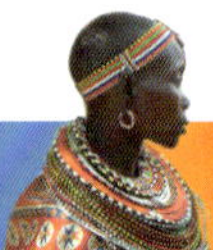

of universal HIV testing and counselling and simplified treatment for HIV/AIDS — need to be applied more widely.

These simplified, low-cost approaches to treatment need to be scaled up so that they are available to all the people in the Region who need them. Research and development is needed to find more effective medicines for diseases such as tuberculosis and other neglected diseases and vaccines for malaria and HIV/AIDS. Meanwhile, countries in the Region need to promote safe sex and more countries need to provide HIV testing and counselling to prevent further HIV infections and reverse the AIDS pandemic. Political will backed by financial support is crucial to scaling up tried-and-tested control methods that are specific to each disease.

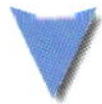

# Chapter 4: *Noncommunicable diseases in Africa*

Noncommunicable diseases and injuries constitute a growing public health problem in the African Region, but at the same time represent one of the most neglected areas of public health. Although the noncommunicable diseases and injuries burden represents 27% of the Region's total disease burden (see Table b), African countries and their partners do not devote resources that are adequate to address the problem. The risk factors for noncommunicable and chronic diseases — such as unhealthy diet and lack of physical exercise, are on the rise in many African countries. The result is that stroke, diabetes, cancer and heart disease — diseases that are seen as affecting mainly wealthy industrialized countries — are becoming increasingly prevalent in Africa and represent an emerging threat.

Chapter 4 looks closely at Africa's growing "double burden" of infectious and noncommunicable disease. It charts Africa's lesser known toll of ill-health, including a growing burden of cardiovascular diseases, malnutrition and obesity, cancer, injuries, blindness, mental illnesses, genetic and oral diseases. Some of these conditions are a consequence of infectious diseases, such as cervical cancer, while others, such as noma, are specific to this Region.

There is a huge unmet need in terms of addressing noncommunicable diseases, mental health and injuries in the African Region. This state of affairs must be rectified. The challenges are many and include a scarcity of resources; inadequate awareness and commitment to this area; and limited data. Donor agencies and research institutions, too, are neglecting the growing burden of noncommunicable diseases and injuries in the Region.

The chapter gives an overview of tried-and-tested solutions for tackling the problems. These include: legislation and marketing which can be particularly effective to control tobacco; mental health legislation; promotion of healthy diets and lifestyles is also an effective, low-cost solution; and low-cost disease management programmes.

Table b

Leading causes of death in the African Region, 2002

| Rank | All ages |
| --- | --- |
| 1 | HIV/AIDS |
| 2 | Malaria |
| 3 | Lower respiratory infections |
| 4 | Diarrhoeal diseases |
| 5 | Perinatal conditions |
| 6 | Cerebrovascular disease |
| 7 | Tuberculosis |
| 8 | Ischaemic heart disease |
| 9 | Measles |
| 10 | Road traffic crashes |
| 11 | Violence |
| 12 | Whooping cough |
| 13 | Chronic obstructive pulmonary disease |
| 14 | Protein–energy malnutrition |
| 15 | Nephritis and nephrosis |
| 16 | Syphilis |
| 17 | War |
| 18 | Tetanus |
| 19 | Diabetes mellitus |
| 20 | Drowning |

Source: *Global Burden of Disease 2002.*

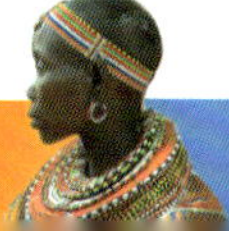

Priority should be given to primary prevention of noncommunicable diseases by tackling risk factors, such as diet, physical activity, alcohol consumption and tobacco use. Secondary prevention should focus on controlling risk factors among those affected, with special emphasis on obesity, high blood pressure, high blood sugar and high blood lipid levels. The third approach is tertiary prevention through proper clinical management of cardiovascular disease, chronic obstructive respiratory disease, diabetes, and cancer. Similar approaches are needed for mental health disorders and oral health.

Government departments, such as health, transport and education, need to work together to introduce measures to reduce the risk of injuries and noncommunicable diseases, such as seat-belt laws and promotion of healthy diets. There also needs to be more collaboration between government, nongovernmental organizations and the media.

Many developed countries are only now realizing the value of health promotion strategies, such as tobacco control. African countries have the opportunity to learn from the mistakes made in developed countries and to act early before the growing epidemic of noncommunicable disease gets out of control.

## Chapter 5: *Health and the environment in Africa*

People living in the African Region face a number of environmental health risks. High levels of air pollution, both within and outside the home, unsafe water supplies, inadequate sanitation and unhygienically prepared food are widespread in many parts of the Region. There are also emerging environmental risks to health in the African Region, such as ecosystem degradation and climate change.

Rapid urbanization has forced millions of people to live in shanty towns without basic services, meanwhile day-to-day environmental threats to people's health are made worse by armed conflict and natural disasters. There is a growing problem of industrial pollution, the management of solid and liquid waste, and of medical waste.

This chapter summarizes trends in the environmental risk factors for health in the Region, it outlines the efforts to tackle them and underscores areas where more needs to be done to tackle these factors. Wider coverage of clean water and sanitation, and wider provision of sewage and waste disposal would be major steps towards a healthier environment (see Fig. d).

The challenges for governments are immense. Widespread poverty limits people's ability to address environmental problems. Success in tackling environmental heath problems depends very much on collaboration between ministries and agencies.

Chapter 5 describes some success stories, where communities have used locally developed technologies and innovations that are effective, affordable and sustainable.

**Fig. d**

Improved water source (% of population without access) in sub-Saharan Africa

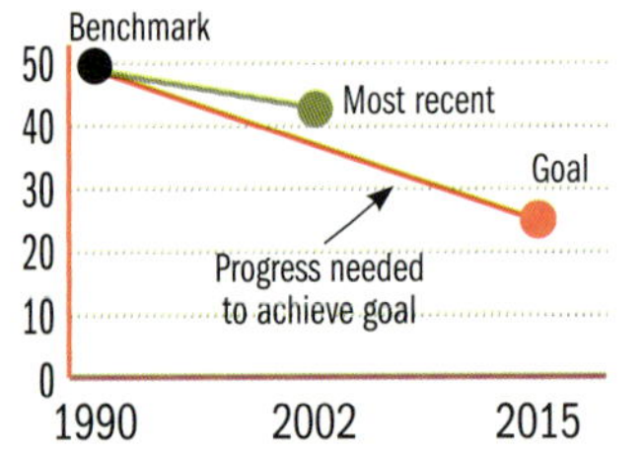


Source: WHO/UNICEF Joint Monitoring Programme for Water Supply and Sanitation — Water for life: make it happen. 2005.

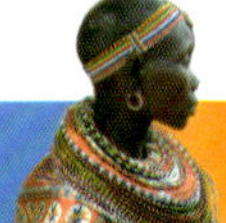

Low-cost, sustainable solutions for water and sanitation need to be scaled up. Countries in the Region and international organizations need to work more closely together to prevent and resolve conflicts. Governments in the Region also need to scale up food safety and hygiene education. Closer cooperation between government ministries and sectors in those countries is also key to making the environment more healthy.

WHO has several strategies to address these issues. For example, WHO's strategy on health and the environment urges governments to develop environmental health policies and to make communities more aware of the relationship between the environment and public health.

Community-management programmes run by WHO and other agencies using the Participatory Hygiene and Sanitation Transformation, Demand-Responsive Approach and Ecological Sanitation, along with the Africa 2000 Water and Sanitation programme, have all shown results. Through the Healthy Settings approach, several countries in the Region are for the first time, addressing complex urban health problems in a holistic way.

WHO programmes aim at empowering people and improving conditions at community and workplace level to prevent and reduce factors that prevent communities and individuals from achieving better economic and positive health outcomes. In this way, WHO helps countries to improve their capacity to plan, implement and evaluate their programmes to inform policies and implementation plans.

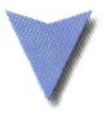

## Chapter 6: *National health systems — Africa's big public health challenge*

One of Africa's major public health challenges is building and reinforcing health systems capable of delivering essential health care to the population. Countries in the African Region have weak and dysfunctional health systems. Several key elements are required for health systems to function properly: adequate numbers of skilled health workers, basic infrastructure and equipment; essential medicines and supplies; and health financing systems. It is also important to establish effective health information systems, including vital registration, to measure the scale of a given health problem in order to gauge the appropriate response.

Health care in these countries is provided by a mix of public and private providers, often resulting in "vertical" or single-disease/issue programmes. Funds for health care come from a variety of public and private sources, including donor funds. Some governments have started to take a "sector-wide approach" to improve

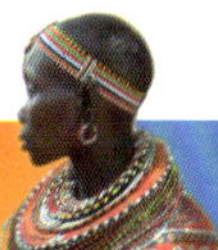

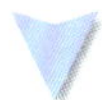



the coordination of those funds so that they can be used more effectively and to avoid duplication.

The chapter closes with one of the report's key messages: that establishing well-functioning health systems is essential to addressing the many health problems described throughout this report. Furthermore, health systems need to be tailored to their specific setting, whether urban or rural.

To strengthen health systems, governments of Member States need to forge strong collaboration with other partners at national and local level, including the private sector, civil society and communities. Universal access to health care can only be achieved by scaling up essential health system interventions. This will be difficult to achieve without adequate investment and without taking the delivery of essential health services as close to the communities as possible through strong and effective district health systems. Stronger health systems can act as a bridge to social stability, peace and prosperity throughout the Region. ■

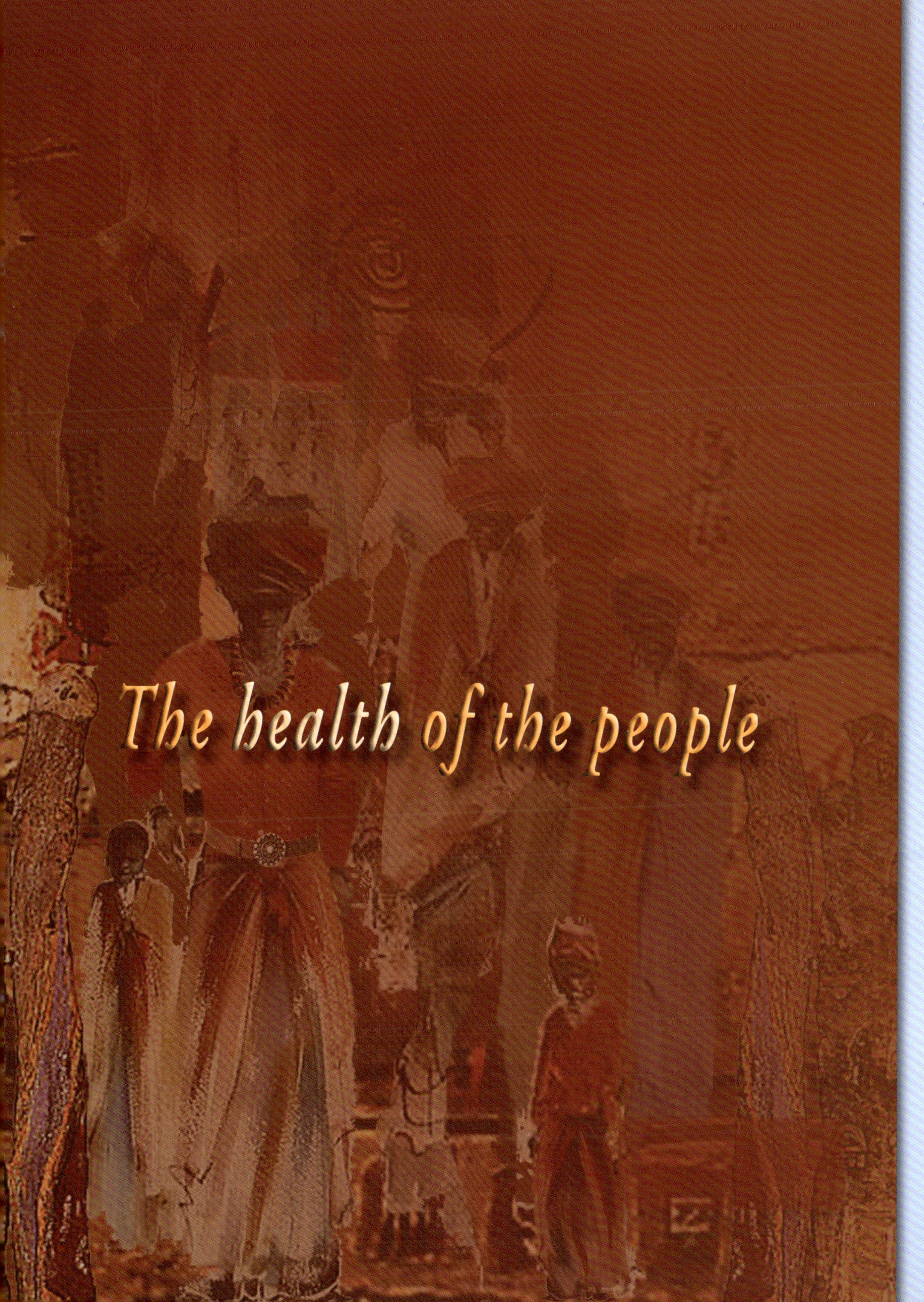



# The health of the people

*Improving the health of the 738 million people in the 46 Member States of the African Region of the World Health Organization (WHO) is absolutely essential, along with education, good governance and sound economic policy. Improvements in health can spur social progress and economic growth, but cannot be achieved without increasing current levels of investment in health in this Region.*

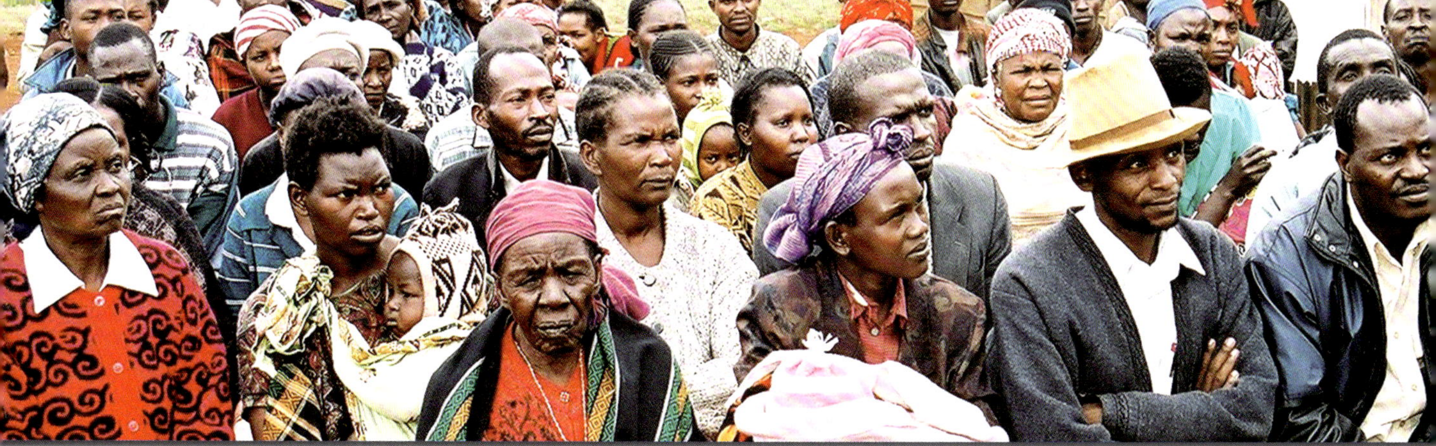

# The *health* of the people

The first African Regional Health Report comes at a crucial time for Africa, a time when the continent has come into sharp focus. Major international efforts have recently got under way to reduce poverty and achieve other Millennium Development Goals (MDGs) in Africa. In July 2005, the Group of Eight (G8) industrialized nations provided debt relief and increased aid to African countries. In December 2005, the 148 Members of the World Trade Organization (WTO) agreed on a package of trade and aid measures intended to help the world's poorest countries. The package is a small first step towards the "trade-for-aid" goal of the Doha Development Round: to abolish tariffs on African products and subsidies paid to farmers in wealthy countries, tariffs and subsidies that make it difficult if not impossible for African farmers to compete internationally.

This report shows that improving the health of the 738 million people (in 2005) in the 46 Member States of the African Region of the World Health Organization (WHO) is absolutely essential, along with education, good governance and sound economic policy. Improvements in health can spur social progress and economic growth, but cannot be achieved without increasing current levels of investment in health in this Region.

The need to invest more in health is not only a moral imperative to alleviate suffering and to address a basic human right to health, but — in today's interconnected, globalized world — it also makes economic sense, and can help pave the way to a more prosperous and secure future for all. At the same time, efforts to improve health need to be closely coordinated and monitored as never before to ensure that funds are used to optimal effect and in an accountable way.

This report provides an overview for governments, civil society and health professionals in Africa, as well as for donors and other members of the international community. It reviews how the health of the people in the African Region has developed over the last 10–15 years and tracks progress — or lack of it — towards achieving the health-related MDGs by 2015. Outlined are the main public health challenges this Region faces as well as the initiatives and programmes intended to tackle these, and their successes to date.

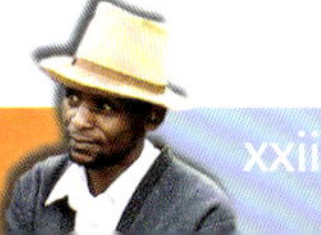

The solutions described in this report draw on the advances in diagnosis, treatment and prevention of major diseases that have led to greater life expectancy in the rest of the world, but from which most people in Africa have yet to benefit. The path to success in providing people in Africa with these basic services is in implementing the solutions and strategies outlined in these pages: strategies that are known to work in this Region, strategies that invest in the welfare of the African people.

The starting point for improving public health is firm political resolve on the part of Member States of the African Region (see map and definition on p. xxv) andtheir partners. In order to make progress, some Member States could increase spending on health, while donor countries could seek ways to provide a more reliable and sustainable flow of aid. In this way, health can be a bridge to economic prosperity for every African nation.

# The challenges confronting Africa

Success in improving public health in Africa depends on renewed efforts and determination to overcome a number of challenges in the African Region.

A child born in Africa faces more health risks than a child born in other parts of the world. Such a child has more than a 50% chance of being malnourished, a high risk of being HIV-positive at birth, while malaria, diarrhoeal diseases and acute respiratory diseases account for 51% of deaths. A child born in the African Region is more likely to lose his or her mother due to complications in childbirth or to HIV/AIDS, while that child has a life expectancy of just 47 years, and is very likely — at least once in his or her short life — to be affected by drought, famine, flood or civil war, or to become a refugee.

People living in the African Region are more exposed to a heavy and wide-ranging burden of disease partly because of this Region's unique geography and climate. These factors make malaria, for instance, more intractable in Africa than it is elsewhere. At the same time, noncommunicable diseases and injuries are emerging as significant contributors to the disease burden.

Nowhere has HIV/AIDS killed such large proportions of the population as it has in Africa. Nowhere has the old scourge of tuberculosis re-emerged to fuel the HIV/AIDS epidemic as it has in the African Region. No other region has witnessed so many armed conflicts and other humanitarian emergencies.

Nowhere is poverty so prevalent. The population of the African Region represents about 10% of the world's population, but an estimated 45% or more of its people live below the poverty line, on less than US$ 1 a day. About 330 million people in this Region — one-third of the world's 1.1 billion poor — are caught in this poverty trap, in which low household incomes lead to low household consumption and, in turn, the countries in which they live have low capacity and low productivity. Agricultural productivity is lower than in other regions due to unreliable water supply, inadequate irrigation and poor soil quality. High transportation costs for the continent's interior, due to the lack of navigable rivers and the slow diffusion of technology, also hamper development.

Nowhere has life expectancy reversed so sharply as in the African Region. Life expectancy at birth in this Region was 45 years in 1970. This rose to 49.2 years in the late 1980s but fell during the 1990s and early 2000s to just 47 years. Overall life expectancy for people born in the African Region in 2002 would be 54 years, if it were not for about six years of life lost due to the sole impact of HIV/AIDS.

The African Region faces some of the same constraints as other regions. International trade agreements that benefit the world's wealthier countries make it difficult for poorer countries to compete in international markets. Only about 10% of research and development funds for medicines and vaccines go into diseases that account for 90% of the global disease burden.

The challenge confronting public health in the African Region today is that most diseases and conditions described in this report are preventable, treatable or both. Most deaths in this Region could be avoided if basic health care — vaccines, drugs, diagnostic methods and the health systems to deliver them — were widely available. This report is about how to make this happen.

## African Region of the World Health Organization

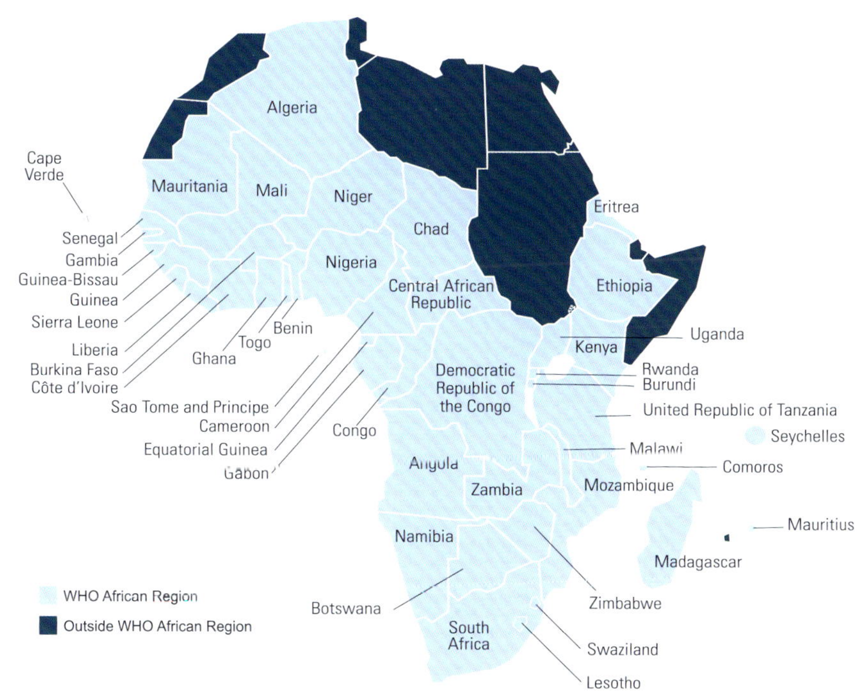


This report is about the 46 Member States of the African Region of the World Health Organization (WHO), as illustrated in this map. The African Regional Office of WHO is based in Brazzaville, the Republic of the Congo. When this report refers to "Africa", it is referring to the continent and islands as a whole. When the report refers to "the African Region" or "the Region", it is as defined by WHO.

It is important to note that the WHO African Region does not include all the countries on the African continent and the Region itself is not limited to all of sub-Saharan Africa.

Please note: the World Bank divides the continent into two regions: North Africa and sub-Saharan Africa, while UNICEF divides it into three regions: Eastern and South Africa, West and Central Africa, and the Middle-East and North Africa.

# Health *and* development in Africa

# *Key messages*

- Health can drive social progress and economic growth
- Ill-health pushes people into the poverty trap
- Severe burden of disease in Africa hampers development
- Current investment in health is inadequate

# *Solutions*

- African governments need to invest more in health
- Africa needs more development support from outside
- Scale up tried and tested public health solutions
- Paradigm shift is needed: need to address underlying determinants of ill-health, such as poverty

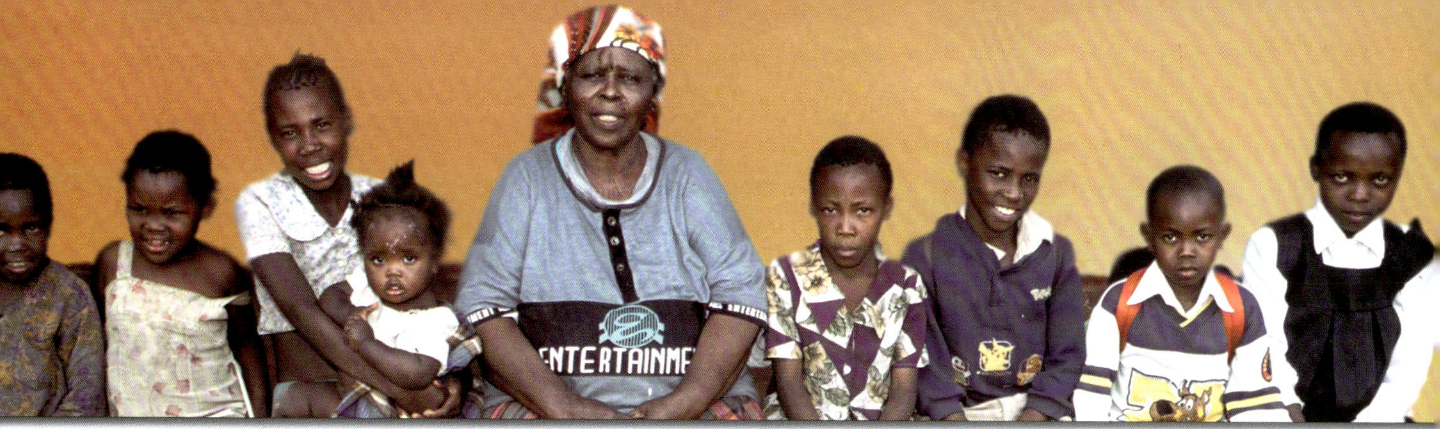

# Health and development in Africa

## The cycle of poverty and ill-health

People living in the African Region face a heavy and wide-ranging burden of disease, which takes its toll on social and economic development and shortens their life expectancy. The HIV/AIDS epidemic as well as the resurgence of malaria and tuberculosis have swept away improvements in life expectancy in some sub-Saharan countries (see Fig. 1.1). Other infectious diseases and — increasingly — noncommunicable conditions are also a severe burden, while the complications of pregnancy and childbirth take millions of lives every year.

The health services that have evolved in countries in Africa are often not able to address adequately this severe burden of disease. These health systems are weak, reflecting the overall state of the economies in the African Region. In many countries out-of-pocket payments are high in proportion to household incomes and are a major factor driving poverty. The cost of treatment for an adult with HIV/AIDS, in addition to lost income due to time off work, can drag a whole household below the poverty line. Therefore, just as health can drive economic growth, ill-health can push people into poverty and make it very difficult for them to escape the poverty trap.

This vicious cycle of poverty and ill-health can be seen in many countries in Africa. Some 76% of the population of sub-Saharan Africa live on less than US$ 2 a day, and 46.5% on less than US$ 1.08 a day (see Fig. 1.2). While poverty has declined in other parts of the world, such as East and South Asia, over the past 20 years, in sub-Saharan Africa the trend has been strongly in the other direction. Between 1981 and 2001 the gross domestic product (GDP) of sub-Saharan countries decreased by 13%, resulting in a doubling in the number of people in the Region living on less than US$ 1 a day from 164 million to 314 million. While Africans represented only 16% of the world's poor in 1985, by 1998 this proportion had risen to 31%. The trend is likely to continue, with poverty expected to decline over the next 20 years in every part of the world except sub-Saharan Africa, where a dramatic increase is expected.

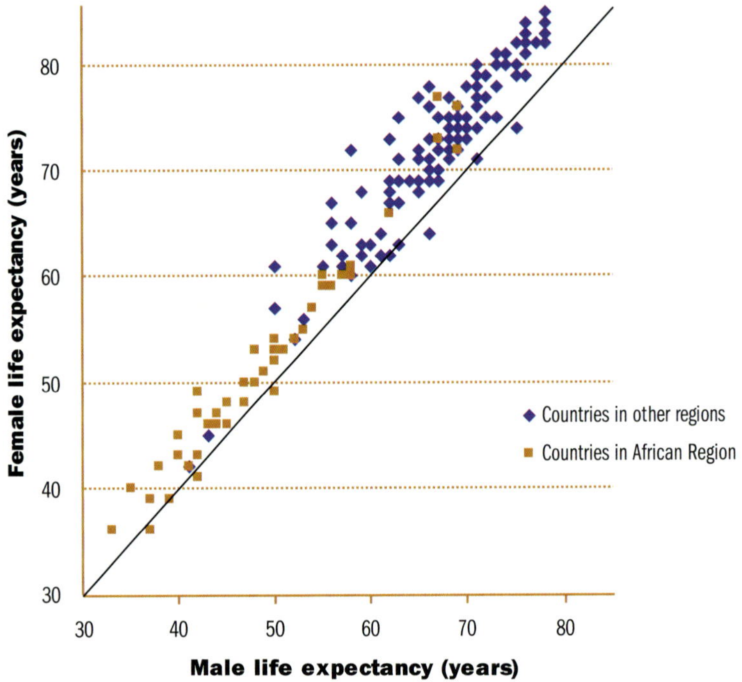



Figure shows low life expectancy in countries in the African Region.

Source: *World Health Statitstics 2005*. Geneva: World Health Organization; 2005.

Progress in human development made by some African countries in the 1970s and 1980s has been sharply reversed by HIV/AIDS and by armed conflict. On top of that, countries in the Region continue to suffer from other emergencies, large-scale migration, famine and economic decline.

Chronic diseases are becoming increasingly prevalent in middle-income countries of the African Region, such as South Africa and Kenya. Furthermore, road traffic collisions place a heavy burden on households and, in turn, regional and national economies. For instance, road traffic collisions cost the Ugandan economy around US$ 101 million per year, which is 2.3% of the country's gross national product (GNP). In addition mental health is one of the most under-resourced areas of public health in the African Region, even though mental health problems are on the rise and mental health services are desperately needed in post-conflict societies to help them achieve stability. In many countries of the Region this area of public health requires more attention than it is currently receiving.

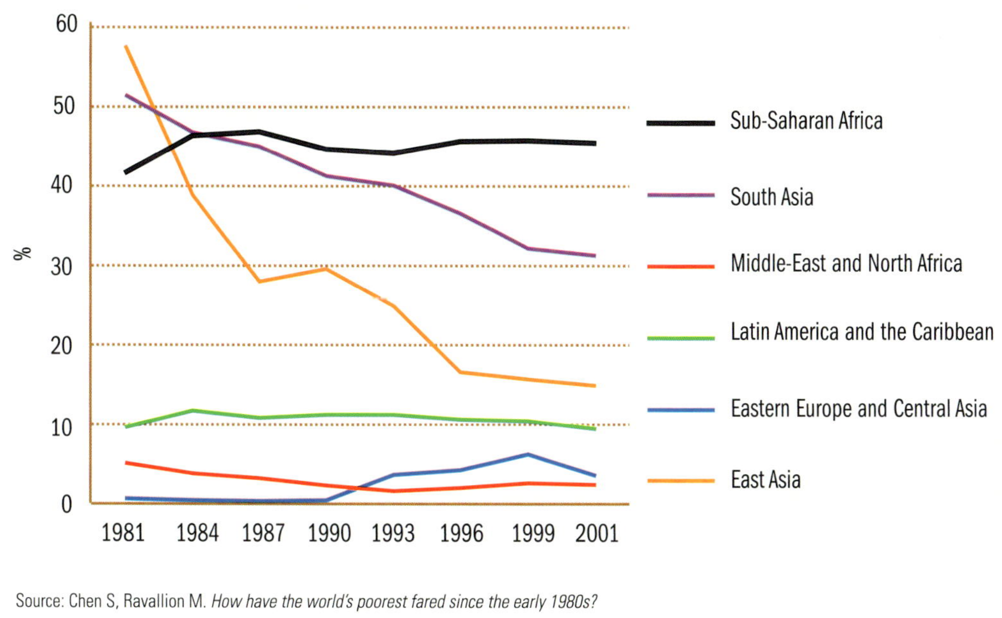



Source: Chen S, Ravallion M. *How have the world's poorest fared since the early 1980s?* World Bank Policy Research Working Paper 3341. Washington, DC: World Bank; June 2004.

Outside the African Region, about two-thirds of deaths are due to noncommunicable diseases. In Africa, by contrast, according to 2002 estimates, 72% of deaths are caused by communicable diseases such as HIV/AIDS, tuberculosis, malaria, respiratory infections, other infectious diseases, and complications of pregnancy and childbirth. These are largely preventable deaths, which account for about 23% of mortality in other regions.

The WHO Commission on Macroeconomics and Health made a powerful case in favour of investment in health — by scaling up known, cost-effective interventions — as an important driver of economic growth. No other region of the world has so much potential to benefit from such investment in health as the African Region.

African economies are growing fast, but not fast enough to achieve the UN Millennium Development Goals (MDGs). The economies of sub-Saharan countries need to grow at an average annual rate of 7% over the next decade to achieve the UN Millennium Development Goal 1 of cutting poverty in half by 2015 (see Box. 1.1), according to the International Monetary Fund. At current rates some countries may succeed, but many will fail. Economic growth and more investment in health will not help countries attain the improvements envisaged by the MDGs alone. More efforts are needed to achieve greater peace and security, good governance, gender equality and sustainable management of the environment.

## Achieving MDG 1: Poverty

MDG 1 aims to halve by 2015 the number of people who were living on less than US$ 1 a day in 1990. The poverty rate and number of poor increased in the 1990s, making sub-Saharan Africa the region with the largest proportion of people living on less than US$ 1 a day. World Bank economists say that projected economic growth over the 2006–15 period marks a reversal of the region's long-term decline but is far short of the growth needed to reduce poverty to half the 1990 level.

Bank economists say, however, that a few countries, such as Uganda and Ghana, have sustained remarkable growth and achieved some progress in poverty reduction and other MDGs. They say there are indications that Cameroon is making progress in achieving the poverty target.

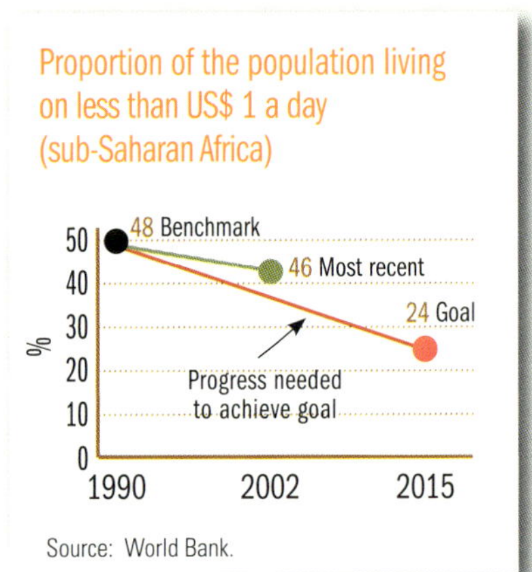


Source: World Bank.

Some countries in the African Region are not far off achieving the MDG targets and may need increased overseas development support to help bridge the gap in economic growth rates. Sub-Saharan countries reported their best economic performance for years in 2004, with an average 5% growth in real GDP, while average inflation fell to below 10% for the first time in 25 years. Oil producers, such as Nigeria and Equatorial Guinea, and post-conflict countries, such as Burundi and Sierra Leone, have seen some rapid though often sporadic growth in recent years.

Economic growth has not always led automatically to improvements in public health in the African Region. Current growth rates are an opportunity for African governments to invest more in health, an investment that would lead to more social and economic stability.

Increased investment in public health can reduce the burden of preventable and treatable diseases that — on macroeconomic level — can be a drag on national economies and — on microeconomic level — a drain on household and individual incomes.

Health must, therefore, constitute a central pillar of any coherent vision of African development, while increased investments in health should include those in health-related sectors, such as water and sanitation, education and environmental protection (see Fig. 1.3)

# Putting health in the development context

Development experts have long recognized health as an important moral and social goal. Health is also a key component of a sound development strategy, along with education, economic growth and good governance. As a form of human capital, health is essential to a productive society. Furthermore, the MDG project of the United Nations fully endorses the central role of health in development.

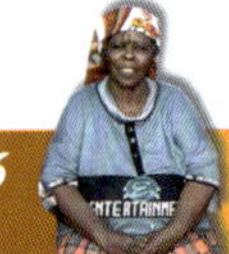

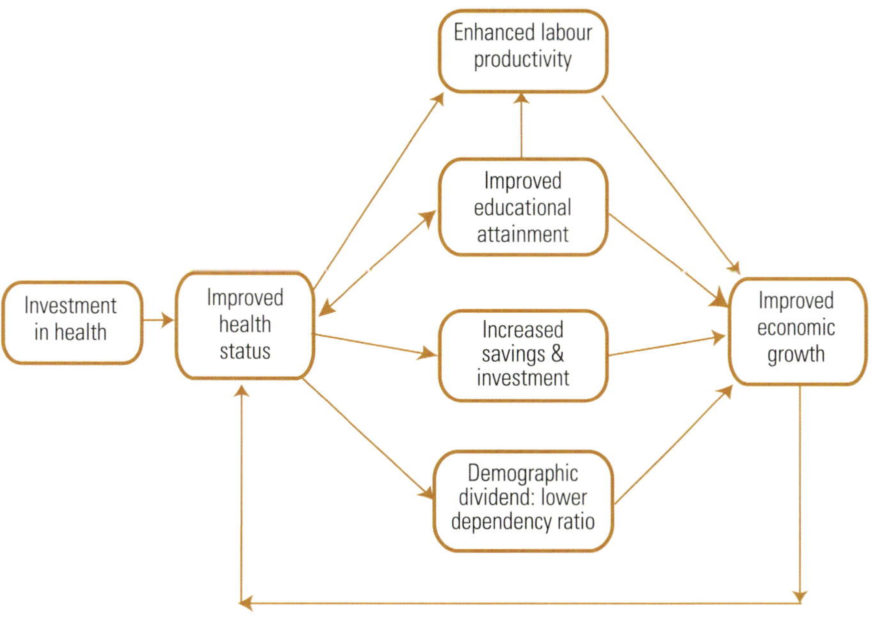


Source: adapted from: Saunders MK, Gadhia R, Connor C. *Investments in health contribute to economic development.* Publisher: Partners for Health Reformplus (PHRplus) E-version: http://www.phrplus.org/Pubs/sp12.pdf

Several studies have sought to quantify the macroeconomic impact of the disease burden (see Table 1.1). The prevalence of HIV/AIDS for adults aged 15-49 years in the African Region is estimated at about 7.2%. In every other WHO region the average was less than 1%. There is general agreement that the economic and social impact of HIV/AIDS in the African Region has been devastating. The epidemic has drastically reduced the workforce in many countries, while the cost of caring for the growing generation of AIDS orphans could slow down long-term GDP growth by as much as 1–1.5% in countries with high prevalence of HIV/AIDS, such as Kenya and South Africa.

Exacerbated by HIV/AIDS, the older scourge of tuberculosis has made a comeback in many parts of the world. Southern Africa has become the epicentre of the dual epidemic and both diseases are causing untold human suffering and reducing household income, in turn slowing economic growth in southern African countries.

Malaria has been dubbed "an African disease" because 90% of cases occur in this continent. Estimates show that countries with endemic malaria have 1.3% less economic growth per annum compared with similar non-endemic countries, and that in Africa the annual cost of lost productivity and providing treatment is US$ 12 billion.

# Efforts to promote development in Africa

There have been many regional and international initiatives to promote development in Africa. Some have focused on health as well as education, governance and sound economic policy, while others have focused entirely on health. In recent years both governments in Africa and donors have pledged to provide more money for health and development.

African governments pledged to raise their spending on health to 15% of their annual national budgets at a meeting in the Nigerian city of Abuja in 2001. A year later, the United Nations called on developed countries to increase their overseas development assistance to 0.7% of their GDP by 2015. European countries have pledged to do this, but only a few have done so. By early 2006, Denmark, Luxembourg, the Netherlands, Norway and Sweden had actually honoured that commitment.

The debt forgiveness granted by the G8 industrialized countries in 2005 to 23 countries in Africa presents an opportunity for the latter countries to invest more in health, as well as in water, sanitation and education. Following pledges by governments in Africa to invest more in health and health-related sectors, mechanisms need to be set up to monitor spending. Below are some of the major regional and international initiatives to promote development in Africa.

## The Abuja Declaration

Leaders of African countries gathered in the Nigerian city of Abuja in April 2001 to declare their continent to be in a "State of Emergency" over the HIV/AIDS pandemic. Governments declared that "containing and reversing the HIV/AIDS epidemic, tuberculosis and other infectious diseases" should constitute their "top priority for the first quarter of the 21st century". Their declaration said that tackling these epidemics was an integral part of poverty reduction and sustainable development as well as peace and security, and that the fight against HIV/AIDS was "the highest priority issue in our respective national development plans". In

Table 1.1

Burden of disease in the African Region 2002

| Burden of disease in DALYs* by cause and mortality stratum in the African Region | | |
|---|---|---|
| | Mortality stratum | |
| | High child, high adult (000) | High child, very high adult (000) |
| 1 AIDS | 14 620 | 49 343 |
| 2 Malaria | 20 070 | 20 785 |
| 3 Respiratory infections | 18 976 | 16 619 |
| 4 Perinatal conditions | 10 869 | 10 485 |
| 5 Diarrhoea | 11 548 | 11 689 |
| 6 **Top five subtotal (1 – 5)** | **76 083** | **108 921** |
| 7 Other communicable diseases | 39 234 | 41 484 |
| 8 Communicable diseases (6 and 7) | 115 317 | 150 405 |
| 9 Noncommunicable diseases | 30 124 | 34 727 |
| 10 Injuries | 14 974 | 15 829 |
| Total **Total (8 – 10)** | **160 415** | **200 961** |

The Member States of the Region have been divided into mortality strata on the basis of their levels of mortality in children under five years of age and in males aged 15–59 years as described on pp. 156–7 of the 2004 *World health report.*

* See glossary for explanation.

Source: *The world health report 2004.* Geneva. World Health Organization; 2004.

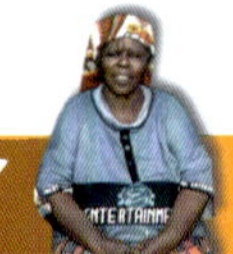

the Declaration, the governments in Africa called for the lifting of all tariff and economic barriers to funding AIDS-related treatment and medicines. For their part, the governments pledged to increase spending on health to at least 15% of their annual budgets.

## NEPAD

The New Partnership for Africa's Development (NEPAD) was launched in 2001 by the Organization of African Unity (OAU) to eradicate African poverty, promote sustainable growth and development, help countries in Africa take a more active part in the global economy and improve the status of women in African society.

In NEPAD's 2002 Health Strategy, African governments identified the "huge burden of potentially preventable and treatable disease" as causing "unnecessary deaths and untold suffering". According to NEPAD, the burden of disease in Africa "continues to block economic development and damages the continent's social fabric". NEPAD recognizes the central role of building and reinforcing health systems to assist in improving health in Africa, but also that health-care services are "too poorly funded". The NEPAD health strategy calls on African governments to honour their pledge to raise health spending to a level of 15% of their annual national budgets.

NEPAD argues that peace and security are vital for development and acknowledges the devastating impact of war on human health and development.

## The United Kingdom's Commission for Africa

According to a report released by the UK's Commission for Africa in March 2005, Africa and its partners have a unique opportunity to act now to promote social and economic development in the continent. The report argues that Africa should drive its own development and that it is already doing so through the African Union and NEPAD. The report states that it is in the interests of the rich countries to support Africa's development agenda to create a more prosperous and secure world.

The one-year Commission brought together by the United Kingdom — mainly made up of African political leaders, public servants and private entrepreneurs — sought wide consultation. The Commission calls for more investment in education and the rebuilding of health systems. To achieve this end, it recognizes that the top priority in health care is scaling up services to respond to the human tragedy of HIV/AIDS.

The Commission for Africa report argues that a stronger investment climate is required to boost the economies of Africa and reduce poverty, and suggests that such a boost might be achieved through stronger public–private partnerships. In addition, it suggests that donors should double their spending on infrastructure — including both rural development and slum upgrading — so that Africa's poorest people will also be able to participate in economic growth. Corruption, customs procedures, bureaucracy and trade tariffs must be minimized to boost trade between African nations, it says.

*NEPAD recognizes the central role of building and reinforcing health systems to assist in improving health in Africa.*

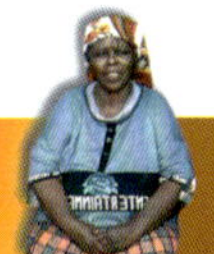

## UN Millennium Development Goals

The United Nations Member States agreed in 2000 to work towards eight Millennium Development Goals (MDGs). These goals set a number of targets to be achieved by 2015. The targets include halving extreme poverty and providing universal primary education. The health goals are to reduce the number of deaths of under-five-year olds by three-quarters, to reduce maternal deaths by two-thirds and to reverse epidemics of HIV/AIDS, malaria, tuberculosis and other infectious diseases. The MDG project has galvanized a global effort to meet the needs of the poorest people in the world.

In 2005, a UN report identified four main reasons why some regions are not making enough progress towards the MDGs. The first was poor governance. The second was national poverty traps, a particular problem in the African Region. The third was the presence of pockets of poverty within countries. The fourth was political neglect. The UN report recommends that every government should adopt and implement a national strategy — with the help of bilateral and multilateral donors and organizations — to help each country achieve the MDGs.

## G8 Summit 2005

The Group of Eight industrialized countries (G8) agreed to cancel the debt of 18 of Africa's poorest countries and to increase aid to developing countries by US$ 50 billion at a summit in Gleneagles, Scotland, in July 2005. Of those, 23 are in Africa. The G8 lamented declining life expectancy in Africa and pledged to continue to support African strategies to improve health, education and food security. The G8 also pledged to support investment in improved health systems, including the training and retraining of health workers to tackle the major diseases affecting Africa, such as HIV/AIDS, malaria, tuberculosis, polio and other neglected diseases. The G8 pledged to give support for investments in water and sanitation and to comprehensive food security and famine prevention programmes. It also pledged to support African countries in building peace and security, promoting good governance, investing in people, and promoting growth and development.



### MDG 8: A global partnership for development

MDG 8 calls for international trade and finance that are more equitable and give a fair chance to poor countries. It calls for sustainable development and youth employment as well as better access to essential drugs and communication technology in developing countries. Progress in these areas depends not only on developing countries themselves, but also hinges on policy changes made by wealthy countries, such as debt forgiveness, commitments to increased aid, freeing of market restrictions and relaxing patent protection for life-saving technology. Some progress has been made in these areas. For example, partial debt relief has been offered to Burkina Faso, Mali, Mauritania, Mozambique, the United Republic of Tanzania and Uganda. Thirty-four of a total of 42 countries in the heavily-indebted poor countries initiative are in the African Region. Donor countries have also agreed to harmonize aid and respect development priorities in recipient countries. However, official development assistance declined in sub-Saharan Africa from US$ 34 per capita in 1990 to US$ 21 in 2001. The goal reminds rich nations of their commitment to give 0.7% of their annual income in aid. By early 2006, only Denmark, Luxembourg, the Netherlands, Norway, and Sweden had actually honoured that commitment. However, increased aid can only lead to progress on the rest of the goals if recipient countries improve governance and commit themselves to a policy of poverty reduction.

# Conclusion: Making it happen

What should be done to ensure that health development in the African Region plays its rightful role in national development efforts? The answer is that there are tried and tested health-care interventions that work, interventions that enable safe childbirth, treat acute respiratory and diarrhoeal illnesses, and prevent HIV transmission and early death from AIDS. There are established methods of preventing malaria transmission and treating tuberculosis. The results of a public heath experiment called the Tanzania Essential Health Interventions Project (TEHIP) suggest that it is possible to achieve dramatic gains in maternal, newborn and child health at little additional cost. Mauritius achieved some of the best reproductive health indicators in WHO's African Region through providing family planning services, strong political commit ment to tackling HIV/AIDS, health promotion, public health education and accurate recording of statistics to gauge changes in health indicators.

African governments can avoid some of the burden of noncommunicable diseases that wealthy, developed countries now face. While the greatest focus is on the diseases that kill the most people, more efforts are needed to improve on outdated methods of control and cure for neglected diseases, such as sleeping sickness, which also hamper development in African countries.

Some countries are already linking public health and economic interests to tackle shortages of essential medicines, while others may follow suit.

For example, some African countries are already using new ways to purchase drugs at reduced prices, such as negotiating low prices for patented antiretrovirals for HIV/AIDS. Other countries are hoping to purchase cheaper generic antiretrovirals from other developing countries, making use of a waiver in international trade law for poor countries that was made permanent at the WTO meeting in December 2005. Farmers in the United Republic of Tanzania are growing the *Artemisia annua* plant to improve domestic supply of antimalarial medicines.

Empowering women is crucial to lifting countries out of poverty and improving the health of the people in the Region. Health systems cannot function without the talents of sufficient health workers. Successful development reform, such as disbursing and spending aid in a more accountable manner, is more likely to happen if it is driven by local priorities.

A concerted effort by African governments and their partners is gathering momentum for change and to help the Region come closer to achieving the MDGs (see Box 1.2). Five key elements are vital for success. First, stronger political will and commitment is essential to ensure solutions are implemented. Second, African nations need to allocate a

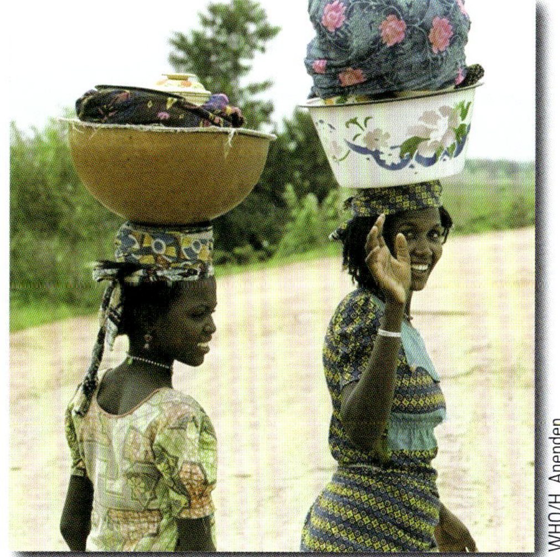

higher percentage of their national expenditure to health and their partners need to increase aid to Africa to address the lack of financial resources. Third, to draw full benefit from that additional donor aid, African nations need good governance to use it wisely. Fourth, adequate numbers of health-care staff are required across the African Region to provide health care, and governments and their partners need to implement adequate programmes to train, retain and utilize these resources better. Fifth, governments and their partners — domestic and international — need to translate good policies into action.

If the African Region is to achieve peace, prosperity and health for all, African nations and their partners need to act now to implement the many known solutions. A paradigm shift is needed. While delivering interventions to prevent and treat disease, governments also need to shift their focus to addressing the underlying factors that determine health, such as poverty and education.

The development challenge that Africa faces is evident from the sheer magnitude of human death and disease that is outlined later in this report. These are not simply catalogues of despair or tales of woe. Within the African Region, solutions to the continent's challenges exist. Africa can overcome its problems through partnerships and political will. ■

## Bibliography

- Ainsworth M, Fransen L, Over M, editors. *Confronting AIDS: evidence from the developing world: Selected background papers for the World Bank Policy Research Report*. Brussels: European Commission; 1998.

- *Abuja Declaration on HIV/AIDS, tuberculosis and other related infectious diseases. 27 April 2001*. Available from: http://www.uneca.org/adf2000/Abuja%20Declaration.htm

- Barro RJ. *Health and economic development*. Washington, DC: World Bank; 1996. Available from: http://www.paho.org/English/DPM/SHD/HP/barro.pdf

- Bloom DE, Canning D, Sevilla J. *Health, human capital, and economic development*. Commission on Macroeconomics and Health Working Paper Series, Paper No. WG1: 8. 2001. Available from: http://www.cmhealth.org/docs/wg1_paper8.pdf

- Bryce J, Boschi-Pinto C, Shibuya K, Black RE, WHO Child Health Epidemiology Reference Group. WHO estimates of the causes of death in children. *Lancet* 2005;365:1147-52.

- *Our common interest: report of the Commission for Africa*. London; Commission for Africa: 2005.

- Global indicators. In: *World development indicators 2005*. Washington, DC: World Bank; 2005. Available from: http://www.worldbank.org/data/wdi2005/wditext/Section6_1.htm

- Global Partnership to Roll Back Malaria. *World malaria report: 2005*. Geneva: World Health Organization and UNICEF; 2005.

- *Health Economics: getting value for money. African Health Monitor Jan-June 2005*. Brazzaville: World Health Organization, Regional Office for Africa; 2005.

- *Human development report 2004: cultural liberty in today's diverse world*. New York: United Nations Development Programme; 2004.

- *Macroeconomics and health: investing in health for economic development. Report of the Commission on Macroeconomics and Health*. Geneva: World Health Organization; 2001.

- *Our common interest: report of the Commission for Africa*. London; Commission for Africa: 2005.

- Peden M, Scurfield R, Sleet D, Mohan D, Hyder AA, Jarawan E, et al. *World report on road traffic injury prevention*. Geneva: World Health Organization; 2004.

- Ranis G, Stewart F, Ramirez A. Economic growth and human development. *World Development* 2000;28:197-219.

- *Regional economic outlook sub-Saharan Africa*. Washington, DC: International Monetary Fund; 2005. Available from: http://www.imf.org/external/pubs/ft/AFR/REO/2005/eng/01/SSAREO.htm

- *Regional HIV and AIDS estimates 2005*. Geneva: UNAIDS; 2005. Available at: http://www.unaids.org/epi2005/doc/report.html

- *Report on the International Conference on Financing for Development, Monterrey, Mexico, 18–22 March 2002*. New York: United Nations; 2002. UN document A/CONF.198/11. Available from: http://www.un.org/esa/ffd/aconf198-11.pdf

- Sachs J, Malaney P. The economic and social burden of malaria. *Nature* 2002; 415:618-85.

- Saunders MK, Gadhia R, Connor C. *Investments in health contribute to economic development*. Bethesda (MD): Partners for Health Reform*plus* (PHR*plus*). Available from : http://www.phrplus.org/Pubs/sp12.pdf

- Subbarao K, Coury, D. *Reaching out to Africa's orphans: a framework for public action*. Washington, DC: World Bank; 2004. Available from: http://siteresources.worldbank.org/INTHIVAIDS/Resources/375798-1103037153392/ReachingOuttoAfricasOrphans.pdf

- *The world health report 2004: changing history*. Geneva: World Health Organization, 2004.

- *The world health report 2005: make every mother and child count*. Geneva: World Health Organization, 2005.

- *The state of the world's children 2005*. New York: UNICEF. Geneva: World Health Organization, 2005.

- UNAIDS epidemic update 2004. Geneva: UNAIDS; 2004. Available from: http://www.unaids.org/wad2004/EPI_1204_pdf_en/EpiUpdate04_en.pdf

- United Nations Development Programme. *Human development report 2002: deepening democracy in a fragmented world* New York: Oxford University; 2002. Available from: http://hdr.undp.org/reports/global/2002/en/

- *World health statistics 2005*. Geneva: World Health Organization; 2005.

- *World report on knowledge for better health: strengthening health systems*. Geneva: World Health Organization; 2004.

# Maternal, newborn and child health

# Key messages

- *Millions of women, newborns and children die every year in Africa needlessly*
- *Most deaths are from treatable, preventable causes*
- *Little or no improvement in maternal, newborn and child health over the last 20 years*
- *Major global effort to address the situation is needed*

# Solutions

- *African governments must take more action to save these lives*
- *Allocation of resources to this area of public health is needed*
- *Scale up tried and tested public health solutions*
- *Educate women and improve their economic and social status*

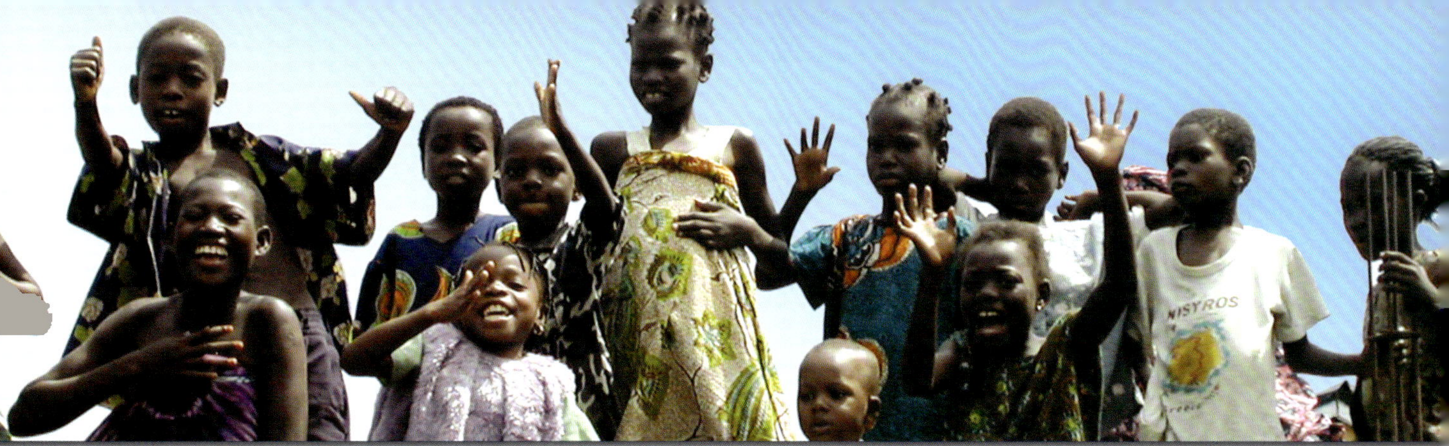

# Maternal, newborn and child *health*

## Africa's "silent epidemic"

**M**illions of women, newborns and children in Africa are dying from preventable causes every year. Millions more suffer ill-health or disability related to pregnancy and childbirth. African women risk death to give life and their offspring have the smallest survival chances in the world. It is the sheer magnitude of this death, disease and disability that constitutes Africa's "silent epidemic". High-level political commitment is vital, but not enough, to make a difference in the lives of these women, newborns and children. More needs to be done to save these lives.

A concerted effort is under way to remedy this situation. The *World health report 2005: make every mother and child count* and World Health Day 2005 were devoted to maternal and child health. Both of these focused on the tragedy that so many mothers, newborns and children die of preventable, treatable causes. In 2004, all 46 Member States of the African Region agreed to improve maternal and newborn health through the adoption and implementation of the Road Map for accelerating the attainment of the Millennium Development Goals (MDGs) relating to maternal and newborn health in Africa. The Region is also making progress in implementing the Integrated Management of Childhood Illness (IMCI) to improve child health.

Nearly 20 years after the launch of a major global campaign, the Safe Motherhood Initiative, there have been pockets of improvement in maternal, newborn and child health in the African Region but no overall reduction in pregnancy- and childbirth-related death and disease.

During the 1990s, the countries with the highest tolls of maternal, newborn and childhood disease and death made the least progress in reducing them, while advances in some countries, such as Botswana, South Africa and Zambia, have been reversed by the spread of HIV/AIDS. In 1960, countries in the African Region accounted for 14% of deaths of children aged under five years globally. In 1980, the proportion was 23% and by 2003 this had increased to 43%.

## Achieving MDG 4: Child health

MDG 4 on child health set the target of reducing by two-thirds the 1990 level of mortality of children aged under five by 2015. The child health goal is measured by three indicators; the under-five mortality rate, the infant mortality rate and the proportion of one-year-old children immunized against measles. Mortality of children aged under five years has improved slightly in sub-Saharan countries, according to the World Bank. *The world health report 2005* found that child mortality in the following 10 countries in the Region had increased: Botswana, Cameroon, Côte d'Ivoire, Kenya, Rwanda, South Africa, Swaziland, the United Republic of Tanzania, Zambia and Zimbabwe. These countries are unlikely to achieve the child health goal.

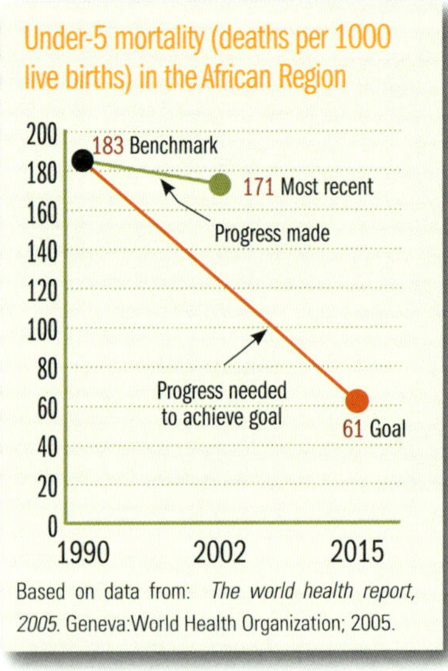


Based on data from: *The world health report, 2005.* Geneva:World Health Organization; 2005.

Fig. 2.1

Causes of maternal mortality in the African Region

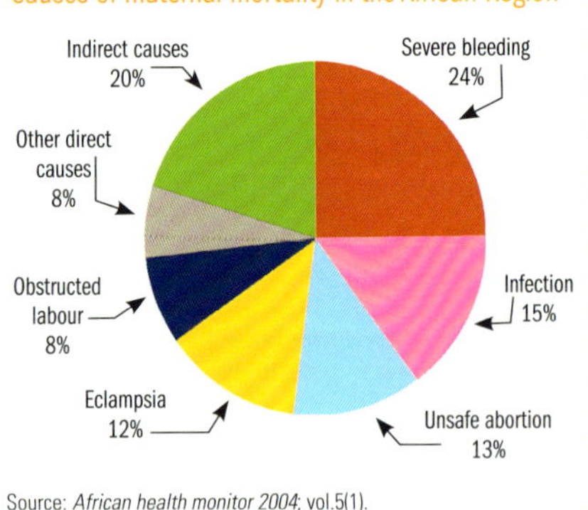


Source: *African health monitor 2004;* vol.5(1).

A few countries in the African Region, such as Cape Verde, Mauritius and Seychelles, have very low maternal, neonatal and child mortality rates that are comparable with those in industrialized countries. If progress is going to be made in improving maternal, newborn and child health in this Region, these successes need to be replicated where possible and primary health-care systems in these countries need to be revived as conduits to deliver essential care and treatment.

## Development goals for maternal and child health

In recognition of the importance of maternal and child health, an MDG has been devoted to each of these. Many countries in the African Region have a long way to go to achieve MDG 4 on child health (see Box 2.1 and Figure) and MDG 5 on maternal health (Box 2.2 and Figure).

In 2000, when UN Member States unanimously adopted the Millennium Declaration agreeing on eight MDGs, some countries in the African Region faced the daunting task of having to catch up with 1990 levels before they could contemplate moving beyond them. Some countries in this Region are still struggling to catch up with those levels of maternal and child health mainly due to HIV/AIDS, which has reversed advances made in the 1970s and 1980s.

## Mothers: the causes and numbers of deaths

The main causes of maternal death are severe bleeding (haemorrhage), infection (sepsis), eclampsia, obstructed labour and unsafe abortion, but increasing numbers of mothers in this Region die from indirect causes, such as HIV/AIDS, tuberculosis, malaria and anaemia (see Fig. 2.1).

Of the 20 countries with the highest maternal mortality ratios in the world, 19 are in Africa and one — Afghanistan — is in Asia. The African Region accounts for about one-tenth of the world's population and 20% of global births, yet nearly half of the mothers who die globally as a result of pregnancy and childbirth are in this Region (see Fig. 2.2).

Pregnancy- and childbirth-related complications were the second-leading cause of death and disability for women aged 15–49 years in this Region in 2002 with an estimated 231 000 deaths, according to WHO data. The leading cause was HIV/AIDS with 866 000 deaths. Apart from the personal tragedy for the children and families concerned, the deaths of so many mothers in pregnancy and childbirth is a disaster for communities and a major setback for the economic and social development of countries.

During the 1970s and 1980s, maternal mortality fell across the Region as countries started establishing primary health care, including antenatal services and emergency obstetric care. Millions more lives could be saved if health systems were capable of ensuring that good quality services are available to everyone who needs them. It is clear, however, that maternal mortality in this Region has hardly improved over the last 15 years. Many women in this Region face an even greater risk of dying as a result of pregnancy or childbirth than they did 15 years ago. A woman in sub-Saharan Africa faces a 1-in-16 risk of dying due to pregnancy or childbirth during her lifetime compared with 1 in 2800 in developed countries.

African women are more likely to suffer debilitating complications linked to pregnancy and childbirth. A study in West Africa showed that for each maternal death, a further 30 women may suffer long-lasting disabilities due to a range of conditions, such as chronic anaemia, infertility and obstetric fistula.

Harmful traditional practices such as female genital mutilation and nutritional taboos also contribute to poor maternal health. Female genital mutilation, which is the partial or total removal of external genitalia is practised in 27 Member States of the 46 in this Region,

## Newborns: the causes and numbers of deaths

The main causes of neonatal death in this Region are: severe infections, birth asphyxia (the inability to breathe normally after birth), preterm birth, neonatal tetanus, congenital anomalies and other conditions (see Fig. 2.3). In developing countries, the children of mothers who die during the first six weeks of their babies' lives are up to 10 times more likely to die within two years than children with two living parents. The reason is that the babies do not get breastfed, the family food supply is threatened and there is no direct care for those children. The dead woman's children are also less likely to get adequate health care and education as they grow up.

While progress was made in improving the health of children aged one month to five years in the 1970s and 1980s, the health of neonates — babies in their first 28 days of life — remained a neglected area of public health. Recent data show that neonates represent about 40% of children who die before their fifth birthday and that 29% of global neonatal deaths occur in Africa. The African Region's neonatal mortality rate is the highest in the world (see Fig. 2.4). For every newborn baby that dies, another 20 face illness or disability from conditions such as birth injury, infection and the complications of premature birth.



### Achieving MDG 5: Maternal health

MDG 5 on maternal health set the goal of reducing the 1990 level of maternal mortality by three-quarters. It is measured by two indicators: the maternal mortality ratio (MMR), which is the number of maternal deaths per 100 000 live births, and by the average proportion of deliveries by skilled birth attendants. The different values of MMR for 1990 and 2000 are due to differences in methodology and not because there has been an increase in MMR since 1990. Estimates for 1990 and 2000 suggest that there has been little change in the levels of maternal mortality ratios in the African Region.

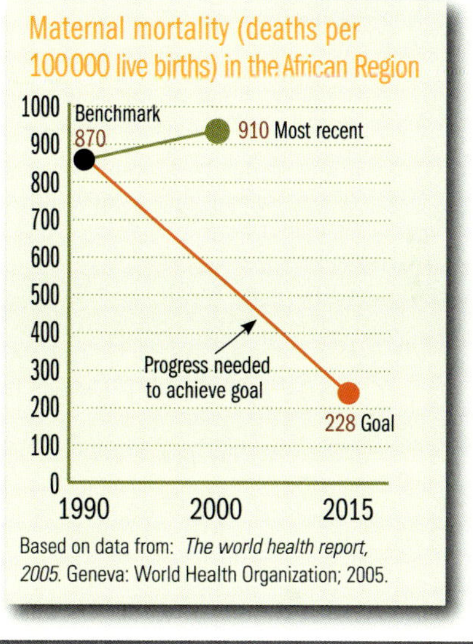


Based on data from: *The world health report, 2005*. Geneva: World Health Organization; 2005.

Fig. 2.2

Global distribution, by region, of maternal deaths, world population and live births, 2000

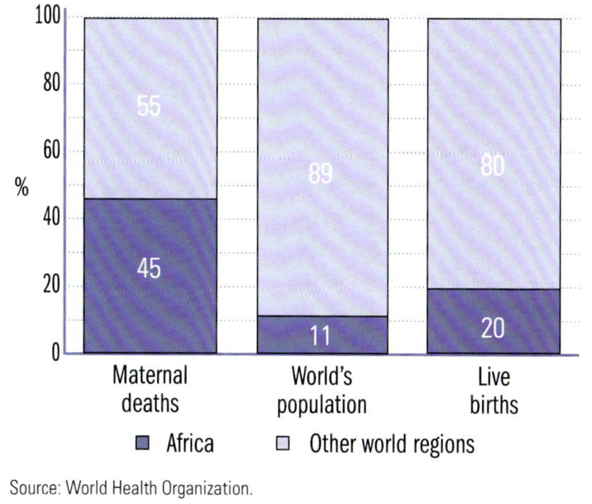


Source: World Health Organization.

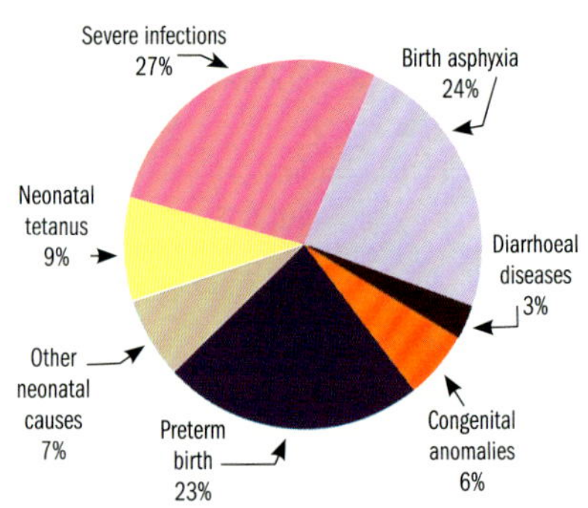

The percentages do not add up to 100% due to rounding.
Source: *World health report 2005*. Geneva: World Health Organization; 2005.

The first global estimates for neonatal deaths were made as late as 1983, while more rigorous estimates were made in 1995 and 2000. There are scant vital data on newborn babies but even less is known about stillborn babies. WHO estimates that the African Region has the highest proportion of stillbirths in the world: 30% of an estimated 3.3 million stillborn babies globally in 2000.

## Under-fives: the causes and numbers of deaths

The vast majority of deaths of children aged under five years in this Region are due to preventable causes. Fig. 2.5 shows that the chief causes are neonatal conditions, acute respiratory infections, malaria, diarrhoeal diseases, HIV/AIDS and measles, all complicated by malnutrition.

The importance of malnutrition as an underlying cause of death for children aged under five years has been recognized for many years and has recently been reconfirmed: 53% of all of these child deaths could be attributed to underweight and 35% of deaths are due to the effect of undernutrition on diarrhoea, pneumonia, malaria and measles.

Deaths of children under five years of age are increasingly concentrated in the African Region, at 43% of the global total in 2003, up from 31% in 1990. Of an estimated 10.6 million children under five years of age who died each year during 2000–03, some 4.4 million died in the African Region, according to WHO estimates. Every day an estimated 12 000 children die in sub-Saharan Africa from easily preventable or treatable illnesses and conditions, such as pneumonia, diarrhoea, measles, malaria and malnutrition.

Fig. 2.6 shows that mortality of children aged under five stagnated between 1990 and 2003 in 29 countries globally, and that 23 of these countries were in Africa. This lack of change occurred in Africa partly because modest reductions in death rates due to improved health care were offset by population growth and the increasing number of births. Lesotho, Malawi, Mozambique and Namibia made slow progress in reducing child mortality, while under-five child mortality fell in a further 10 countries in this Region. However, the number of under-five deaths has since increased, and during the 13-year period there has been no overall reduction in child mortality in this Region.

# Preventing millions of deaths

The tragedy of maternal, neonatal and child mortality today is that the vast majority of these deaths can be prevented by making sure pregnant women and children have access to good quality health care. Considerable progress has been made across much of the African Region in terms of providing antenatal care. In the 1990s, the level of

Fig. 2.4

Neonatal mortality rate in the WHO regions
(per 1000 live births)



Source: *World health statistics, 2005*. Geneva: World Health Organization; 2005.

antenatal care rose by 4% to a currently estimated 70% of women in sub-Saharan Africa receiving at least one antenatal consultation. Millions more lives could be saved if health systems were developed to ensure that services are of high quality and extended to everyone who needs them. This means providing every woman with skilled care during childbirth and emergency obstetric and neonatal care if complications arise. It also means ensuring children's access to quality services for prevention and treatment of childhood illnesses.

## The obstacles

Inadequate education, illiteracy and the women's lack of economic power compounded by their low social status contribute to women's low utilization of available health services. Other major factors that have led to inadequate coverage of maternal health services are poverty, weak health systems and the shortage of skilled health workers. According to the latest estimates,

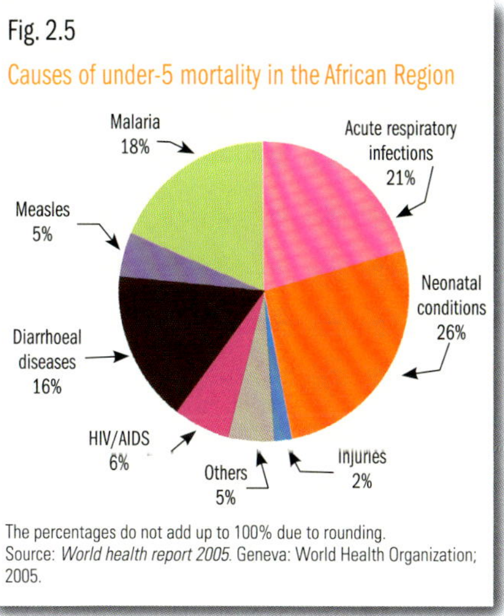


Fig. 2.5

Causes of under-5 mortality in the African Region

The percentages do not add up to 100% due to rounding.
Source: *World health report 2005*. Geneva: World Health Organization; 2005.

Fig 2.6

Patterns of reduction of under-5 mortality rates, 1990-2003

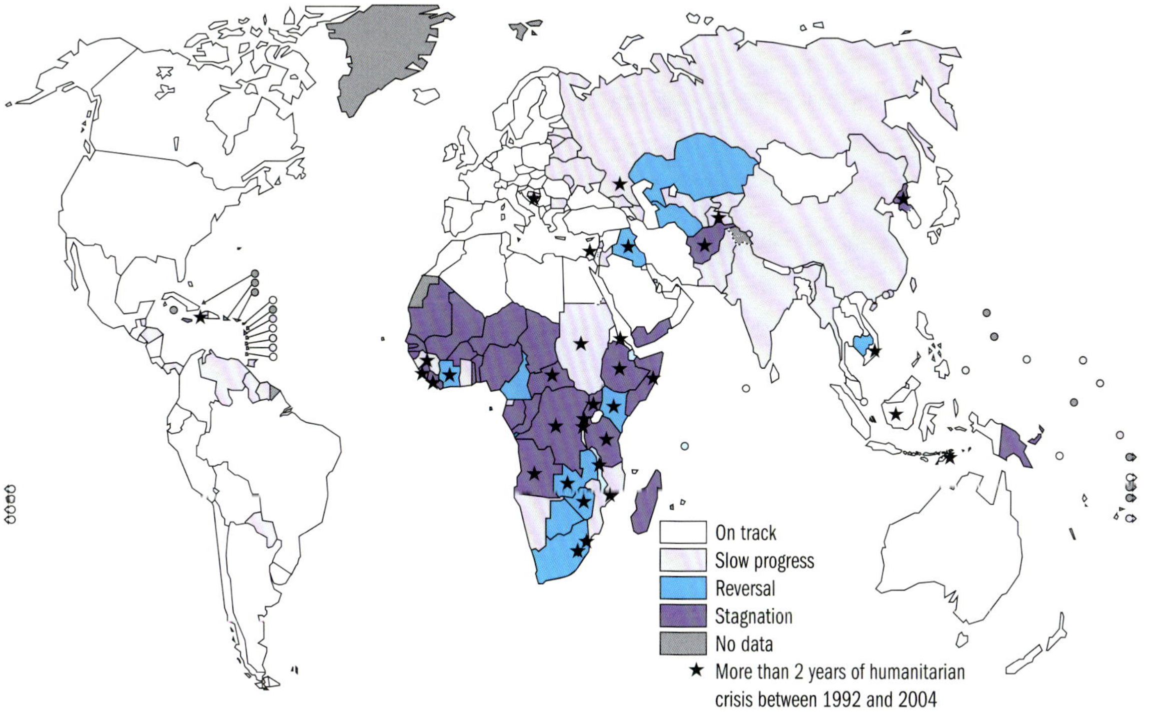

Source: *World health report 2005*. Geneva: World Health Organization; 2005.

skilled attendants assist in only 43% of the deliveries in the African Region. The remaining births are assisted by traditional birth attendants, relatives and neighbours, while some mothers give birth alone.

In some parts of the African Region, about one-third of pregnant women are adolescents. Adolescent mothers face a greater risk of death in pregnancy and childbirth than women aged 20 or over. Their babies are particularly vulnerable to premature birth, low birth weight and risk dying in the first month of life. In some countries in this Region, adolescents represent 40–60% of mothers who die in pregnancy and childbirth. If these adolescents had access to family planning services many deaths and much ill-health could be avoided.

## Conflict and emergencies

Over the last two decades, the African Region has seen more armed conflict and humanitarian emergencies than any other. Between 1992 and 2004, 22 of 33 humanitarian crises globally that lasted two or more years occurred in Africa alone, according to the Consolidated Appeals Process for humanitarian disasters. These crises have taken a major toll on human life and disrupted routine health services. Conflict situations fuel sexual violence and rape, which have reproductive and mental health repercussions and which require specialized clinical and psychological care.

Pregnant women and their infants are often the most vulnerable members of displaced and refugee populations. Emergencies, such as floods and other natural disasters, and armed conflict also result in the destruction of hospitals and loss of medical staff.

In humanitarian emergencies, pregnant women still need routine antenatal care and skilled assistance when they give birth, and if there are complications they need back-up services, including emergency obstetric and neonatal care. After giving birth, women need access to child care and family planning services. In the vast majority of cases these services are not available.

A bitter testament to the impact of conflict on maternal and child health is the example of Sierra Leone. After a devastating 1991–2001 civil war, the West African country was estimated to have the highest maternal mortality ratio in the world with 2000 deaths per 100 000 live births in 2002. It also had a stillborn rate of 50 per 1000 births and a neonatal mortality rate of between 42 and 56 per 1000 live births. Since 2000, Sierra Leone has been at the top of the list of the 20 countries worldwide with the highest maternal mortality ratio.

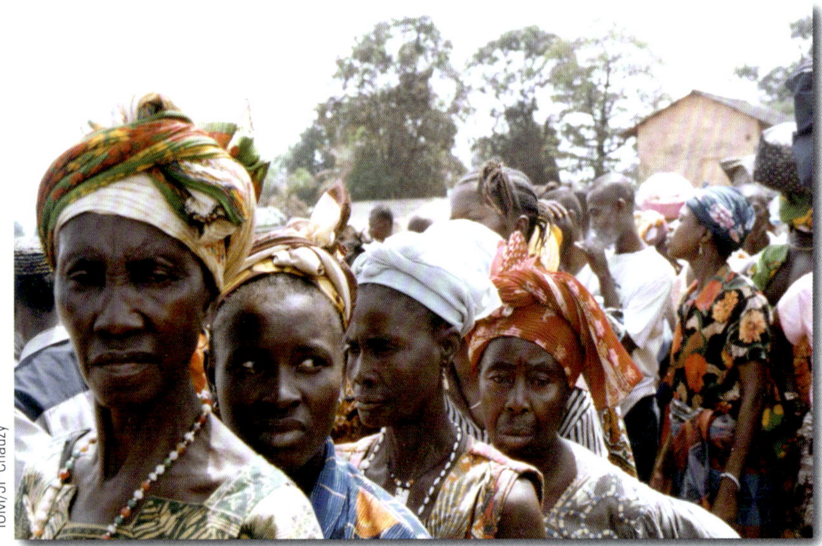

IOM/JP Chauzy

Women displaced by conflict, in a camp in Freetown, Sierra Leone.

## HIV/AIDS

HIV/AIDS has had a dire impact on maternal and child health over the last two decades. In some African countries an estimated 20–30% of pregnant women are infected with HIV, while transmission rates from mother to child range from 25% to 40%.

In Botswana, South Africa, Zambia and Zimbabwe, the spread of HIV/AIDS has in part reversed progress made in maternal, newborn and child health. HIV/AIDS has, in turn, spurred the re-emergence of tuberculosis and complicated forms of malaria, and all three diseases have become the biggest indirect causes of maternal and neonatal death in this Region.

## Inadequate resource allocation

Despite numerous maternal and child health campaigns, political commitment in the African Region has not been sufficient to make a difference to the lives of mothers and their children. Many governments in this Region are aware of the magnitude of the problem but are prevented from allocating adequate resources to maternal, newborn and child health care by poverty, indebtedness, armed conflict or humanitarian emergencies.

Also donors are not always prepared to provide substantially more aid for this area of public health. As a result, efforts to reduce the toll of maternal and child death and disease in this Region have had limited success.

## Weak health systems

Public health experts broadly agree that widespread exclusion from good quality health care and the absence of well functioning public and private health systems — whether through the absence, destruction or neglect of those health systems — are at the root of the problem: that millions of mothers, newborns and children aged under five die every year of preventable causes.

It is vital to scale up health-care services, but if the resulting services are of insufficient quality people will not benefit from improved coverage. In some parts of this Region antenatal care has been scaled up and extended to a large proportion of pregnant women, but the quality of this care is so poor that it barely makes a difference. For instance, Chad and Zimbabwe are among the 12 countries with the world's highest maternal mortality rates. Each has a rate of 1100 maternal deaths per 100 000 live births, yet Zimbabwe's antenatal services have a 82% coverage rate compared with only 51% in Chad. The indicators of the quality of antenatal care reflect how well this care screens for major complications of pregnancy and childbirth, and prevents them.

Health systems also serve to gather reliable data. One of the main challenges for improving the health of women, newborns and children is gathering data to measure progress. Many countries with the highest burden of maternal, newborn and child death and disease lack reliable data which they need to gauge an adequate response. WHO helps such countries develop information systems to collect reliable data.

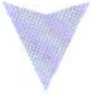

*Many countries with the highest burden of maternal, newborn and child death and disease lack reliable data which they need to gauge an adequate response.*

# Efforts to tackle the problem

More than a decade of research has shown that modest, low-cost measures can significantly reduce the health risks that women face when they become pregnant; for instance, educating the woman to look after herself and recognize danger signs that indicate when she should seek help at a health facility. These measures also include providing basic and regular antenatal care to check blood pressure, weight gain and renal function, diagnose anaemia and treat infections. Breastfeeding is one of the best ways to ensure the baby's survival.

## Safe motherhood

The Safe Motherhood Initiative, launched in Nairobi, Kenya, in 1987 by international agencies, placed maternal health — previously regarded as a private or family matter — firmly on the global public health agenda. The initiative has succeeded in drawing more attention to maternal health over the last two decades. Critics, however, argue that it failed to bring about a broad-based improvement in this area of public health because countries were not given the technical assistance they needed to translate its recommendations into practice. Moreover, donors and humanitarian agencies failed to coordinate efforts well enough to fill the gaps in public health services in the African Region, leading to a patchwork approach.

Another major initiative, the UN International Conference on Population and Development in Cairo, Egypt, in 1994 urged all countries to address the human rights issues relating to maternal and child health. It called on them to provide public information on sexual and reproductive health, to protect pregnant women and to criminalize violence against women, and it condemned the harmful traditional practice of female genital mutilation. The most important outcome of this conference was the commitment by governments to provide universal access to reproductive health care including family planning information and services by 2015.

WHO launched the Making Pregnancy Safer (MPS) initiative in 1999 to assist countries to strengthen their health systems to improve access to skilled care, including access to emergency obstetric and newborn care. The aim is to ensure that mothers and their newborns have timely access to the care they need through strengthening the health system and appropriate community involvement. WHO started working with Ethiopia, Mauritania, Mozambique, Nigeria and Uganda in 2002 to implement the MPS initiative and later that year 34 more Member States in the African Region requested similar assistance.

To advocate more effectively for the continuum of care that is needed for improved Maternal and newborn and child health, the three initiatives that address newborn and child health (the Healthy Newborn Partnership established in 2000, the Child Survival Partnership created in 2004; and the Safe Motherhood and Newborn Health also created in 2004) were merged in 2005 to form the Partnership for Maternal, Newborn and Child Health.





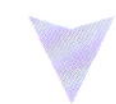

# Prevention of mother-to-child transmission of HIV

Countries in the African Region started introducing the Prevention of Mother-to-Child Transmission of HIV (PMTCT) programme in 2002. This programme aims to prevent HIV-positive mothers from infecting their babies during pregnancy, delivery and afterwards. Its goal is also to prevent men and women from becoming infected with HIV and to prevent unwanted pregnancies in HIV-positive women.

A successful pilot project conducted in a clinic in Zimbabwe in 2001 showed that PMTCT programmes are more effective if clinical treatment given to HIV-positive mothers is combined with psychosocial support for those mothers and their families (see Box 2.3).



## Psychosocial support for HIV-positive mothers and families

The modest two-room Zengeza clinic in the Zimbabwean city of Chitungwiza is playing a pioneering role in helping expectant mothers and their families cope with the discovery that they are HIV positive. This is one of a growing number of antenatal clinics in the African Region that have started to provide counselling and psychosocial support to HIV-positive mothers in addition to clinical treatment as part of their programmes to prevent transmission of HIV from mother to child.

A recent study found that mothers who received counselling and psychosocial support at Zengeza were better equipped to cope with being HIV positive than those who did not. Staff and activists are now calling for all antenatal clinics in Zimbabwe to adopt this approach. They say it has led to an increase in voluntary HIV/AIDS counselling and testing, and higher awareness levels in the community at large — a major step to curbing the spread of HIV/AIDS. The only problem, they say, is that not enough men participate in the counselling sessions.

Gladys Nyamunokora, 35, said the programme had helped her to build up the courage to disclose her HIV-positive status to her husband and to discuss this openly with him. The study showed that mothers like Gladys are better informed about HIV/AIDS than those who do not receive counselling.

"When I found out I was HIV positive I was shattered, ashamed and afraid," said Gladys. Like other mothers in Zimbabwe and other African countries, Gladys discovered she was HIV positive when she sought antenatal care. She was four months pregnant with her third child.

"I had a lot of questions. 'How will I disclose my status to my husband? Who will look after my children and my unborn baby? How long will I live?' I isolated myself and felt hopeless. Every day I contemplated suicide."

An HIV-positive diagnosis is devastating for pregnant women, leaving them feeling even more vulnerable, but Gladys was lucky enough to attend the clinic in 2002, when it started offering counselling and psychosocial support.

The clinical treatment was a success and Gladys's daughter was born free of HIV. Two years later after regular counselling sessions and receiving psychosocial support at the clinic, Gladys said: "The pain and sadness will never go away completely, but now I know how to cope with them when they resurface. The counselling and social support from the caregivers and counsellors gave me hope".

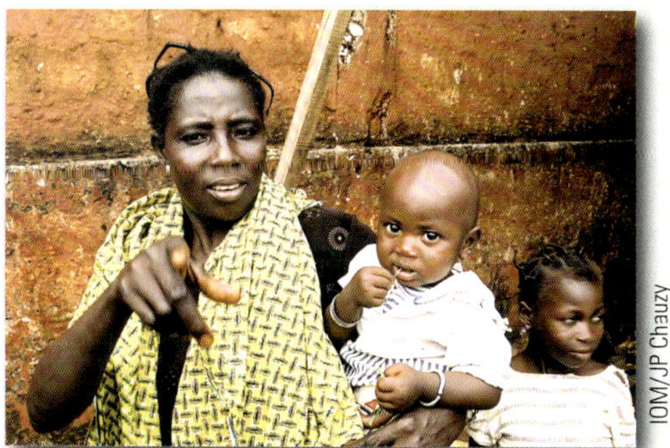

Coping strategies are important for women who are at risk of becoming infected with HIV.

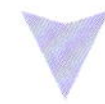

*Developed in the 1990s by WHO and UNICEF, the Integrated Management of Childhood Illnesses (IMCI) strategy is being implemented in 44 of the 46 countries of the African Region to reduce the growing number of child deaths attributable to a few preventable, treatable illnesses. The idea of IMCI is to improve the prevention or early detection and treatment of the main childhood killers in developing countries.*

## Repositioning family planning

The African Region has some of the highest fertility rates in the world — 4.9 children per woman on average — and a low prevalence of contraceptive use of 17%. In contrast, global fertility has dropped from 4.5 to 2.8 children per woman since the 1970s. The low use of contraception is not the only reason for this. High fertility rates drop in societies where people are convinced that their children have good chances of survival. The high fertility in this Region increases the life-time risk a woman faces of dying from pregnancy and childbirth-related complications

In the African Region, where women are at greater risk of dying in pregnancy or childbirth than anywhere else in the world and where they have some of the highest fertility rates in the world, family planning is essential. However, over the last 10 years it has become a neglected area of public health because of conflicting priorities, insufficient high-level political commitment and lack of donor interest. One of the challenges here is overcoming religious barriers and cultural beliefs that encourage high fertility and create misconceptions that prevent men and women from using effective family planning methods or prevent providers from suggesting certain family planning methods as options.

Countries need to address reproductive health to come closer to achieving the Millennium Development Goals on maternal and child health. In 2004, the 46 ministries of health in the African Region adopted a 10-year framework called Repositioning Family Planning. This aims to provide guidance on how to revitalize the family planning component of national reproductive health programmes. WHO's Regional Office for Africa is working with countries to help strengthen their family planning services.

## Managing childhood illnesses

Improved child survival became a global phenomenon largely due to the success of oral rehydration therapy for diarrhoeal diseases and immunization. Another key strategy for improving child health is the Integrated Management of Childhood Illnesses (IMCI). Developed in the 1990s by WHO and UNICEF, this strategy is being implemented in 44 of the 46 countries of the African Region to reduce the growing number of child deaths attributable to a few preventable, treatable illnesses.

The idea of IMCI is to improve the prevention or early detection and treatment of the main childhood killers in developing countries. Six conditions account for about 70% of all deaths.  These are: acute respiratory infections — mostly pneumonia — as well as diarrhoea, malaria, measles, HIV/AIDS and neonatal conditions.

IMCI training guidelines are designed to be adapted to the situation in each country. In addition, some countries are training health workers to address the problem of HIV/AIDS in children. Health workers have also been trained to support and counsel HIV-positive mothers on appropriate infant nutrition in over 20 countries in this Region. It is estimated that 6% of deaths of children aged under five years in Africa are due to HIV/AIDS.

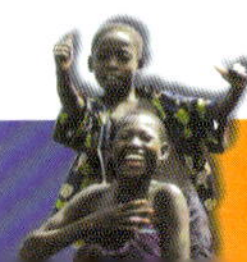

There have been reductions in child mortality in some countries that have implemented IMCI. Malawi and Mozambique have managed to lower their child mortality rates over the last 10 years. The United Republic of Tanzania reduced the mortality of children aged under five years by 13% over the two-year period from mid-2000 to mid-2002 in two districts, where IMCI was part of a comprehensive strategy to improve access to health care (see Box 2.4).

The Global Strategy on Infant and Young Child Feeding (GSIYCF) adopted by the World Health Assembly in 2002 is also a step towards addressing malnutrition in children under five years of age. WHO is supporting 17 countries in this Region in developing and implementing a GSIYCF plan to address the problem of malnutrition.

## Increasing skilled attendance at birth

Traditional birth attendants, who have no formal training, are often the only people available to assist with a birth in the African Region. These women can play an important role in educating mothers about nutrition, breastfeeding and childcare, but studies show that in countries where births are increasingly attended by skilled health workers, maternal and newborn deaths decline.

WHO has developed a set of technical and managerial guidelines and tools for the Integrated Management of Pregnancy and Childbirth (IMPAC). Countries can adapt these guidelines to provide better access to quality maternal and newborn care services. The tools can be used to improve the health workers' skills, fine tune the organization of maternal, newborn and child health-care service delivery and promote health education and community involvement in pregnancy and childbirth.

Maternal mortality in Botswana has declined since independence in 1962 with the training of skilled birth attendants and implementing other recommended guidelines. In 2000, 94% of births in this southern African country were attended by skilled health workers compared with an estimated level of 43% across the African Region. The prevalence of contraceptive use in Botswana was 39% compared with an average of 17% in this Region. The maternal mortality ratio in Botswana was 100 deaths per 100 000 live births — one of the lowest in this Region — and neonatal mortality was 40 per 1000 live births.

## Immunizing more women and children

Immunization can do much to improve child, newborn and maternal health, but its potential has still not been exploited to the full in the African Region, where vaccine-preventable diseases remain a major cause of death and disease. In 2001, WHO and other partners from the Global Alliance for Vaccines and Immunization (GAVI) launched a new initiative, Reaching Every District, to make routine immunization more widely available. So far the approach has been implemented in 26 countries in this Region.

## Caring for sick children in the United Republic of Tanzania

The Tanzanian district of Morogoro introduced free child health care and the Integrated Management of Childhood Illness strategy as part of the Tanzania Essential Health Interventions Project (TEHIP) 10 years ago. Since then, fewer children are dying of preventable and treatable causes, but challenges remain.

Zena Juma first took her sick child, Abduli Yahya, to a private clinic believing she would get better service there than in a public clinic. The boy showed no improvement, so she brought him to Morogoro Regional Hospital. On arrival at the clinic where health workers use the IMCI guidelines to manage sick children, Zubeda Dihenga, paediatric nursing officer, immediately diagnosed the little boy with severe dehydration after pinching his tummy. His skin remained bunched where she had pinched it. The child had a listless unblinking stare, and the sides of his mouth were cracked.

The child was then given an oral rehydration solution, and put on a drip while some tests were done to give a diagnosis of what was ailing him. "I just hope he will be better. I hope this hospital does something for my child," Juma said.

Meshack Massi, head doctor at Morogoro Regional Hospital, said that there were many benefits to using the Integrated Management of Childhood Illness (IMCI) approach. "IMCI is a strategy where children are treated immediately according to symptoms that they exhibit," Dr Massi said. "In the rural areas where they don't have access to laboratories, the doctors or medical personnel know that the biggest child killers are diseases with symptoms and signs of fever, diarrhoea or a cough. I am happy to say that we have since seen a reduction in child morbidity and mortality."

Habiba Ramadhani did not know about the free medical care for children under five years. Her son, Juneydi Maulidi, fell sick with malaria at the beginning of the month. She took him to the village dispensary, which is about 40 km away from Morogoro town. Medical personnel at the dispensary prescribed antibiotics and paracetamol for the four-year-old boy although tests showed he had malaria.

"They didn't have medicine and asked us to buy some from the pharmacy," 22-year-old Ramadhani said. "He got worse over the month and we decided to bring him to the bigger hospital."

When they got to the clinic at Morogoro, where IMCI is implemented, Ramadhani's child  was immediately seen by a clinical officer, and was diagnosed as having anaemia and admitted to hospital. As she waited for a relative to donate some blood so that her son could get a transfusion, Ramadhani said she was not aware of any free medical services for children aged under five years.

Ramadhani had to get a relative to donate some blood to replace the blood that her son would use up. There is a perennial shortage of blood in most Tanzanian hospitals and family or friends have to give blood if their sick relative is to receive any.

A woman in the same ward as Ramadhani had not been so lucky. Nineteen-year-old Geroda Robert's baby had just died a few minutes earlier. She and her family live in a remote village in Morogoro. Her one-year-old child fell sick but they could not get her to a doctor quickly because a neighbouring river had flooded and was impassable. They were marooned in their village until the river subsided. They came as quickly as they could to the dispensary where they were referred to Morogoro Regional Hospital, but the baby died soon after arrival.

Sifa Juma is a 27-year-old mother of four children whose ages range between nine years to four months. She stays at home to care for them while her husband buys tomatoes from village farmers and sells them in Morogoro town. Her two youngest children have benefited from the recent introduction of free medical care in the district.

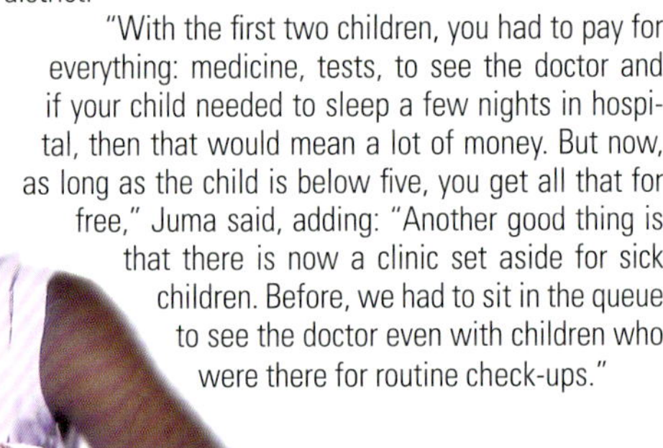

"With the first two children, you had to pay for everything: medicine, tests, to see the doctor and if your child needed to sleep a few nights in hospital, then that would mean a lot of money. But now, as long as the child is below five, you get all that for free," Juma said, adding: "Another good thing is that there is now a clinic set aside for sick children. Before, we had to sit in the queue to see the doctor even with children who were there for routine check-ups."

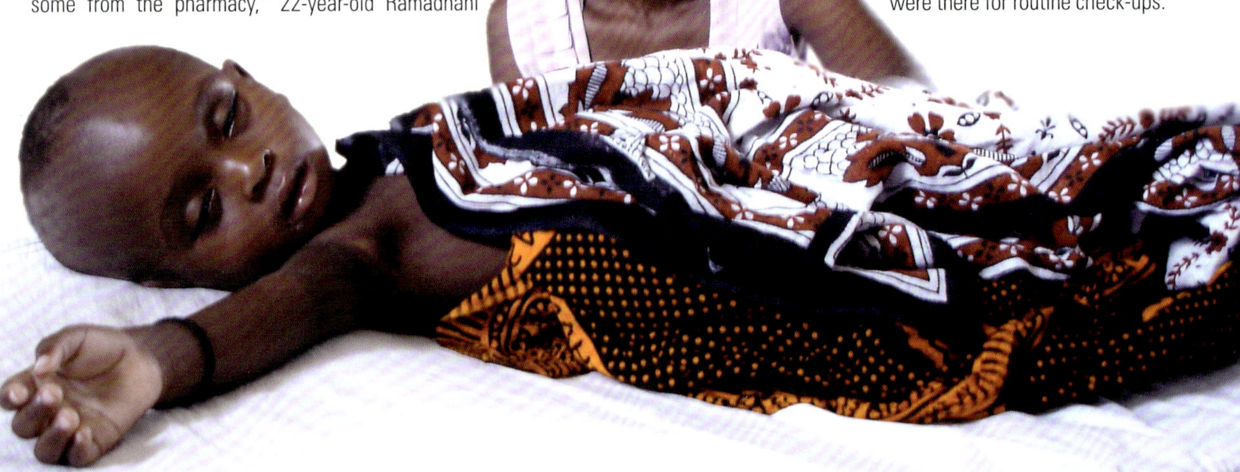

Helen Nyambura

Zena Juma watches her sleeping son Abduli Yahya.

As a result, routine vaccination coverage, as measured by coverage of DPT3 (diphtheria toxoid, tetanus toxoid and pertussis vaccine) improved from 2002 to 2005. This can be seen in overall national immunization coverage as well as in the numbers of districts that have achieved DPT3 coverage of 80% and higher. WHO/UNICEF data for 2005 show that coverage continued to improve and that the average regional DPT3 coverage was 69% at the end 2003 (see Fig 2.7)

By the end of 2004, hepatitis B vaccine was introduced in the routine immunization programme in 24 countries in the African Region, *Haemophilus influenza* type B (Hib) vaccine in 11 countries and yellow fever vaccine in 21 countries. Thirty-four countries in this Region have been granted immunization system support (ISS) by GAVI. The ISS fund has provided them with resources to strengthen their immunization systems, so that they can introduce new vaccines. The countries also received ISS to improve injection safety by providing autodisable syringes for three years as well as safety boxes for the collection of the syringes once they have been used.

Routine immunization plays a role in the prevention of vitamin A deficiency. Thirty-two countries in the African Region have a policy on using vitamin A in routine immunization, while 36 countries have used vitamin A supplementation during polio and/or measles supplemental immunization activities.

The African Region's accelerated measles control initiative has seen significant success over the last five years. The average routine measles vaccination coverage for the Region stood at 69% in 2003, up from 54% in 1999. Thirty-seven countries in this Region reported routine measles coverage of 60% or more. Since 2001, at least 26 countries have conducted mass immunization campaigns and instituted case-based measles surveillance.

Since 1999, countries that have conducted these accelerated measles control activities have documented a more than 95% decline in measles cases. The overall reduction in measles deaths for the African Region is estimated to be more than 50% compared with 1999 estimates. If the project continues in current areas and expands into new ones, it will help to achieve the 2005 World Health Assembly (WHA) goal of a 90% reduction in global measles deaths by 2010.

A total of 139 million children in 31 countries were vaccinated between January 2001 and December 2004. An additional 75 million children were targeted for vaccination in 2005. These campaigns will help the African Region achieve its goal of vaccinating 200 million children by the end of 2005. From the beginning

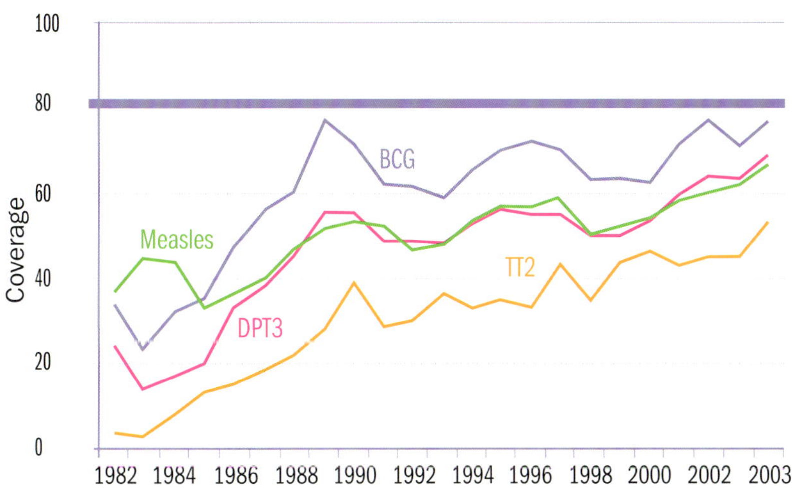

Fig 2.7

Immunizaton coverage with EPI (Expanded Programme on Immunization) vaccines, African Region, 1982–2003



Figure shows coverage for BCG (tuberculosis), DPT3 (diphtheria, pertussis or whooping cough, and tetanus), TT2 (tetanus toxoid) and measles.

Source: *Communicable diseases in the WHO African Region 2003*. Division of Prevention and Control of Communicable Diseases. WHO Regional Office for Africa; 2004

of 2006, all countries in this Region — except Liberia and Nigeria — were due to conduct nationwide catch-up measles campaigns targeting children aged 9 months to 15 years.

Most countries have integrated their supplemental measles immunization activities into their measles immunization strategy, such as the provision of vitamin A supplementation, de-worming medicines, insecticide-treated nets for malaria control and oral polio vaccine. The savings that resulted have allowed health authorities to spend more on expanding the reach of these important public health interventions. The efficiency and success of integrating supplemental activities in immunization programmes has increased donor interest, and it has helped to boost multisectoral collaboration and partnerships on an unprecedented scale.

## Conclusion: scaling up success

In much of the African Region, there has been little or no improvement in maternal, newborn and child health since the end of the 1980s. In some parts, some of the gains of the post-independence years have been reversed. However, there are interventions that work in the African setting and the key to success is scaling these up effectively.

Cape Verde, Mauritius (see Box 2.5) and Seychelles have improved maternal and newborn health through public health education including education for girls, family planning and strong political commitment to HIV/AIDS prevention and care. Similar best practices implemented in Uganda's Soroti district in 2001 with the adoption of the Making Pregnancy Safer initiative have also reaped positive results. There, community involvement, improved communications and transport, training to produce more skilled birth attendants and upgrading of health facilities led to a reduction in maternal and neonatal deaths over a period of 18 months.

Some countries in the African Region have found successful ways to address the challenges they face in financing health care for maternal, newborn and child health. For example, Mali and Mauritania have both developed community financing schemes to subsidize maternal health-care services (see Box 2.6).

Another success story is improved access to antenatal care. Many countries reached the relatively high level of 70% of women in sub-Saharan Africa receiving at least one antenatal consultation in the 1990s. Some African countries are already building on this by using antenatal consultations not only to prepare the mother for the birth but as a platform to provide other essential screening and care, such as for HIV/AIDS, tuberculosis and malaria.

A further key to success in the African context is boosting community involvement. Many people in African countries do not go to a health facility when they need care. Increasing the quality of care at health facilities alone would not reduce the maternal, neonatal and child mortality rates significantly. Essential health



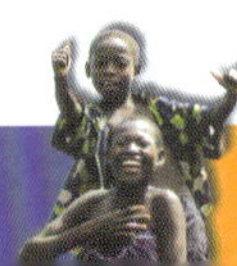

## Giving birth in Mauritius

Gone are the days when deliveries were performed at home by traditional midwives in the Indian Ocean island of Mauritius. Now, 99% of births are carried out by skilled attendants, many in hospitals or clinics. Mothers like Geeta Ramdin, a 25-year-old mother from the island, receive a high standard of antenatal and postnatal care, and if complications arise, emergency obstetric care is available.

Geeta went to her local clinic in the fourth month of pregnancy to begin monthly checks of her weight and blood pressure, and for blood and urine tests. Testing for HIV is recommended, but only done with the patient's consent, which Geeta readily gave. She was advised to have a balanced diet and take regular exercise. In the seventh month she was referred to a hospital for more comprehensive tests, including an ultrasound scan of her baby.

All was going fine. When her contractions started three days before the birth was due, doctors at the hospital said she was not dilated enough and eventually decided to do an emergency Caesarian. Obstructed labour can result in the death of the baby, the mother or both, and accounts for 12% of maternal deaths in the African Region. Geeta was fortunate enough to have access to a well-equipped hospital, able to provide her with a straightforward Caesarian delivery.

Nurses helped her to express breast milk to feed Shaksh immediately after the birth. Once Geeta recovered, she started breastfeeding Shaksh herself: "I was overjoyed to be able to hold my baby in my arms," she said. Six weeks later, Geeta took Shaksh to the health centre for a check-up. Shaksh, who is now a healthy one-year-old toddler, has had a full course of routine vaccinations.

Over the last four decades the infant mortality rate — that of babies aged less than one year — has dropped sharply in Mauritius from 60 per 1000 live births in 1962 to 12.4 in 2003. The maternal mortality ratio in 2003 was 21 per 100 000 live births, on a par with the level in developed countries.

A WHO report found that Mauritius owed this success to strong political commitment to building health systems, providing primary health care and having an efficient drug supply system. The report also found that free education — resulting in today's 95% literacy rate — and free health care were also key. Public health experts believe that health districts in other African countries that are the same size as Mauritius can emulate some of these successes.

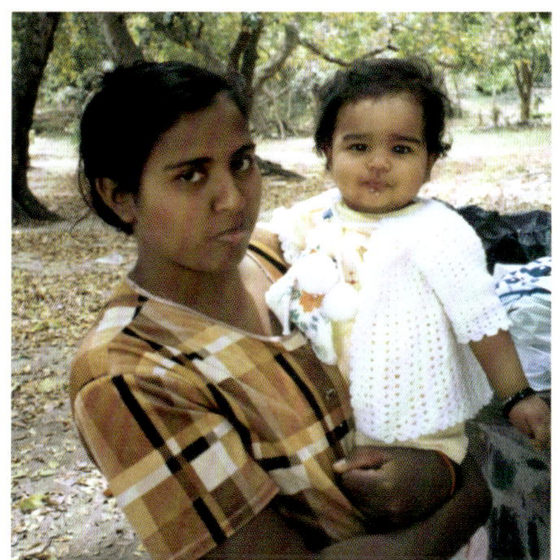

Geeta Ramdin and one-year-old Shaksh.

care needs to be brought closer to the community. One way to do this is to deliver more services through community providers, for example by supporting community-based family planning services to improve utilization of contraception.

Scaling up health systems is vital but will not be effective if many people — particularly girls and women — remain uneducated about their health. Lack of education and illiteracy are major challenges in this Region and can be overcome by taking a multisectoral approach that calls for investment in girls' education as well as an improved public health infrastructure.

Governments and international agencies need to deliver essential and sustainable maternal, newborn and child health care to the people who need them. Unless current efforts are stepped up, most countries in the African Region will have little or

## Innovative financing to provide maternal care in Mali and Mauritania

Families in the African Region cannot always afford antenatal, delivery and postnatal care, and their lack of financial access to these sometimes life-saving services contributes to the high rates of maternal and newborn deaths. Mali and Mauritania have developed community cost-sharing schemes to relieve poor families of this financial burden and to subsidize care in a bid to reduce high rates of maternal and neonatal mortality. Mali introduced a community-funded scheme in 2002 to provide 35 of 57 community health centres with staff trained to deliver babies and perform emergency obstetric surgery as well as to supply the centres with emergency kits, containing anaesthetic and other medicines for mothers who need a Caesarian. The cost is shared between community health associations, development partners and the government, while patients also make a small contribution.

WHO and Malian officials have praised people's willingness to contribute financially to improve their own maternal, newborn and child health and say the scheme needs to be extended to general hospitals and villages, where the majority of maternal and newborn deaths occur. Such deaths often result from delays in transportation and seeking help from traditional healers before taking mothers to a clinic.

Mauritania has introduced a health insurance scheme called the Obstetric Package in the capital, Nouakchott, and several other districts, to cover the costs of antenatal, delivery and postnatal care. Each pregnant woman and her family contribute US$ 0.26 to cover the costs of antenatal, delivery and postnatal care. The remaining costs are covered by French development aid, WHO and the Nouakchott health district. The scheme has helped to finance the training of nurses in emergency obstetrics and the hiring of doctors to perform Caesarians. Community members are trained to manage funds to cover the cost of ambulances.

Mauritania was one of the five countries in WHO's African Region to join the Making Pregnancy Safer programme in 2002 in a drive to halve its high maternal death rate by 2010. This year the authorities plan to extend the cost-sharing system to four other regions of the country.

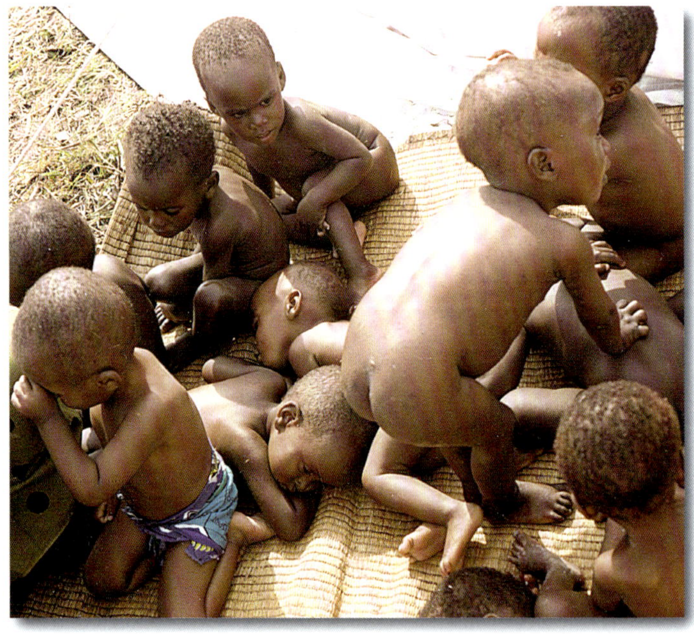



The future prospects for children depend on decisions made today.

no chance of substantially reducing the toll of avoidable maternal, newborn and child death and disease in the foreseeable future. Rapid progress is needed to come even close to achieving the target reductions envisaged by the MDGs on maternal and child health. The Road Map and the IMCI strategy are there to accelerate progress towards these goals. This ambitious MDG project can only succeed in the African Region if governments and donors pledge substantially more funds and if their joint efforts to improve maternal, newborn and child health are tightly coordinated in a way that can be sustained in the long-term. ■

## Bibliography

- Black RE, Morris SS, Bryce J. Where and why are 10 million children dying every year? *Lancet* 2003;361:2226-34.

- *Communicable Diseases in the WHO African Region 2003*. WHO Regional Office for Africa, Brazzaville: 2004.

- *Family and reproductive health: 2002 in brief. Making the difference throughout the lifespan*. Brazzaville: WHO Regional Office for Africa; 2004. WHO Regional Office for Africa document AFR/RHR/04/01.

- Hyder AA, Wali SA, McGuckin J. The burden of disease from neonatal mortality: a review of South Asia and sub-Saharan Africa. *BJOG*;110:894-901.

- Lawn J, Shibuya K, Stein C. No cry at birth: global estimates of intrapartum stillbirths and intrapartum-related neonatal deaths. *Bulletin of the World Health Organization* 2005;83:409–17.

- Maruping A. Policy interventions for reducing maternal and newborn mortality in adolescents. *African health monitor* January–June 2004:11-4.

- *Maternal mortality in 2000: estimates developed by WHO, UNICEF and UNFPA*. Geneva: Department of Reproductive Health and Research, World Health Organization; 2004.

- Murray C and Lopez A, *Health dimensions of sex and reproduction: the global burden of sexually transmitted diseases, HIV, maternal conditions, perinatal disorders, and congenital anomalies*; Harvard School of Public Health, Cambridge (MA), 1998.

- Phumaphi J. Fighting the "silent epidemic". *Bulletin of the World Health Organization* 2005;83:247–8.

- Prual A, Bouvier-Colle MH, de Bernis L, Breart G. Severe maternal morbidity from direct obstetric causes in West Africa: incidence and case fatality rates. *Bulletin of the World Health Organization*. 2000;78:593-602.

- *Road map for accelerating the attainment of the Millennium Development Goals relating to maternal and newborn health in Africa*. Brazzaville: WHO Regional Office for Africa. Document AFR/RC54/R9.

- Schellenberg JRA, Adam T, Mshinda H, Masanja H, Kabadi G, Mukasa O, et al. Effectiveness and cost of facility-based Integrated Management of Childhood Illness (IMCI) in Tanzania. *Lancet* 364;2004:1583-94.

- *The world health report 2002: reducing risks, promoting healthy life*. Geneva: World Health Organization; 2002.

- *The world health report 2005: make every mother and child count*. Geneva: World Health Organization; 2005.

- *World health statistics 2005*. Geneva: World Health Organization; Geneva: 2005.

# Infectious diseases in Africa

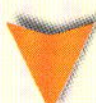

# Key messages

- Infectious diseases are a major obstacle to development
- Geography and climate are conducive to infectious diseases
- HIV/AIDS increases occurrence of other infectious diseases, particularly tuberculosis
- Health worker shortage is hampering health-care efforts

# Solutions

- Wider application of tried and tested public health interventions
- Scale up simplified, low-cost approaches to treatment
- Research and Development to find more effective medicines and vaccines
- Promotion of safe sex, and HIV testing and counselling to prevent further HIV infections and reverse AIDS pandemic

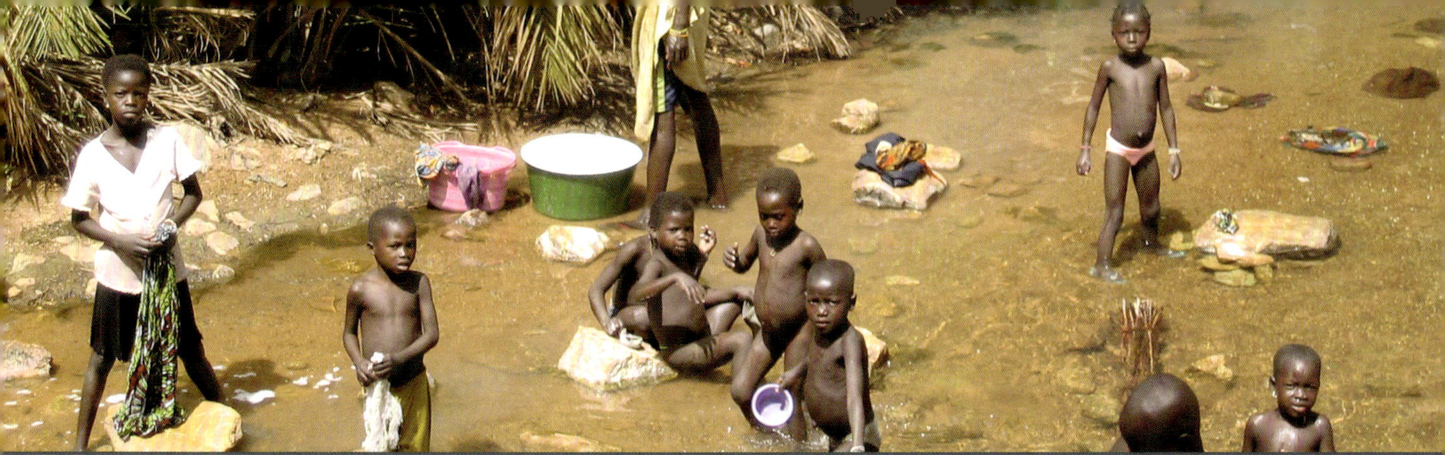

# Infectious *diseases* in Africa

## Major obstacle to development

**M**any people in Africa have yet to benefit from the improvements in diagnosis, prevention, treatment of common diseases and of living standards that have contributed to greater life expectancy in most of the rest of the world over the past half century. Unlike other regions of the world, the African Region still largely attributes its slow progress in terms of human development to the ravages of infectious diseases.

People in Africa suffer from a vast range of preventable and curable infectious diseases. HIV/AIDS, tuberculosis and malaria alone are estimated to kill about three million people every year in the Region. Africa's children bear the brunt of ill-health caused by measles, waterborne infections and parasitic diseases. The result is hardship, impoverishment, countless lives lost and reduced productivity. The diversion of scarce resources into tackling these diseases spins countries on an inescapable cycle of poverty and ill-health.

One reason for limited progress in the control of infectious diseases in Africa is cost. Many African countries cannot always afford to diagnose and treat common infections adequately. Expenditure on health is rarely as much as 5% of a country's gross domestic product, and often is as little as 2%. Average public spending on health is about US$ 10 per person per year, while patients and their families must cover the remaining costs, and these can be substantial. A realistic estimate of the cost of providing minimum health care to people in Africa is about US$ 34 per person per year. In contrast, high-income countries spend US$ 2000 per person, or more.

## HIV/AIDS, tuberculosis and malaria

The devastating impact of HIV/AIDS, tuberculosis and malaria — known as the "big three" — on people in developing countries has earned them their own Millennium Development Goal: MDG 6. Meeting this goal in the African Region is proving difficult and may be impossible without adequate funding.

Of the major contributors to short lifespans in the Region, more than six are infectious diseases: HIV/AIDS, tuberculosis, malaria, diarrhoeal diseases, acute respiratory infections and vaccine-preventable diseases. Concerted efforts to control infectious diseases in Africa have resulted in some spectacular gains against leprosy, river blindness (onchocerciasis), poliomyelitis and guinea-worm disease (dracunculiasis), while other efforts — such as those targeting the "big three" — have had little impact, despite recent improvements in prevention and treatment techniques.

HIV/AIDS is the leading cause of death and disease for adults in the Region, while malaria is the leading cause of death and disease for children aged under five years. The HIV/AIDS epidemic affects southern African countries most.

Malaria has been a constant scourge in countries south of the Sahara for centuries and, despite decades of control efforts, Africa has more than 90% of the global disease burden. Young children and pregnant women in rural areas suffer most from the complications of malaria and are most likely to die from the disease. Despite intense efforts and increased funding, the populations that are most at risk still lack adequate access to effective prevention and treatment.

With the advent of curative drugs over 50 years ago, tuberculosis came to be perceived in wealthy industrialized countries as a disease of the past. Yet, tuberculosis is on the rise in the Region with over one million new cases notified in 2003. To achieve MDG 6, case detection (Fig. 3.1) and treatment for tuberculosis need to reach many more people, particularly those who are also infected with HIV. MDG 6 will not be reached until HIV/AIDS transmission is almost interrupted in the 24 high-burden countries of the African Region. Under the "3 by 5" initiative, there are 34 high-burden countries globally.

## Challenges for disease control

Infectious diseases continue to exact a heavy toll on African countries for a number of reasons. Vectors, such as mosquitoes and flies,

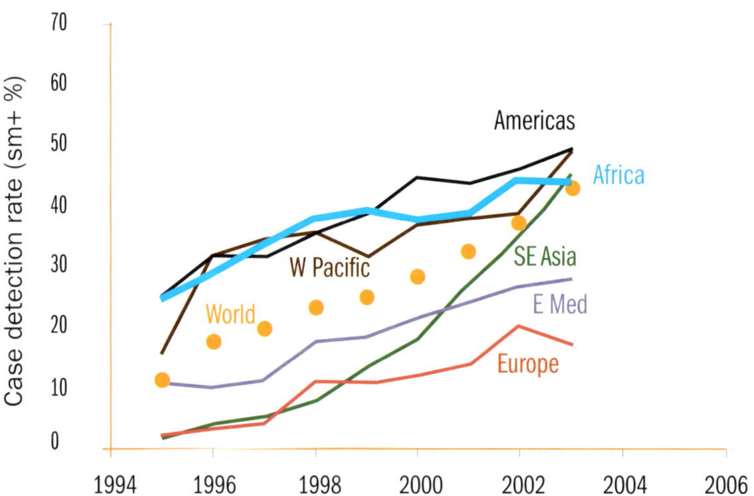

Fig 3.1

Regional progress towards 70% case detection of tuberculosis: Europe low, SE Asia acceleration, Americas high



Source: Communicable diseases in the WHO African Region 2003. Division of Prevention and Control of Communicable Diseases. WHO Regional Office for Africa; 2004.

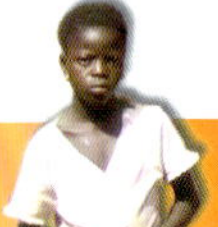

have developed resistance to insecticides and this has reduced the impact of control measures for vector-borne diseases. For many diseases — notably HIV/AIDS and malaria — there are no vaccines. Another reason why control strategies may not succeed is that some pathogens quickly become drug resistant. Also, the type and severity of infectious diseases in Africa are altering due to changes in human behaviour. Outbreaks of lethal viral fevers are examples of the unpredictable consequences of changing patterns of land use. People are thrown into close contact with infectious agents by urbanization, conflict, migration, tourism and trade.

Africa's climate and geography are conducive to the spread of infectious diseases. Mosquitoes that transmit malaria breed all year round in the hot, humid climate that dominates large swathes of the continent. In areas of scrubland, sandflies transmit leishmaniasis. Blackflies that transmit river blindness (onchocerciasis) breed on the rocks of fast-running river water. Tsetse flies transmit sleeping sickness (trypanosomiasis) and ordinary flies transmit trachoma, which causes blindness. Dogs, cats and bats transmit rabies, which can be fatal for humans. Freshwater snails carry schistosomes, the parasites that cause schistosomiasis (bilharziasis).

People living south of the Sahel region and in parts of the Great Lakes region and southern Africa are at risk of epidemic meningitis. Forests harbour rare but headline-grabbing haemorrhagic fever viruses, such as Marburg and Ebola. By cutting down the trees surrounding a village, people can expose themselves to an outbreak of one of these highly fatal diseases. Mosquitoes that transmit malaria are capable of breeding in a footprint filled with water. Other mosquitoes transmit yellow fever, lymphatic filariasis (see Fig. 3.2) and some of the haemorrhagic fever viruses. Hepatitis, typhoid and diarrhoeal diseases — including cholera and bacillary dysentery — are also frequent in cities.

Schistosomes are transmitted via freshwater snails, while worms such as roundworm, hookworm and tapeworm are soil-transmitted. Schistosomiasis has a major impact on the healthy development of children and the quality of life of adults. Some 160 million people in Africa are infected with schistosomes. Schistosomiasis also contributes to anaemia among pregnant women. Worms of all species are particularly problematic for children aged 5–14 years. Studies show that heavy infestations may impair the cognitive function of these children.

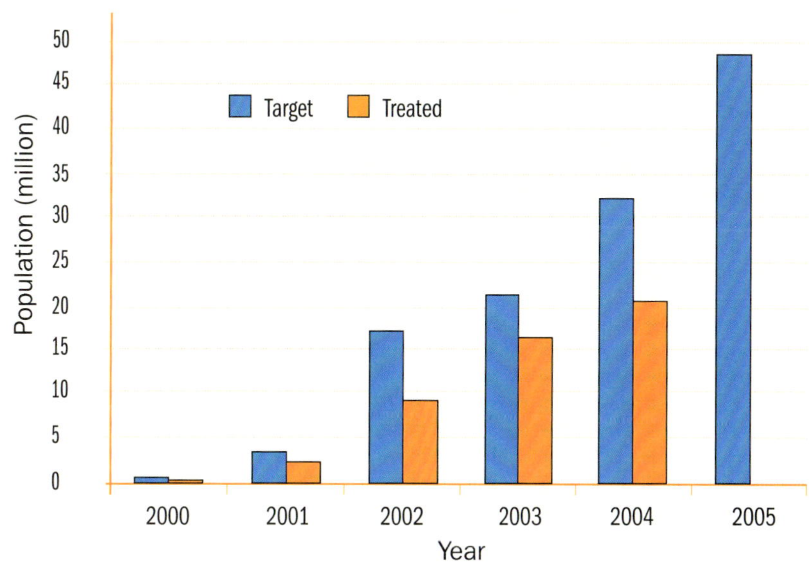

Fig 3.2

Mass drug administration for elimination of lymphatic filariasis: Population targeted versus number treated



Source: Roungou JB, Mubila L, Dabiré A, Kinvi EB, Kabore A. Progress in lymphatic filariasis elimination in the African Region. *Communicable Diseases Bulletin for the African Region.* 2005 Mar; 3:10-1.

The good news is that highly effective and affordable de-worming drugs exist that are safe for all groups at risk, including pregnant women. Large-scale control is technically feasible, but sustaining this control is a challenge. Worms have proved hard to combat where water supplies are poor and sanitation inadequate. Intestinal worms tend to persist as long as people live in extreme poverty,



## Guinea-worm disease and leprosy in Nigeria

### Guinea worm eradication: a major public health success

Control of dracunculiasis, also known as guinea-worm disease, in the African Region has been hailed as a major public health success, but sustaining this success remains a challenge. People become infected with guinea worm by drinking water containing water fleas that are infected with guinea-worm larvae. These larvae are reintroduced into water sources by people who are infected with the disease and who dip their feet in water. Guinea-worm disease can be prevented by filtering water with simple material, such as cloth. Global control efforts have been successful, with an estimated 97% reduction in cases from 1986 to date. Most remaining cases are in 13 African countries, where the final phase of eradication is proving difficult.

Despite years of control efforts and a measure of progress, residents in the village of Ikija in south-western Nigeria are still becoming infected, though not as much as in the past. "There was a time when we had people removing hundreds of worms from their legs. Now, the situation has really improved," said village head Isaiah Sobowale.

"Our river is basically stagnant water. We fetch water there around 5 am. After that, there is nothing left until the next morning. Officials treat the water regularly, but we need a better water supply," said farmer Lekan Fabowale, adding that shallow wells become infected quickly and what the village needed was a deep borehole.

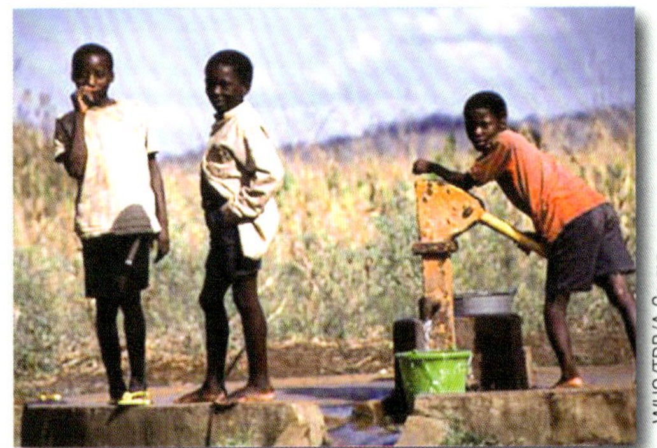

A safe drinking-water supply is necessary for the control of guinea worm.

WHO/TDR/A Crump

### Curing and reintegrating people with leprosy

There are 90% fewer cases of leprosy today than 20 years ago globally, but it is proving hard to reach the last remaining cases. In the African Region seven countries have not yet reached the global elimination target of less than one case per 10 000 people. Nigeria reached that target in 2003, but is still struggling to overcome discrimination against people with obvious signs of the disease and to address the disability it causes.

"Attempts to treat leprosy in Nigeria are hampered by stigma, socioeconomic problems and physical disability, which makes it difficult for many patients to seek help despite the fact that treatment is free," said Dr MO Lawal, the Leprosy Programme Manager in the Ministry of Health in Oyo State.

The Nigerian Government established a National Tuberculosis and Leprosy Control Programme in 1988. Lawal said that there is a long-term government plan to close down leprosy colonies and to provide a community-based treatment programme. Many people with leprosy have already left the colonies. Some live in roadside huts and beg passing motorists for alms. "My father said I could not leave education. I said, 'I must go and beg because I am a leper'. Later, I tried to get an education, but they would not accept me because I had leprosy," said Alhaji Shedu Abdullahi, the chairman of Integration, Dignity, Economic and Advancement, a non-governmental organization which supports people with leprosy in Nigeria.

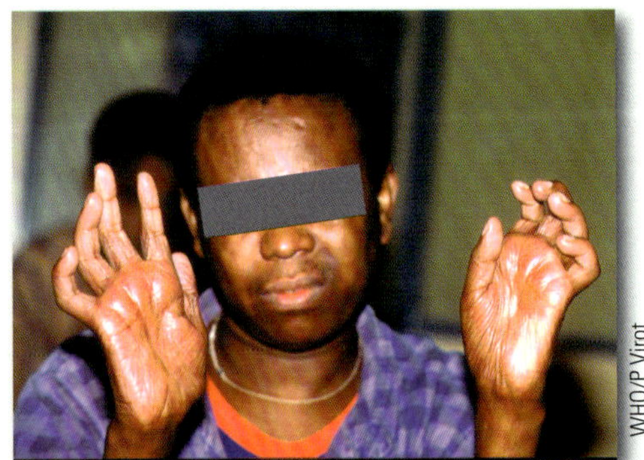

People with leprosy can suffer long-lasting disability.

WHO/P Virot

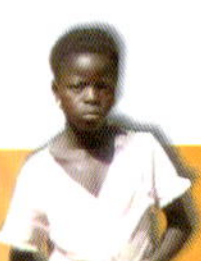

and improvements in nutrition and sanitation could be more effective than drug treatment in the long run.

Lessons from the successful efforts to control infectious diseases elsewhere in the world can be applied in Africa, although the continent faces different obstacles. Africa's geography, climate and political turmoil complicate the task. However, there are parts of the African Region where some infectious diseases are being tackled successfully.

# Diseases for which control has been successful

Infection control has been successful in African countries where diseases have characteristics that make them easier to control and where these characteristics have been countered with timely and effective interventions. Diseases that are transmitted by an insect vector can be controlled as long as an effective insecticide exists and/or humans can protect themselves from contact with the vector. One simple method is sleeping under a mosquito net to avoid the night-biting mosquitoes that transmit malaria. A cheap, effective and easily administered vaccine is an invaluable tool that can render a viral pandemic, such as polio, within reach of complete eradication as is the case today.

It has proved possible to limit the spread of diseases that follow a long course but that are not easily transmissible, such as leprosy, and to limit the spread of diseases that can be controlled by simple measures, such as filtering drinking-water to prevent guinea-worm disease. These simple solutions need to be tirelessly applied to make disease control sustainable and to lead to long-lasting improvements in public health (see Box 3.1).

## Leprosy

Leprosy is close to being eliminated — reduced to a prevalence of below one case per 10 000 people — in Africa despite traditional perceptions that it is both incurable and highly infectious. Since the disease is so disfiguring, people with leprosy have traditionally suffered social stigma and exclusion. Effective treatment exists, but case-finding can be difficult and, even today, the remaining patients scattered over large areas of the African Region have poor access to diagnosis and treatment. The Regional Strategy for Leprosy Control is a simple and effective approach, relying on early detection of cases and cure with multidrug therapy.

The prevalence of leprosy has dropped sharply because of successful application of this strategy (Fig. 3.3). Patient numbers reported to WHO's African

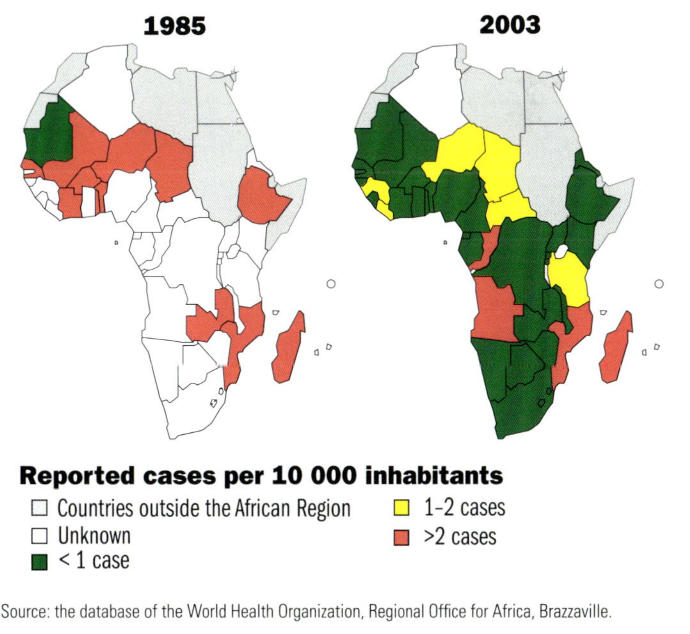

Fig 3.3

Prevalence of leprosy in the African Region, by countries, 1985 and 2003



Source: the database of the World Health Organization, Regional Office for Africa, Brazzaville.

Regional Office declined by over 60% from 127 500 in 1991 to 51 200 in 2003. Treatment coverage soared from 28% to 98% during this period. Over this 12-year period, a total of more than 800 000 cases were cured using multidrug therapy and no resistance has been reported. The Central African Republic, Comoros, the Democratic Republic of the Congo and the United Republic of Tanzania are approaching the elimination target. Angola, Madagascar and Mozambique still have areas that are highly endemic. Twenty-four-month multidrug therapy is effective and in routine programmes the relapse rate is only 0.1% per five-year period.

People with leprosy are no longer as stigmatized as they used to be, while medical treatment is now available to them. After these people have been cured, it is easier for them to integrate back into the community. However, in countries that are approaching elimination, it is difficult to reach the last few patients living in isolated communities. Active surveillance is needed to ensure that these people are diagnosed and treated.

## River blindness

Abandoned villages along valuable stretches of river bear silent testimony to the dilemma people face between having enough to eat and being able to see. River blindness, or onchocerciasis, is a parasitic disease caused by worms that are transmitted by a blackfly that breeds in turbulent river water. Seventeen million people living in West and Central Africa are estimated to be infected. Chronic infection gradually causes skin changes and blindness. People who become blind with onchocerciasis have a life expectancy only one-third of that of sighted people in the same area.

The Onchocerciasis Control Programme began in 1974 by using chemical and biological larvicides to kill blackfly larvae on virtually every infested river in 11 West African countries. It has become one of the Region's biggest and most successful public health campaigns. A total of 1.2 million square kilometres in West Africa are now completely free of onchocerciasis. Fertile land has been resettled and about 40 000 new cases of blindness per year have been prevented. As the adult worms responsible for the disease live for 10–15 years, control measures have to continue for at least this time. Large-scale vector control — using aircraft to spray larvicides on rivers — has been replaced by mass treatment of people living in endemic areas with ivermectin, once or twice a year to prevent blindness and reduce residual transmission. The African Programme for Onchocerciasis Control — which was launched in 1995 — has treated 34 million people in 16 countries to date. These programmes are exemplary cases of scale matching needs in terms of infectious disease control,

WHO/H.Anenden


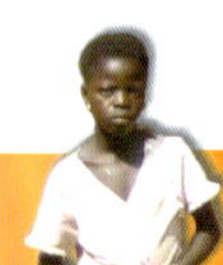

with three decades of sustained efforts tackling this persistent parasitic disease and achieving measurable gains. By helping to eliminate river blindness as a public health problem, WHO and other partners have made a major contribution to reducing poverty in the African Region. Sustaining this historical success, however, remains a challenge.

## Poliomyelitis (polio)

When the Global Polio Eradication Initiative was launched in 1988, wild poliovirus was endemic in 125 countries and paralysed more than 1000 children a day. By vaccinating two billion children against the disease, this enormous public health campaign has reduced the number of cases to less than 1000 per year globally, most of which are in Africa.

In 2004, there were 935 cases of polio across over 12 countries in the African Region, 84% of which occurred in Nigeria. This was a 100% increase in the number of cases recorded in 2003. This setback, however, has to be seen in the context of tremendous progress overall. Despite outbreaks in Angola, Cape Verde and the Democratic Republic of the Congo in 2000, 31 countries have maintained a polio-free status for more than three years. Polio vaccination resumed in 2004 in Nigeria after 11 months' suspension, and cases are subsequently decreasing. In addition to mop-up campaigns following sporadic cases, routine immunization is needed to prevent the wild poliovirus from re-establishing itself.

Each country must continue surveillance for cases of acute flaccid paralysis, which can be caused by other viruses, and test stool specimens to rule out polio as a cause. This surveillance also helps to assess the coverage of other immunizations, and measure progress towards eradication of polio. Countries must show they are continuing surveillance and stool testing to confirm that there have been no cases of polio for three consecutive years, the point at which eradication can be declared and the countries certified polio free. In 2005, 35 of the 46 countries in the African Region achieved certification surveillance standards. The eventual eradication of polio in the Region depends very much on the quality of work performed by the 16 laboratories in the Regional Polio Laboratory Network in the African Region. All members of the network kept their WHO accreditation status in 2005 — a necessary step towards a polio-free Region.

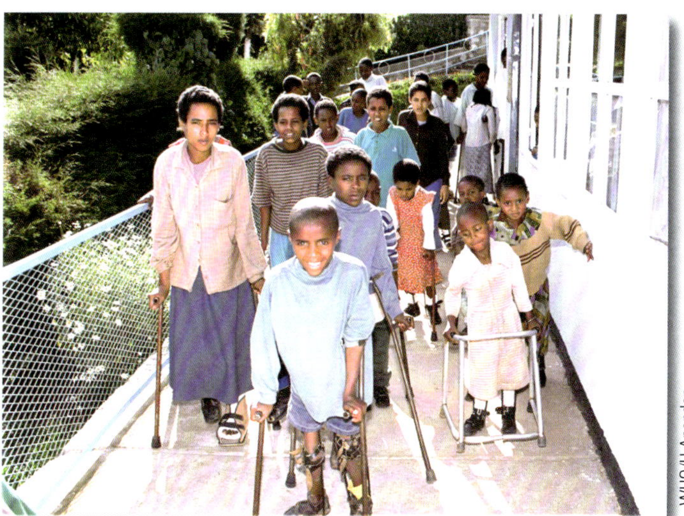

It has been an uphill struggle to eradicate polio.

# Diseases of major public concern

In contrast to the diseases which have been controlled with relative success, some diseases have persisted despite control measures and are of major public concern. HIV/AIDS, tuberculosis and malaria have become more prevalent in Africa during the last 20 years. In the case of HIV/AIDS, the failure to control the epidemic is largely due to the lack of a vaccine and the inability to change human behaviour. Tuberculosis is re-emerging where it is spurred by the HIV epidemic. The persistence of malaria is due to inadequate vector control and drug resistance.

## HIV/AIDS

Africa is the region of the world most affected by the HIV/AIDS pandemic. It has about 11% of the world's population but is home to more than 60% of all people in the world living with HIV infection. In 2005, an estimated 25.8 million people were living with HIV/AIDS, 3.2 million people became infected with the virus and 2.4 million people died of AIDS in the Region. In 16 countries in Africa, at least 10% of the population is infected.

Heterosexual transmission of HIV is the predominant mode in Africa. Some 57% of infected adults are women. Of young people who are infected, 75% are women and girls (see Fig. 3.4). Many factors contribute to the spread of the virus, namely commercial sex, sexual violence, population mobility, poverty, social instability, lack of education, high levels of sexually transmitted infections, stigma and discrimination.

The HIV epidemic has had disastrous effects on African society through its destruction of individuals, families, health systems and the public sector. Nevertheless, countries in the Region have made efforts to prevent the spread of HIV. Most countries are mounting an intersectoral response to the epidemic, in which different ministries and agencies are working together. These responses are led by national AIDS councils many of which are chaired by heads of states, such as in Angola and Burundi. Mass media and information campaigns for the general public are also being implemented in many countries, including programmes targeting young people and other vulnerable groups,

The past decade has seen real advances in the treatment of HIV/AIDS and its complications.

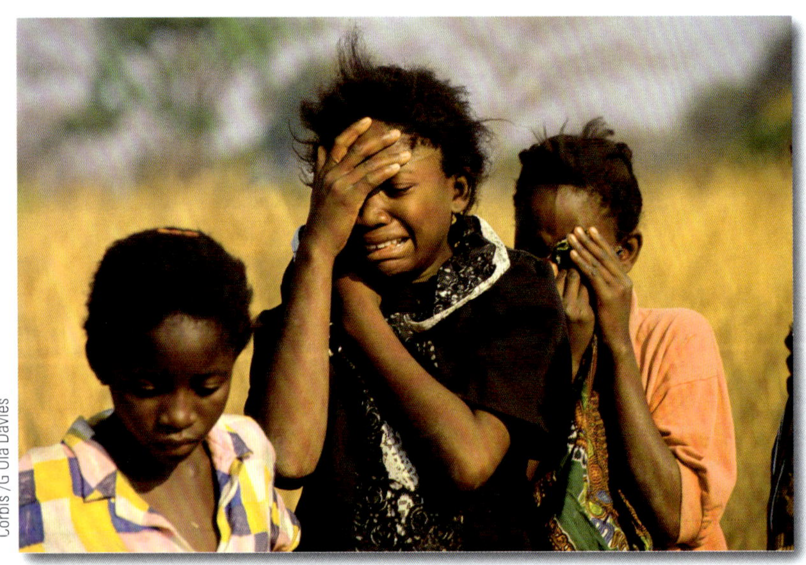



Girl weeping after their mother died of HIV/AIDS

Antiretroviral (ARV) drugs lower the level of HIV in the blood and postpone the development of opportunistic infections, allowing people to regain a good quality of life. ARV medicines are also extremely effective in preventing mother-to-child transmission of HIV during pregnancy and birth, and — as the price of these drugs has decreased — their widespread availability is a realistic target even for poor countries.

WHO and UNAIDS declared the lack of access to ARV medicines to treat HIV/AIDS in developing countries a public health emergency in 2003. Since then, the two agencies and their partners have campaigned to scale up ARV treatment as part of the "3 by 5" initiative to put three million people with HIV/AIDS on antiretroviral therapy (ART) by the end of 2005. By December 2005, the number of people living in sub-Saharan Africa receiving ART had increased more than eight-fold to 810 000 from 100 000 over the two-year period. Of the three million people targeted by "3 by 5", 2.3 million live in sub-Saharan Africa. WHO and its partners have

**Fig. 3.4**

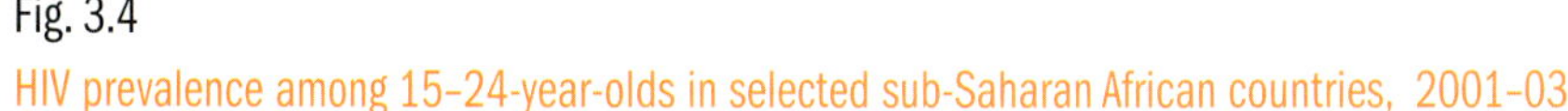

HIV prevalence among 15–24-year-olds in selected sub-Saharan African countries, 2001–03

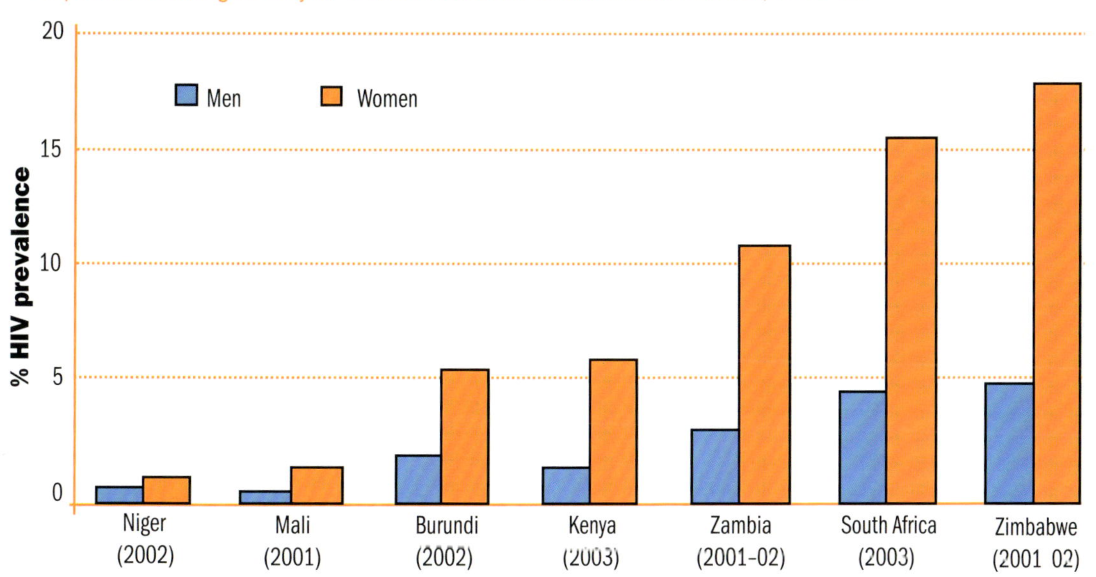


Sources: Burundi (Enquête Nationale de Séroprévalence de l'infection par le VIH au Burundi. Bujumbura, Décembre 2002). Kenya (Kenya Demographic and Health Survey 2003). Mali (Enquête Démographique et de Santé. Mali 2001).  Niger (Enquête Nationale de Séroprévalence de l'infection par le VIH dans la population générale agée de 15 à 49 ans au Niger (2002)). South Africa (Pettifor AE, Rees HV, Steffenson A, Hlongwa-Madikizela L, MacPhal C, Vermaak K, Kleinschmidt I: HIV and sexual behaviour among young South Africans: a national survey of 15-24 year olds. Johannesburg: Reproductive Health Research Unit, University of Witwatersrand, 2004).  Zambia (Zambia Demographic and Health Survey 2001-2002).  Zimbabwe (The Zimbabwe Young Adult Survey 2001-2002) .

## Activists give hope to people with HIV in Burundi

Testing positive for HIV in the 1980s or 1990s in Burundi was like a death sentence. In the absence of treatment and with the common belief that it was a punishment sent by God, many people succumbed to despair, abandoned by their families, who were unaware of the reality that HIV/AIDS is a treatable and preventable disease.

Three associations have been set up in Burundi to educate people more about the disease, to fight discrimination against people with HIV/AIDS and to provide support for them: the Burundian Society for Women Against AIDS in Africa (SWAA) formed in 1992, the Association for the Support of HIV Positive People (ANSS) and the Réseau Burundais des Personnes vivant avec le VIH/SIDA (RBP+ Network of HIV-positive people). These associations encourage Burundians to be tested for HIV, give hope and strength to HIV-positive people to stand up for their rights and, among their many other public health activities, raise awareness about the dangers of HIV.

Years of lobbying has produced results. Activists have started discussing on television what it means to be HIV positive — which had been a major taboo. The Burundian Government responded by proposing a new law against discrimination of HIV-positive people. This was adopted by the national assembly in March 2005. Adrienne Munene, who is in charge of counselling with RBP+, said that the law would help people such as an HIV-positive nurse, who was hired in 2000 by a private health centre in Bujumbura but never given a contract. "They kept telling her that she was not like others," Munene said.

Activists have also lobbied hard for treatment for people with HIV and persuaded the government to waive taxes on antiretroviral drugs. The government has also agreed to subsidize these drugs with help from the Global Fund to Fight AIDS, Tuberculosis and Malaria, and it has also negotiated with pharmaceutical firms to reduce the cost of therapy from US$ 96 to US$ 30 per person per month.

Today more than 4000 Burundians receive free antiretrovirals. HIV-positive people in that country expect to live longer thanks to support they receive from their associations and to subsidized treatment. But despite their achievements, these associations are overstretched. Dr Marie Jose Mbuzenakamwe, ANSS Coordinator, said they cannot cope with increasing demand for testing and support. She believes that all health facilities should provide HIV services so that these patients have access to treatment without travelling long distances.

The National AIDS Council has already identified hospitals and associations to help with distribution of antiretrovirals and related services but not all have adequate facilities and human resources. There is a shortage of diagnostic kits and associations fear that if donor funding dries up patients will be cut off from a drug supply.

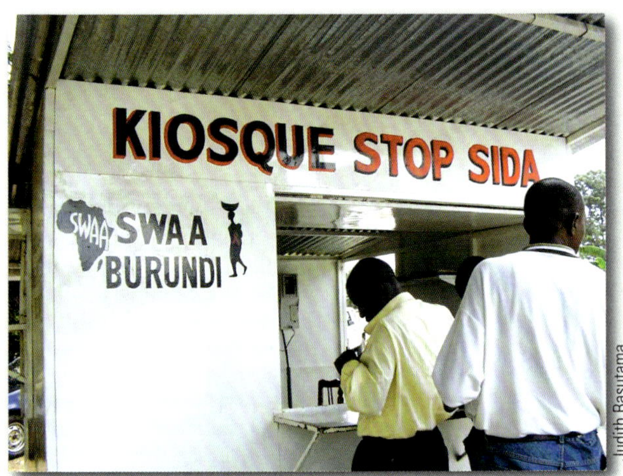


This kiosk is run by the Burundian Society of Women Against AIDS in Africa (SWAA). People come here to buy condoms and booklets on HIV. They can also watch videos on HIV/AIDS here at certain times of the day.

helped 24 high-burden countries in the Region to train more staff to deliver ART. ART coverage is expected to increase further due to solid commitment from those involved, in particular, people living with HIV/AIDS and their governments (See Box 3.2). Rapid expansion of treatment to many more people with HIV/AIDS is expected to contribute further to the lowering of ARV prices (See Box 3.3).

At least 90% of people living with HIV/AIDS across the African Region do not know that they are HIV-positive, and HIV tests are often expensive and not always available. But now that ARVs are becoming more widely available, more people will be encouraged to come forward to be tested for HIV. To encourage people to do this and to make testing services more widely available, WHO and UNAIDS have developed regional guidelines on voluntary counselling and testing (VCT)

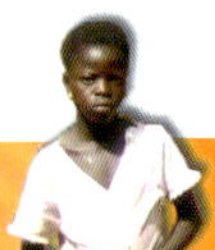

and have issued a policy statement on the provision of HIV testing and counselling services.

Twenty-eight countries — including 21 high-burden countries — have developed plans to scale up ART with the support of WHO and its partners, and 20 countries have developed plans to monitor and evaluate ART as they roll out the treatment. Botswana, Côte d'Ivoire and Lesotho are expanding people's access to treatment by taking the logical first step of providing universal HIV testing and counselling. VCT guidelines have been developed in at least 29 countries, including all 24 high-burden countries. These are the countries where HIV prevalence of women attending antenatal clinics is above 1% and where prevalence of HIV/AIDS among high-risk groups is 5% or more.

The Region is also making progress in rolling out a simplified public health approach to ART delivery based on the Integrated Management of Adult and Adolescent Illness (IMAI) approach. Thirty-three countries have developed and adapted their own simplified guidelines, based on the IMAI model, for delivering and rolling out ART to more people in need. These tools are continuously being updated based on the best available international evidence. Moreover, Regional Knowledge Hubs for HIV/AIDS Treatment and Technical Resource Networks of experts in ART have been established for East/Southern and West/Central Africa.



## How Cameroon secured lower prices for antiretrovirals

Negotiating more affordable prices for antiretrovirals has helped many poor countries deliver more of these life-saving drugs to more people who need them. Meanwhile, generic pharmaceutical companies who manufacture copies of the original patented drugs have helped to push prices further down.

UNAIDS, WHO and other UN agencies established the Accelerating Access Initiative in 2000 with seven pharmaceutical companies: Abbott Laboratories, Boehringer Ingelheim, Bristol-Myers Squibb, GlaxoSmithKline, Gilead Sciences, Merck & Co., Inc. and Roche.

The combination of the UN initiative and pressure from generic manufacturers of antiretrovirals has helped Cameroon obtain these drugs at prices that have decreased from US$ 10 000 per patient per year to about US$ 300 in the space of a few years.

Cameroon has also removed import duties and taxes on essential medicines, a further obstacle to providing the life-saving medicines. The Cameroon experience shows the simple steps that can be taken to provide antiretrovirals to people in need even with limited resources.

First, Cameroon negotiated with drug manufacturers to lower the price of antiretrovirals to US$ 50 per patient per month in early 2001, then the country won a further reduction to US$ 40 in mid-2002. By early 2003 — with generic competition growing — the price dropped further to about US$ 30 per month for the first-line regimen. If a patient does not respond to the first-line regimen, they are given second-line treatment.

Some countries — including Botswana, Burkina Faso, Burundi, Ethiopia, Mali, Mauritania, Senegal and Zambia — provide first-line treatment free to patients, while others such as Cameroon charge US$ 8–9 a month and the government covers the remaining costs. Since October 2004, Cameroon has been able to offer its citizens first-line regimen at US$ 6–9 per month and second-line at US$ 14–20 per month.

WHO and partners are helping at least 16 countries in the Region to improve laboratories to provide HIV testing and CD-cell count services. With an increase in demand for ARV medicines, WHO and its partners are training staff in 31 countries in the Region to develop procurement and supply management plans and helping countries across the Region to monitor HIV drug resistance, as part of efforts to provide appropriate treatment and care for everyone in need.

While progress has been made in the fight against HIV/AIDS in the African Region, significant challenges remain. The scarcity of diagnostic services and surveillance mechanisms makes it difficult to measure the incidence and prevalence of opportunistic infections. The most widespread opportunistic infection is *Pneumocystis jiroveci* pneumonia, which is responsible for the vast majority of AIDS-related deaths in children. Following studies in Côte d'Ivoire, UNAIDS has recommended trimethroprim–sulfamethoxazole prophylaxis for HIV-infected adults and children.

Some people have called for universal prophylaxis for HIV-positive children to prevent deaths from opportunistic pneumonia. Plans are also under way to implement preventive programmes for children in Senegal and Uganda. A vaccine for HIV and an effective microbicide gel to protect women have yet to be developed. The most powerful rallying point for HIV activists has been their campaign for access to ARVs, as these drugs are the only way to reduce complications of HIV/AIDS, prolong life and prevent mother-to-child transmission.

WHO's African Regional Office declared 2006 "the year of HIV prevention in the African Region". The aim of the campaign is to make media, governments and people in the Region as well as development partners, other stakeholders, and the global HIV prevention and control community more aware of the HIV/AIDS epidemic.

The need for further rapid scale-up of HIV/AIDS treatment and prevention in the Region raises many issues: how do countries sustain rapid expansion of treatment in the long-run without neglecting overall health system development? How can prevention be better funded and scaled up to make testing and counselling services more widely available? How can countries galvanize support from all government sectors for these public health efforts to prevent and treat HIV/AIDS, a disease that affects all public and private sectors.

## Tuberculosis

Tuberculosis is one of the world's oldest infectious diseases. Although there has been an effective, affordable and accessible cure for the disease since the 1950s, the disease still kills over 1.6 million people every year globally. In the African Region alone, there are an estimated 2.4 million new tuberculosis cases and half a million tuberculosis-related deaths every year. In 2003, the Region — which is home to 11% of the world's population — accounted for 24% of notified cases. Nine of the 22 high-burden countries that are responsible for 80% of all new tuberculosis cases are in this Region: the Democratic Republic of the Congo (DRC), Ethiopia, Kenya, Nigeria, Mozambique, South Africa, Uganda, the United Republic of Tanzania and Zimbabwe. Eleven of the 15 countries with the highest incidence are also in the Region: Botswana, Kenya, Lesotho, Malawi, Namibia, Sierra Leone, South Africa, Swaziland, Uganda, Zambia and Zimbabwe.

The incidence of tuberculosis in the Region has increased in tandem with the HIV/AIDS epidemic. People with HIV easily contract tuberculosis

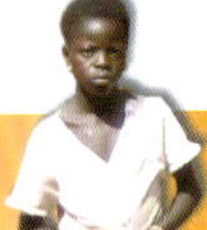

infections because of their weakened immune systems and go on to develop active tuberculosis. People with healthy immune systems recover easily from primary tuberculosis infection and have only a 10% chance of re-developing tuberculosis in their lifetime. In contrast, it is estimated that one-third of people who died of tuberculosis in 2003 in the African Region, were HIV positive.

On average, about one-third of tuberculosis patients notified in countries in the African Region are co-infected with HIV, and in most countries in southern Africa — such as Lesotho, Malawi, South Africa, Swaziland, Zambia and Zimbabwe — over two-thirds of children and adults with tuberculosis are co-infected with HIV. Tuberculosis is increasingly occurring in younger, economically productive members of society in this Region, especially girls and women, closely resembling the trend of HIV prevalence.

The recommended method for diagnosing tuberculosis is through sputum smear microscopy. The need for specialized equipment and skilled personnel to perform this test places limitations on the availability of diagnostic services. This has been complicated further by the fact that sputum microscopy in tuberculosis/HIV co-infected people is not as effective in picking up tuberculosis as in people who are not infected with HIV. With an increasing number of tuberculosis cases that are due to co-infection with HIV, more and more cases of tuberculosis are not being picked up. As a result of co-infection, tuberculosis is occurring increasingly in people aged 15–49 years. Children under five years of age are the most susceptible members of a population to tuberculosis due to HIV infection, while those aged 3–15 years are relatively resistant. The risk of an HIV-positive mother transmitting HIV to her child is 25–48% in the absence of treatment to prevent mother-to-child transmission and these HIV-positive children have a high risk of contracting tuberculosis.

Unfortunately, tuberculosis is difficult to diagnose in children, as its signs and symptoms are not specific. Also, because the tuberculin test in HIV-positive children is often negative, many children with tuberculosis are not diagnosed and do not receive treatment. Furthermore, children do not produce much sputum on demand, and microscopy tends to yield negative results due to relatively small numbers of active bacilli. It is estimated that only half of existing infectious tuberculosis cases in Africa are being detected and put on treatment. Among those put on treatment, about a fifth of them are lost to follow up before completing treatment.

The DOTS strategy, the most effective approach for combating tuberculosis, has been successfully implemented in the African Region. The strategy depends on government commitment, high-quality microscopy for diagnosis, reliable supply of high quality short-course anti-tuberculosis drugs administered under appropriate conditions, including direct observation of drug taking at least for the initial intensive phase of treatment as well as a system to monitor and evaluate case-finding and treatment outcomes.

Close supervision means better cure rates, fewer relapses and prevents drug resistance. However, the growing shortage of trained health workers in the African Region is making this very difficult to achieve. A course of treatment lasts six to eight months. This lengthy time frame is a burden on both patients and the health-care provider system. New shorter-course drugs are urgently needed.

BCG (bacille Calmette–Guérin) vaccination is routinely given to newborns in the African Region. However, even though the BCG vaccine protects people against severe forms of tuberculosis, it has only a minimal effect in preventing pulmonary tuberculosis and therefore does little to reduce the global burden of tuberculosis. A new more effective vaccine is clearly needed.

Multidrug-resistant strains are not yet a significant problem in the African Region, but occur nevertheless in some places. Thus multidrug-resistant tuberculosis needs to be contained and treated, and the interaction with the HIV epidemic needs to be studied further. Interventions for people infected with both tuberculosis and



## HIV and tuberculosis in South Africa

HIV/AIDS and tuberculosis are compounding one another to devastating effect in parts of the African Region. The realization that it will be impossible to curb the spread of HIV and reduce mortality from AIDS without tackling tuberculosis has led to an upsurge in initiatives to treat the two diseases in tandem and to support people infected with both.

It was estimated that in 2003 more than 100 000 people were co-infected with HIV and tuberculosis in South Africa, the highest number in any country in the world. The country has the thirteenth-highest prevalence of tuberculosis cases globally and an estimated 61% of these people in South Africa with tuberculosis are also infected with HIV.

The Massive Effort Campaign, a non-profit organization, tries to combine efforts to combat tuberculosis, HIV and malaria. "Tuberculosis is now the most important killer of people with HIV/AIDS in South Africa. Yet, it is an easily treated and curable disease: the drugs and diagnosis are free and accessible everywhere in the country," said the campaign's regional coordinator, Patrick Bertrand.

The ProTEST Initiative, sponsored by WHO–UNAIDS, has provided the anti-tuberculosis drug isoniazid to HIV-positive people to prevent them from developing active tuberculosis. ProTEST has run pilot programmes in the Eastern Cape, KwaZulu-Natal and the Central and Western Cape. Another initiative, the Raphael Centre in Grahamstown, Eastern Cape, was set up and is run by volunteers. The centre provides residents of the local townships with counselling, support and practical assistance to help them comply with treatment and come to terms with the diagnosis of both diseases. The Raphael Centre also provides on-the-spot HIV testing, one of the first steps recommended by ProTEST to combat the dual epidemic.

Xoliswa Mjuleni, who visits the centre regularly, found out she was HIV positive in 1999. Initially she was terrified but after she started going to the centre she gained confidence, new friends and "a reason to live". "We support each other. It doesn't always help having someone who has not experienced it telling you HIV is not the end of the world. It is so much better to have someone who knows exactly what it is like to live with HIV, someone who has the same problems, the same pain."

The challenges in treating the dual infection are many. The standard tuberculosis smear test is often negative in HIV patients which can delay starting treatment under tuberculosis protocols. Delays in test results can prove fatal and many tuberculosis patients are reluctant to be tested for HIV because of the stigma associated with the disease. WHO and national guidelines recommend first treating patients with the six-month course of directly observed tuberculosis treatment before moving on to antiretroviral (ARV) drugs for HIV/AIDS. For tuberculosis patients with advanced clinical symptoms of AIDS, the alternative is to give two months of tuberculosis treatment then start on ARV drugs. But for some patients the only option is to begin tuberculosis and ARV treatment simultaneously, which can mean taking 10 to 12 pills three times a day.

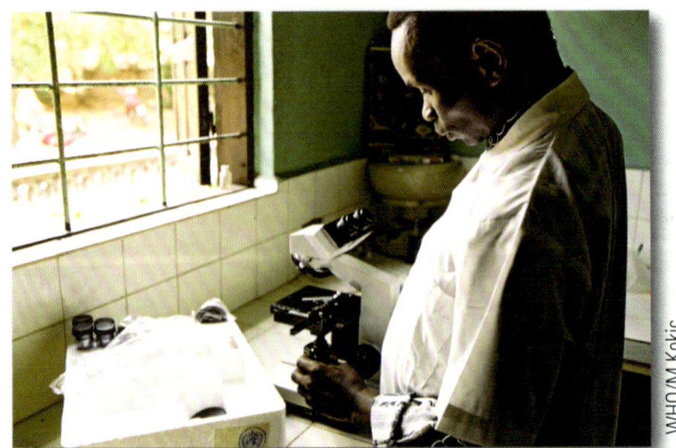

Skilled microscopists are an essential part of tuberculosis control efforts.

HIV, such as chemoprophylaxis with isoniazid for 6–12 months, have proved to be effective in reducing the incidence of tuberculosis in HIV-positive people. This intervention is being provided in some countries, but has not yet been implemented on a wide enough scale for significant impact (see Box 3.4). The battle against tuberculosis has not yet been won in the African Region and was declared a public health emergency by the Regional Committee in 2005.

## Malaria

Malaria causes untold human misery as well as economic and social devastation in the African Region, where it is endemic in 42 of the 46 Member States. Estimates show that countries in Africa with endemic malaria have 1.3 percentage points less economic growth per annum compared with similar non endemic countries, and that the annual cost of lost productivity and providing treatment for malaria in the Region is about US$12 billion.

Africa accounts for over 90% of an estimated 300–500 million clinical cases of malaria that occur in the world every year. Children in Africa account for some 90% of nearly one million malaria-related deaths estimated to occur annually in children worldwide. Malaria contributes significantly to anaemia in pregnant women, and malaria-related anaemia is estimated to cause 10 000 maternal deaths each year. In addition, malaria contributes to low birth weight in newborns.

At a meeting in Abuja, Nigeria, in 2000, African heads of state and government acknowledged the heavy disease burden due to malaria and agreed to reduce its impact through universal implementation of tried and tested interventions. They pledged to provide access to treatment to at least 60% of people with symptoms of the disease within eight hours of onset by 2005 and to halve the number of malaria deaths in the Region by 2010. Also by 2005, they pledged to provide at least 60% of pregnant women in endemic areas with preventive doses of antimalarial drugs and to ensure access to insecticide-treated nets for at least 60% of vulnerable population groups, particularly children aged less than five years and pregnant women. This concerted effort, however, faced major challenges and these goals were not met. Among those challenges, climate change has helped to expand mosquito habitats, insecticide resistance has made it more difficult to control the vectors, and the emergence and spread of drug-resistant parasites has rendered affordable treatments that were once effective, completely useless.

Other factors also make it difficult to overcome malaria. Concurrent infections with HIV have also increased the overall malaria disease burden. Malaria has re-emerged in areas where conflict and civil unrest have destroyed health systems and/or driven refugees from non-endemic areas into areas that are highly malarious, sparking epidemics.

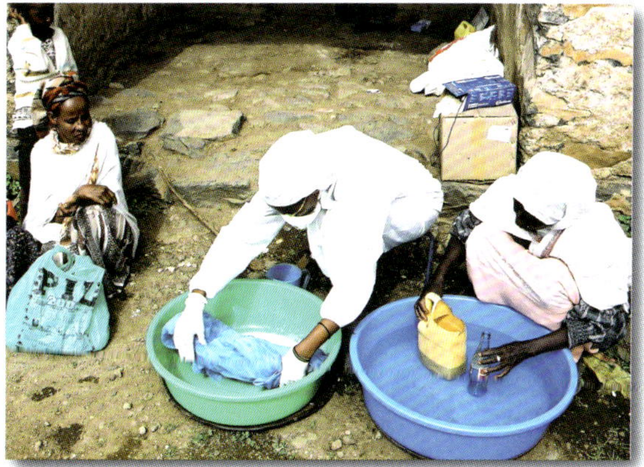

Treating mosquito nets with insecticide increases their efficiency.

Environmental control, such as the removal of standing water, and the use of bednets are two effective means of controlling malaria, but the scale of the need for simple interventions such as these is daunting. Insecticide-treated nets have been shown to reduce transmission of malaria by 50% and the need to re-apply the insecticide has been circumvented by development of nets with insecticide incorporated into the fibres and which do not require re-treatment. Eight and a half million insecticide-treated nets were distributed in 2003, bringing the total number in Africa to 20 million. But with 650 million people at risk of infection, and the fact that most insecticide-treated nets only last up to about three years, many people are still not being protected from the malaria-bearing mosquitoes that bite at night.

It seems unlikely that all the Abuja targets will be met as fewer than 5% of the population at risk and only 3% of children under five years old were sleeping under ITNs, according to the *World malaria report 2005.*

Studies done in Kenya showed insecticide-treated nets significantly improve the health of pregnant women and children, and that the benefits were extended through decreased transmission to households that did not have nets. The best argument for persisting with this simple but effective means of malaria control is illustrated in countries such as Eritrea, where nets are distributed free of charge (Fig 3.5).

Since the Second World War, attempts to control mosquitoes have been less successful in Africa than in the Americas. Indoor residual spraying with DDT and other insecticides can be an effective method for mosquito control, especially during epidemics and emergencies. WHO recommends that countries select insecticides according to local needs. At least 10 African countries include indoor residual spraying as part of their malaria control efforts.

From the 1970s to the 1980s, malaria was reasonably well controlled in much of East Africa, as cheap and affordable drugs such as chloroquine and sulfadoxine–pyrimethamine were readily available. Today cheap and effective treatment for malaria with one drug — known as monotherapy — is no longer an option for most countries in Africa because of drug resistance. Chloroquine, amodiaquine and sulfadoxine–

## Fig. 3.5

Trends in incidence of malaria cases and distribution of insecticide-treated nets (ITNs), Eritrea (1997–2004)

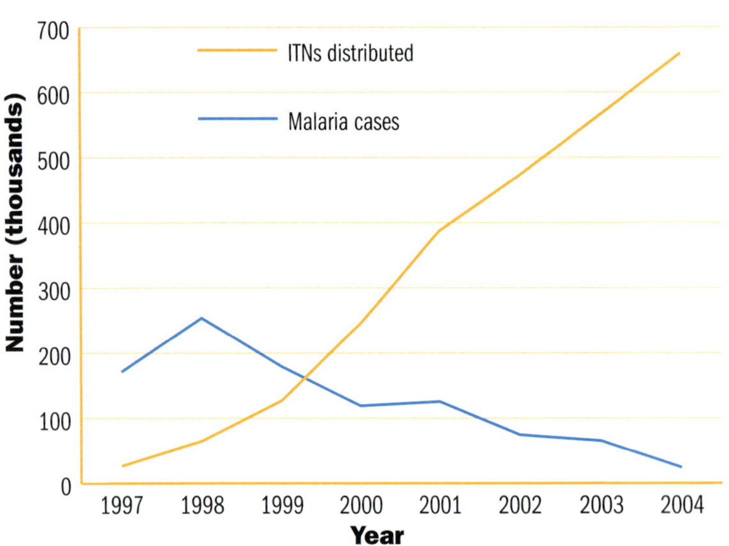


Source: the database of the World Health Organization, Regional Office for Africa, Brazzaville.

pyrimethamine are still effective medicines for malaria in other parts of the world but now fail widely in Africa. That leaves many countries with little choice but to purchase drugs that are more effective but also more expensive (see Box 3.5).

No resistance to artemisinin combination medicines has been reported to date, but many African countries simply cannot afford the US$ 2 per adult it costs for a



## Treating malaria in Ethiopia

Like many countries in the African Region, Ethiopia faces a malaria treatment crisis due to increasing resistance of the malaria parasites to common drugs. Recent experience shows the benefits of switching from old drugs to new effective combination therapies, which are currently more expensive.

When Ethiopia adopted the antimalarial artemether–lumefantrine for first-line treatment, the impact on the remote district of Kafta Humera Wereda was dramatic. "The people were fed up taking the old drugs and them not working, again and again," said Seyoum Dejene, an Ethiopian doctor working there. "The people like it: they call Coartem a 'miracle drug'," he said, referring to one brand name of artemether–lumefantrine.

More than 100 000 migrant workers pour into Kafta Humera Wereda every year from August to November to help with the harvest, adding to a resident population of 65 000. These months coincide with the peak of the malaria season, which starts as the rains end in September. Many migrants from the highlands — where malaria is not endemic — do not have natural immunity to the disease. They sleep outside with no protection from the mosquitoes and have poor access to health services, and so many get sick. The presence of so many migrant workers can trigger a malaria epidemic, as these people are more susceptible than the resident population.

In 2003, about 45 000 people died in a malaria epidemic in Ethiopia largely because of parasite resistance to old antimalarial drugs. Jo Mesure, former medical coordinator of Médecins Sans Frontières (MSF) in northern Ethiopia, recalled how until 2004, when the government approved artemether–lumefantrine for first-line treatment, staff had to give people two drugs, sulfadoxine–pyrimethamine and chloroquine, to treat suspected falciparum malaria, knowing that these drugs were ineffective. Artemether–lumefantrine is one of a group of drugs, known as ACTs or artemisinin-based combination therapies, which are the only antimalarials that currently face no resistance. But at US$ 0.60 to treat a child and US$ 2 to treat an adult, these cost 10 times more than the older drugs.

According to Mesure, the effect of the change in drug policy was immediate and dramatic. Manica Balasegaram, who led an MSF study to inform the Ethiopian national drug policy, agreed: "Before we started the project we had reports from the health staff of people being treated seven to eight times with SP (sulfadoxine–pyrimethamine) — it just was not working."

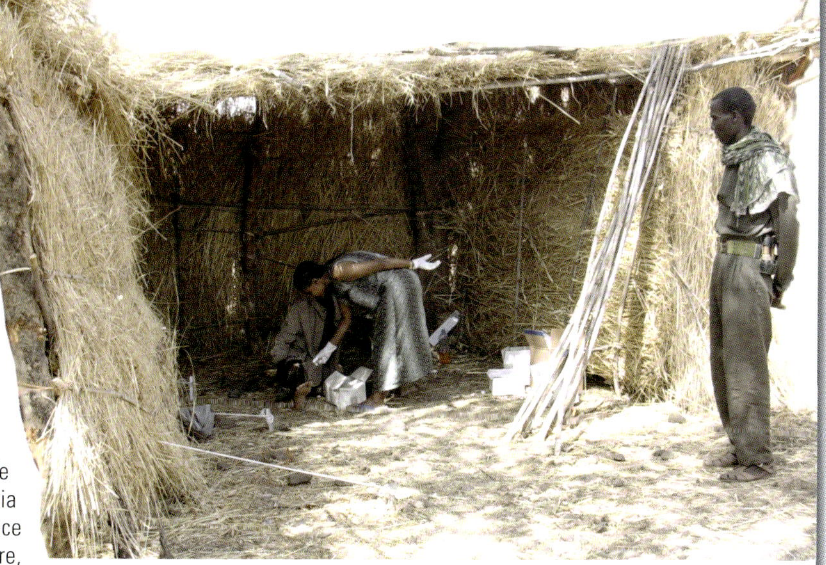

Patient in Kafta Humera Woreda receiving artemether-lumefantrine for treatment of malaria.

Manica Balasegaram

course of artemether–lumefantrine, the only fixed-dose artemisinin-based combination currently on the WHO Essential Medicines List. A recent trial in Mbarara, Uganda, showed that unsupervised administration of artemether–lumefantrine was as efficacious as directly supervised treatment, offering some hope for the feasibility of widespread use in a Region where public health efforts are often hampered by a shortage of trained health workers. Drug resistance and the change in drug policy (Fig. 3.6) in about 18 countries all at once in 2004 has led to a surge in global demand for artemisinin and some efforts are under way to increase supply. For example, farmers, in the United Republic of Tanzania have started to grow the shrub from which artemisinin is obtained. The active ingredient is being extracted, made into pills abroad and being shipped back to the United Republic of Tanzania and other African countries. The plan is eventually to produce tablets locally to meet domestic demand.

Another area of concern for malaria control is drug quality and regulations. Countries in Africa are improving drug regulations to adapt to the use of the new antimalarial drugs and meet international standards. Countries are also working on their pricing policies as expensive drugs could be re-sold on the street or counterfeited. When the street value is high, deaths increase either way. This is because the malaria parasites develop resistance when some patients fail to complete their course of treatment and because hoarding or reselling drugs encourages incorrect use. People unsuspectingly buy counterfeit drugs because they may be cheaper.

In areas where malaria is endemic, fever is often attributed to malaria and people often take antimalarial drugs without being diagnosed properly. It is essential to balance the provision of timely access to drugs with specific diagnosis, but this balance is difficult to achieve when countries lack sufficient numbers of adequately trained health workers in communities where the burden of disease is greatest.

## Fig 3.6

Status of malaria drug policy change and implementation in the African Region as of July 2005

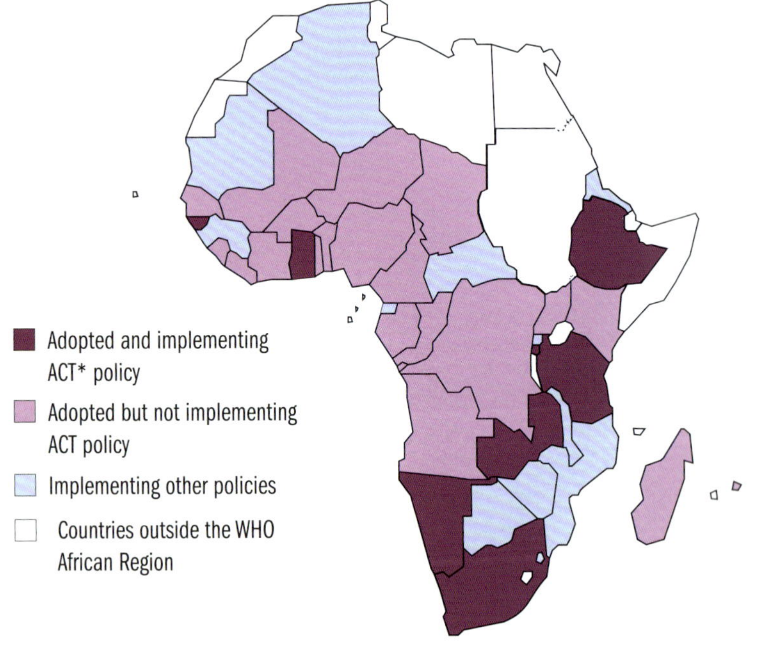


* Artemisinin-based combination therapy drugs (ACTs).

18 countries in the African Region have switched their malaria drugs policy to ACTs

Source: the database of the World Health Organization, Regional Office for Africa, Brazzaville.

Intermittent preventive treatment — in the form of two or three doses of sulfadoxine–pyrimethamine during pregnancy — reduces maternal anaemia and the risk of low birth weight in newborn babies. Intermittent preventive treatment of pregnant women has been implemented in Kenya, Malawi, Uganda, the United Republic of Tanzania, Zambia and Zimbabwe.

Insecticide-treated nets, intermittent preventive treatment during pregnancy and artemisinin combinations for diagnosed infections cost US$ 2–8 per person per year, depending on how many of these three simple antimalarial measures are applied, according to WHO's Regional Office for Africa. In many African countries, some people cannot afford to pay this much for only one of the many health problems they encounter, and that is why subsidized treatment is needed to make progress. Fewer than 5% of the population at risk and only 3% of children under five years old were sleeping under ITNs, according to the *World malaria report 2005*.

Coverage for intermittent preventive treatment for pregnant women in the Region is low, and the number of people receiving effective antimalarial medicines within 24 hours of onset of symptoms also remains low and is made worse by increasing drug resistance. A total of 33 of the 42 malaria-endemic countries in the Region have adopted artemisinin combinations as first-line treatment, but only nine of these are currently implementing such treatment policies.

# Diseases that are prone to cause epidemics

The last two decades have seen the re-emergence in Africa of diseases that are prone to cause epidemics as well as new diseases, all of which require rapid and appropriate response. Countries of the African Region started implementing integrated disease surveillance and response (IDSR) systems as an important step to tackling outbreaks of diseases — such as cholera, meningitis, Lassa fever, yellow fever, hepatitis E, dysentery, plague, malaria and leptospirosis — that can trigger epidemics. These surveillance systems have led to improved epidemiological reporting and outbreak detection, as well as better laboratory confirmation, data analysis and use of information.

Thirty-nine of the 46 Member States have developed integrated disease surveillance and response guidelines. A review of 15 countries in the Region in 2004 showed that a median of 82% of districts were submitting epidemiological reports on time and that 50% of districts notified suspected disease outbreaks within two days. These initial findings show significant progress.

WHO's Office for the African Region is helping countries build and reinforce these systems. A comprehensive regional database for communicable diseases has been set up and by the end of 2004, 26 countries were submitting monthly disease surveillance reports on time. WHO has established a rapid response network of 54 experts to provide technical support to countries in the event of an outbreak or epidemic. Emergency stocks of drugs, vaccines, equipment and reagent have also been made available to countries in need.

WHO has in recent years helped to establish a network of national public health laboratories in Member States to improve each country's outbreak investigation and report those to the Region's central epidemiological database. In 2004, all major outbreaks in the Region were confirmed through this regional public health laboratory network. WHO has also helped train staff from Member States to run integrated disease surveillance and response systems. The main challenge in future will be to scale up these systems to every district in every Member State and to ensure the delivery of timely analysis of data and use of surveillance information as the basis for effective health interventions. Another challenge is to sustain the commitment of national authorities and partners to providing adequate resources and funding for these systems.

## Neglected diseases

Neglected diseases — such as sleeping sickness, visceral leishmaniasis and Buruli ulcer — continue to take their toll in the African Region, but they no longer figure on the disease-control agenda of the developed world. Progress has stalled on drug research and development to treat these diseases, but they still have a considerable impact on human development in the Region and have become worse while efforts have focused on other diseases.

Raising the profile of neglected diseases is the first step towards curing them. Renewed awareness of these diseases and their devastating impact is as badly needed in the Region as the final stages towards attaining the much-publicized goal of eradicating polio. The Drugs for Neglected Diseases Initiative was launched in 2003 to promote the development of drugs for diseases such as sleeping sickness, which affects 500 000 people in 36 African countries, but for which the only effective drug is highly toxic and must be given intravenously. Buruli ulcer is another disease that does not attract adequate funds to fight it but happens to be the most common mycobacterial infection after tuberculosis and leprosy. Buruli ulcer cases have been found in 30 countries worldwide, 17 of which are in the African Region, according to the Global Buruli Ulcer Initiative. Surgery can be used to treat Buruli ulcer, but it has recently been shown that the drugs used for treating other mycobacterial diseases, such as leprosy and tuberculosis, have some effect on the ulcers. Of 1450 new drugs that have gone on the global market since the 1970s, only 13 target the diseases that mainly affect poor people in the tropics of which Africa has by far the greatest share, according to the Drugs for Neglected Diseases Initiative.

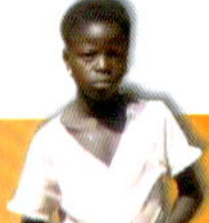

# Conclusion: Learning from past success

The examples of successful disease control: smallpox, leprosy, polio, guinea-worm disease and river blindness show that the huge burden of infectious diseases in Africa can be reduced by better use and wider application of current knowledge and techniques. Political will backed by financial support are the crucial prerequisites to scaling up the tried and tested control methods that are specific to each disease. Effective disease control is eminently feasible given a judicious mix of environmental control, mass chemotherapy, vaccination, case detection, treatment and prevention strategies. For HIV/AIDS, there has been significant progress in improving access to ARV medicines. In the first half of 2005, most African countries reported that demand for ARV treatment was outstripping their capacity to supply it, and stressed their urgent need for increased resources and technical support to maintain their momentum in scaling up this treatment.

Interventions need to be implemented on a large scale and be above critical levels of coverage; they also need to be sustained in order to have an impact. More research and development leading to good vaccines for malaria and HIV and to a more effective vaccine for tuberculosis would prevent the greater part of infectious-disease-related deaths in the African Region and go a long way to meeting MDG 6 (see Box 3.6). More aid is needed for this research and development, as well as for capacity building in public health. The World Bank estimates that it will take a ten-fold increase in current aid levels to bridge the financing gap of US$ 25-40 per person per year it estimates are needed for basic public health in the low-income countries of Africa. Meanwhile, more use of available solutions is also an imperative: better distribution of insecticide-treated nets; very high coverage of routine immunization with recommended vaccines; effective drugs for malaria where and when they are needed; universal testing for HIV; prevention of mother-to-child transmission; and targeted HIV prevention for high-risk and vulnerable groups, such as sex workers.

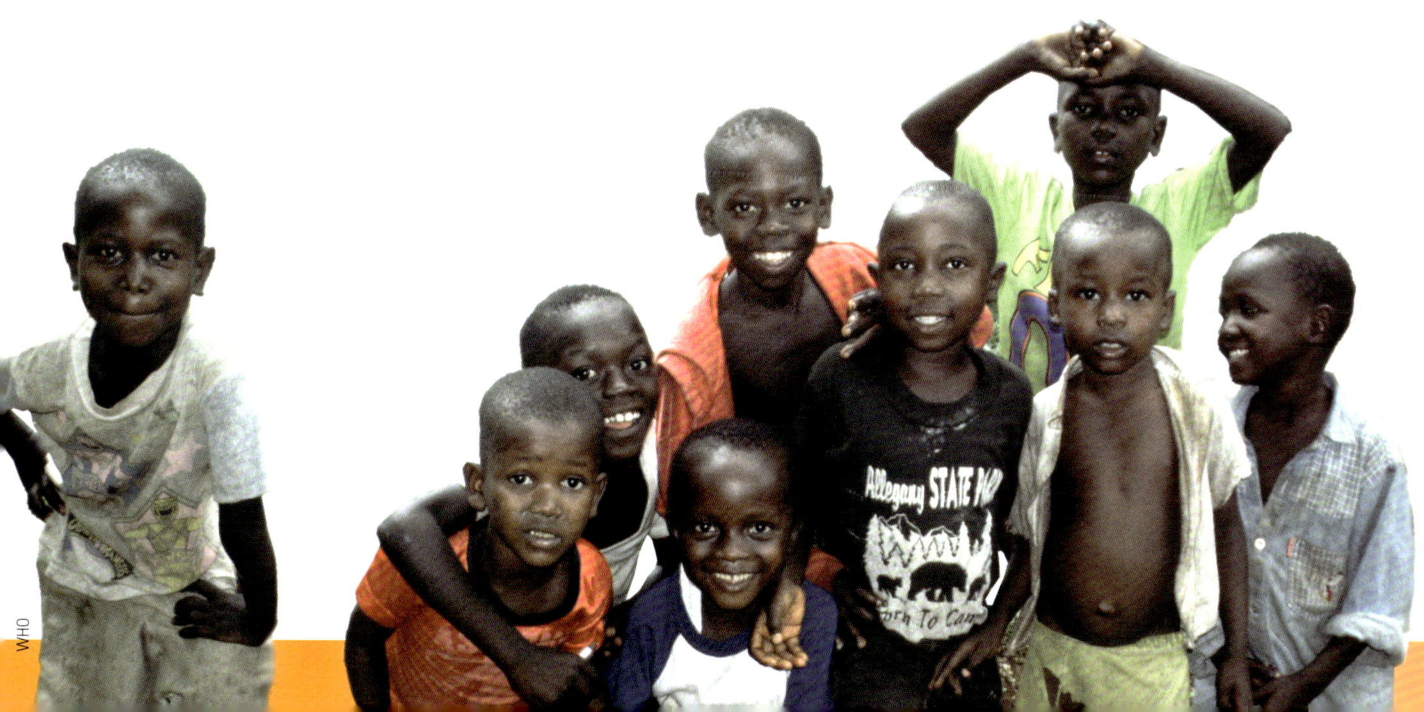

Finally, more collaboration is needed to provide adequate food and clean water, and to promote safe sex. This combined effort would bring the African Region closer to achieving the Millennium Development Goals than any disease-specific intervention. ■



## MDG 6: HIV/AIDS, malaria, and other diseases

The MDG 6 target for HIV/AIDS — the leading cause of morbidity and mortality in the African Region — is to halt and reverse the spread of the virus by 2015. Progress is measured by HIV prevalence among pregnant women aged 15–24 years, condom use and the number of children orphaned by the epidemic. The MDG 6 target for malaria, tuberculosis and other major infectious diseases is also to halt and reverse their spread by 2015. Progress is measured by prevalence and deaths associated with malaria and the proportion of the population in endemic areas using effective malaria prevention and treatment measures. For tuberculosis, progress towards the target is measured by prevalence and deaths due to tuberculosis and the proportion of cases detected and cured under the DOTS strategy.

The HIV/AIDS epidemic is most severe in southern Africa, with more than 15% prevalence among pregnant women aged 15–24 years in eight countries in 2003–2004. According to the World Bank, the epidemic in sub-Saharan Africa has risen steadily from a prevalence of just under 3% in 1990, taken as the baseline for measuring progress on the MDGs, to just over 7% in 2000. In 2005, HIV prevalence of adults aged 15–49 was estimated at 5.8%. This lower estimate for the African Region is partly due to an expansion of surveillance in rural areas where prevalence is lower. There are no clear signs that HIV prevalence is declining in southern Africa, where exceptionally high infection levels continue in some countries.

A major obstacle to tracking progress towards achieving the target of reducing the burden of malaria is the limited availability of data. Most people with malaria in Africa are treated at home. Therefore, reported cases from countries are not a reliable way to measure prevalence. Better data collection is needed to measure progress in fighting malaria.

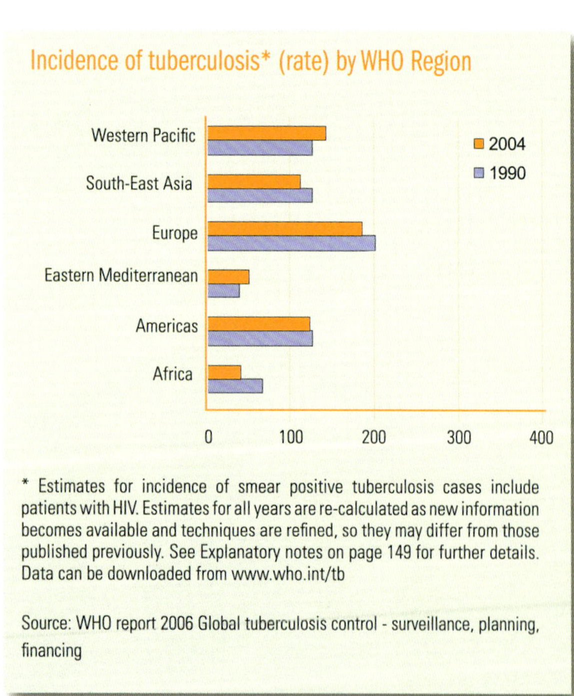


* Estimates for incidence of smear positive tuberculosis cases include patients with HIV. Estimates for all years are re-calculated as new information becomes available and techniques are refined, so they may differ from those published previously. See Explanatory notes on page 149 for further details. Data can be downloaded from www.who.int/tb

Source: WHO report 2006 Global tuberculosis control - surveillance, planning, financing

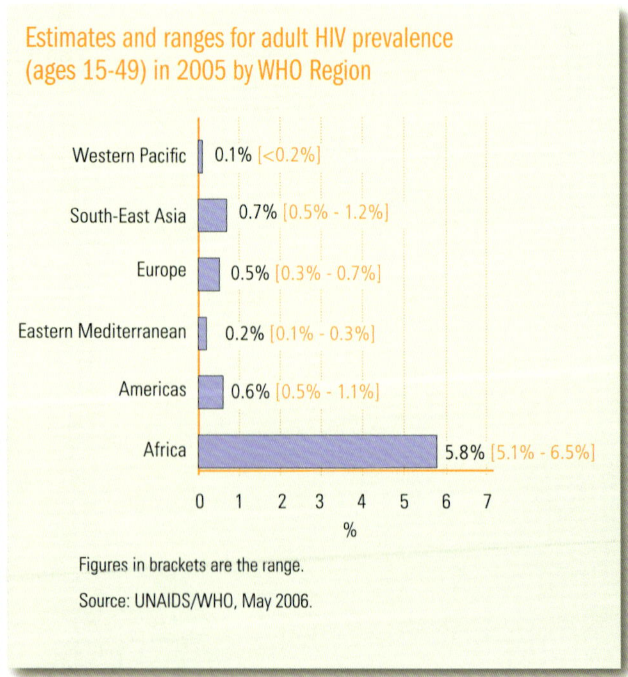


Figures in brackets are the range.

Source: UNAIDS/WHO, May 2006.

## Bibliography

- *2004 report on the global AIDS epidemic: 4th global report*. Geneva: Joint United Nations Programme on HIV/AIDS (UNAIDS) 2004. UNAIDS document UNAIDS/04.16E. Available from: http://www.unaids.org/bangkok2004/GAR2004_html/ GAR2004_00_en.htm

- *2006 report on the global AIDS epidemic: a UNAIDS 10th Anniversary Special*. Geneva: Joint United Nations Programme on HIV/AIDS (UNAIDS) 2004. Available from: http://www.unaids.org/en/HIV_data/2006GlobalReport/default.asp

- *Africa malaria report 2003*. World Health Organization/UNICEF 2003. http://www.rbm.who.int/amd2003/amr2003/amr_toc.htm

- *AIDS in Africa: three scenarios to 2025*. Geneva: Joint United Nations Programme on HIV/AIDS (UNAIDS); 2005. UNAIDS document UNAIDS/04.52E. Available from: http://www.unaids.org/en/AIDS+in+Africa_Three+scenarios+to+2025.asp

- Ainsworth M, Fransen L, Over M, editors. *Confronting AIDS: evidence from the developing world: Selected background papers for the World Bank Policy Research Report*. Brussels: European Commission; 1998.

- Ait-Khaled N. e Enarson D. Tuberculose Manuel pour les étudiants en Médecine. World Health Organization et L'Union Internationale Contre la Tuberculose et les Maladies Respiratoires. Available from: http://www.tbrieder.org/publications/ students_fr.pdf

- Anti-tuberculosis drug resistance in the world report no. 3. Available from: http://www.who.int/tb/publications/who_htm_ tb_2004_343/en/

- Bide L, Regional Advisor, Leprosy Elimination Programme, DDC Division, AFRO. *Annual leprosy situation reports*.

- Chitsulo L, Engels D, Savioli L, Montresor A. The global status of schistosomiasis and its control. *Acta Tropica* 2000;77:41-51

- Cohen D. *Human capital and the HIV/AIDS epidemic in sub-Saharan Africa*. Geneva: International Labour Organization; 2002.

- *Communicable diseases in the WHO African Region 2003*. Division of Prevention and Control of Communicable Diseases. WHO Regional Office for Africa; 2004.

- *Global tuberculosis control: surveillance, planning, financing*. Geneva: World Health Organization; 2005. WHO document WHO/HTM/TB/2005.349.

- Global Partnership to Roll Back Malaria. *World malaria report: 2005*. Geneva: World Health Organization and UNICEF; 2005

- *HIV/AIDS Epidemiological Surveillance Report for the WHO African Region*: 2005 Update. Harare, Zimbabwe; December 2005. World Health Organization, Regional Office for Africa.

- *HIV/AIDS and work: global estimates impact and response 2004*. Geneva: International Labour Organization; 2004.

- *Human development report 2003. Millennium Development Goals: a compact among nations to end human poverty*. UNDP. New York: Oxford University Press; 2003. Available from: http://hdr.undp.org/reports/global/2003/

- *Interim Policy on Collaborative TB/HIV activities*. WHO/HTM/TB/2004.330; WHO/HTM/HIV/2004.1. Geneva: World Health Organization; 2004. Available from: http://whqlibdoc.who.int/hq/2004/who_htm_tb_2004.330.pdf

- *Macroeconomics and health: investing in health for economic development. Report of the Commission on Macroeconomics and Health*. Geneva: World Health Organization; 2001.

- Piola P, Fogg C, Bajunirwe F, Biraro S, Grandesso F, Ruzagira E, et al. Supervised versus unsupervised intake of six-dose artemether-lumefantrine for treatment of acute, uncomplicated *Plasmodium falciparum* malaria in Mbarara, Uganda: a randomised trial. *Lancet* 2005;365:1467-73.

- *Progress on global access to HIV antiretroviral therapy: an update on "3 x 5"*. Geneva: UNAIDS and World Health Organization; 2005

- *Progress on global access to HIV antiretroviral therapy: A Report on "3 x 5" and Beyond*. Geneva: UNAIDS and World Health Organization; 2006

- Roungou JB, Mubila L, Dabiré A, Kinvi EB, Kabore A. Progress in lymphatic filariasis elimination in the African Region. *Communicable Diseases Bulletin for the African Region*. 2005 Mar; 3: 10-1.

- Roungou J. Regional Advisor Annual Reports, Other Tropical Diseases (OTD) DDC Division, WHO Regional Office for Africa. *Annual reports, other tropical diseases*.

- Sachs J, Malaney P. The economic and social burden of malaria. *Nature* 2002;415:618-85.

- Steketee RW, Nahlen BL, Parise ME, Menendez C. The burden of malaria in pregnancy in malaria-endemic areas. *American Journal of Tropical Medicine and Hygiene* 2001;64:28-35.

- Stephenson LS, Latham MC, Ottesen EA. Global malnutrition. *Parasitology* 2000;121 Suppl:S5-22

- *Strategic Framework to reduce the burden of TB/HIV.* Geneva: World Health Organization; 2002. Available from http://www.who.int/docstore/gtb/publications/tb_hiv/2002_296/pdf/tb_hiv_2002_296_en.pdf

- *TB/HIV Clinical Manual.* Second Edition. Geneva: World Health Organization; 2004. Available from http://whqlibdoc.who.int/publications/2004/9241546344.pdf

- *Treatment of Tuberculosis. Guidelines for National Programmes.* Geneva: World Health Organization; 2003. Available from http://www.who.int/tb/publications/cds_tb_2003_313/en/

- *UNAIDS/WHO AIDS epidemic update: December 2005.* http://www.unaids.org/epi/2005/doc/EPlupdate2005_html_en/epi05_05_en.htm

- *UNECA Compact For African Recovery: Operationalizing the Millennium Partnership for the African Recovery Programme.* Addis Ababa: United Nations Economic Commission for Africa. Available from: http://www.uneca.org/cfm/compact_for_african_recovery.htm

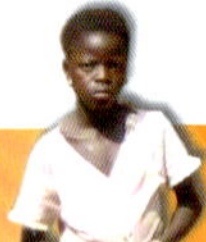

# Noncommunicable diseases in Africa

# Key messages

- Noncommunicable diseases and injuries constitute a growing public health problem in the African Region
- African countries do not devote adequate resources to address noncommunicable diseases
- Donor agencies and research institutions are neglecting the growing burden of noncommunicable diseases and injuries
- Risk factors for noncommunicable and chronic diseases are on the rise in many African countries

# Solutions

- African governments should act fast to avoid the mistakes of wealthy industrialized countries
- Scale up key, low-cost health solutions, particularly prevention and health promotion to whole population
- Legislation can improve mental health care and control of noncommunicable diseases
- All government departments and nongovernmental organizations should work together to ensure a comprehensive approach to the problem

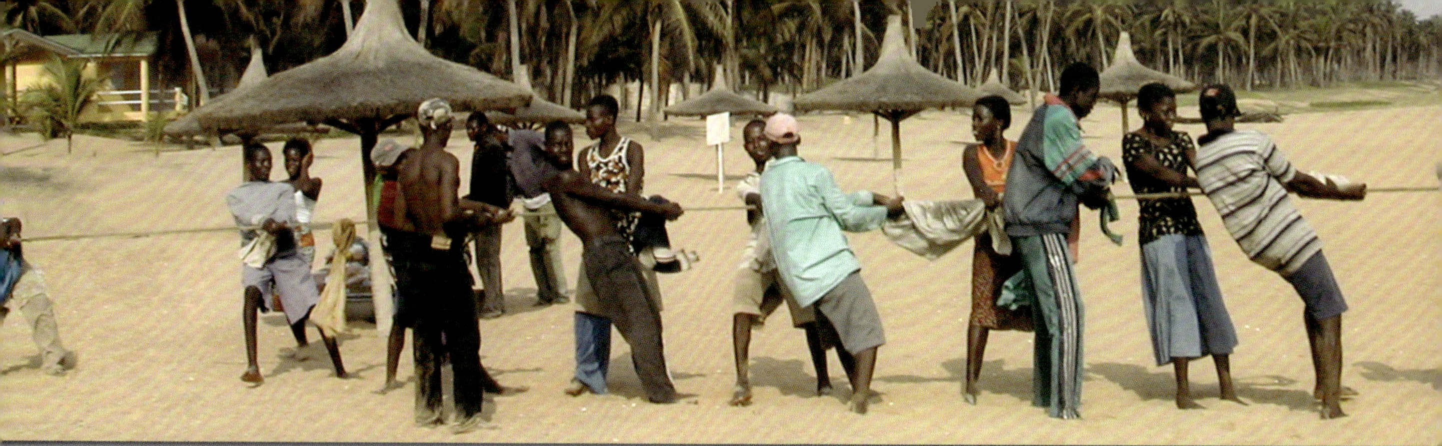

# *Noncommunicable diseases* in Africa

## An emerging threat

Noncommunicable diseases such as stroke, diabetes, cancer and heart disease — usually thought of as "Western diseases" — are becoming increasingly common throughout the African Region. Injuries have also become a significant public health problem. But these chronic diseases and injuries tend to be overshadowed by other headline-grabbing illnesses such as HIV/AIDS and are given low priority and few resources (Fig. 4.1).

In fact, twice as many deaths from cardiovascular disease now occur in developing countries as in developed countries. In South Africa noncommunicable diseases were the number one cause of death in 2000, accounting for 37% of deaths and 21% of years of life lost due to premature death (see Table 4.1).

Furthermore, complications — especially stroke, cardiac and renal failure — and certain forms of cancer, such as cervical cancer, occur at younger ages and in larger numbers in the Region than in developed countries. The average age at death from cardiovascular disease is at least 10 years younger in low-income settings than in developed countries and as a result adults are hit in their most productive years.

## Africa's double burden

Health systems in the African Region are straining under a double burden: a high mortality and morbidity due to communicable diseases coupled with increasing rates of noncommunicable diseases including mental illness and injury. Health systems developed to provide acute, episodic care in some countries are inadequately designed and resourced to care for people with chronic conditions.

The most common noncommunicable diseases are linked to a few common and modifiable risk factors: high blood pressure, high cholesterol levels, tobacco use, excessive alcohol use, inadequate intake of fruit and vegetables and being overweight, obese or physically inactive. Indeed, 75–85% of new cases of coronary heart disease can be explained by these risk factors. In the African Region these risk factors are increasing and they are linked to urbanization and globalization. As people move out of villages into towns and cities, a traditional diet rich in fruit and vegetables is gradually being replaced by one rich in calories from animal fats and low in complex carbohydrates.

This dietary change is combined with a decrease in physical activity as people move away from traditional farming into sedentary jobs. Global marketing of tobacco, alcohol, and fatty, sugary and salty foods has reached into all but the most remote parts of the Region.

Fig 4.1
Burden of noncommunicable diseases and injuries in DALYs* by cause in the WHO African Region, estimates for 2001
Noncommunicable diseases and injuries represented 27% of the total burden of disease in the WHO African Region in 2001

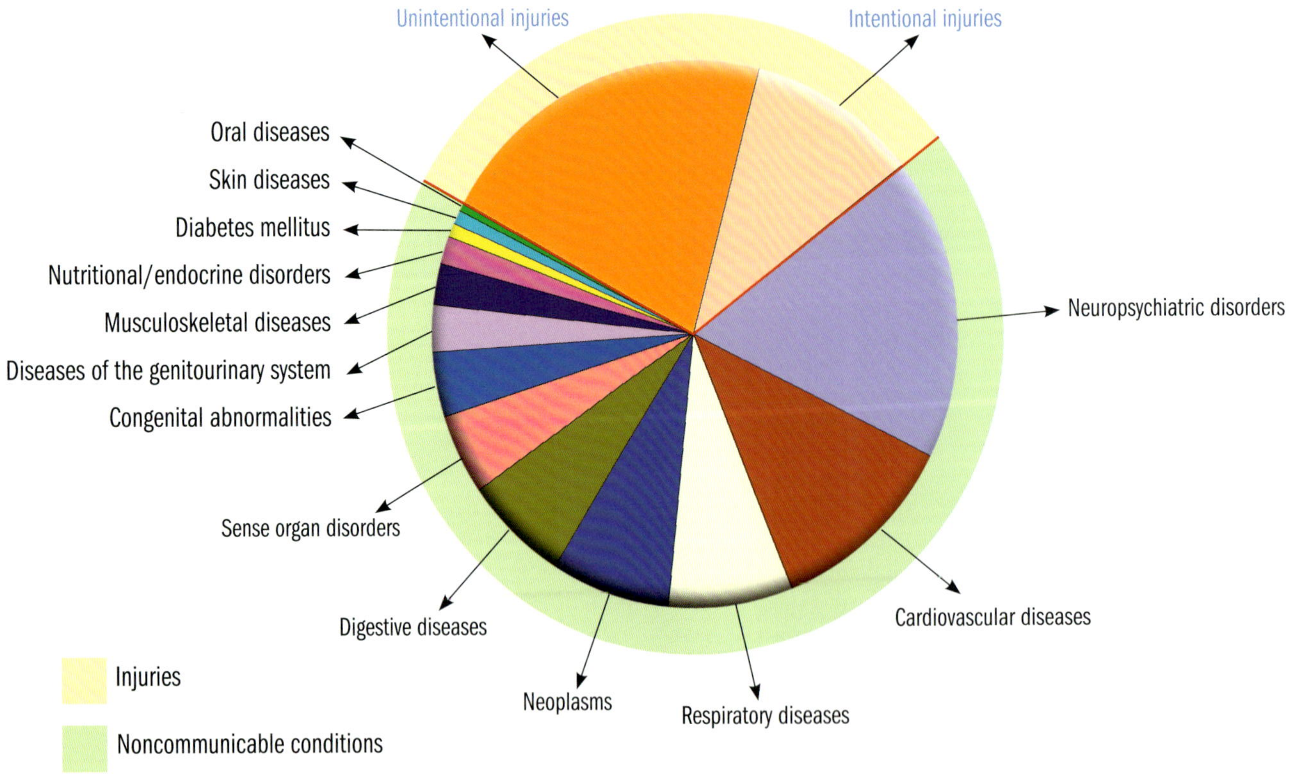

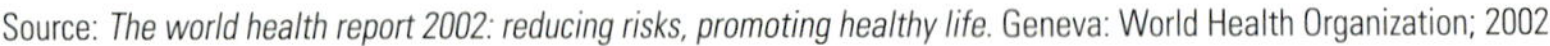


Source: *The world health report 2002: reducing risks, promoting healthy life.* Geneva: World Health Organization; 2002.
* Disability-adjusted life years

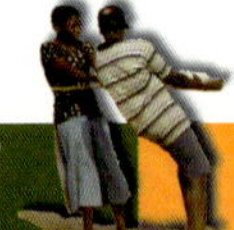

A survey carried out in Algeria in 2003 illustrates the extent of the problem. Of the 4000 people surveyed from both urban and rural areas: 12.8% were current daily smokers, 5.1% were current alcohol consumers, 55.8% consumed less than five servings of fruit and vegetables per day, 25.6% were mostly inactive, 16.4% were obese, 29.1% had high blood pressure, 2.9% had high blood sugar and 36.5% had high cholesterol.

Other surveys done in Cameroon, the Republic of the Congo, Eritrea and Mozambique have produced similar results, though alcohol consumption is much higher in these countries.

# Africa's lesser known toll of ill-health

## Cardiovascular diseases

*The world health report 2001* showed that cardiovascular diseases alone accounted for 9.2% of the total deaths in Africa in 2000 compared with 8.15% in 1990. More than 20 million people have hypertension in the African Region — with a prevalence ranging from 25% to 35% in adults aged 25–64 years and a clear upward trend over time.

In general, people living in urban areas are more likely to be at risk of cardiovascular diseases than those in rural areas. A study of more than 1000 men and women in Ghana found that the prevalence of hypertension was 33% in semi-urban villages compared with 24% in rural areas. Detection, treatment and control of high blood pressure was found to be poor overall, but was particularly bad in rural areas.

If hypertension is left untreated it increases the risk of stroke and cardiovascular disease. Globally 15 million people suffer a stroke every year. Of these, five million die and another five million are left permanently disabled. The African Region is one of the most heavily affected areas in this respect. For example, mortality rates from stroke were up to 10 times higher in the United Republic of Tanzania than in the United Kingdom. This high incidence of stroke is believed to be due to untreated hypertension. The ageing of populations in the Region may lead to a large increase in incidence of stroke in the coming years.

## Obesity and undernutrition: an African paradox

Africa is a vast continent containing extremes of poverty and wealth. Undernutrition is still the most important underlying factor causing high infant and child mortality in the Region. According to the Demographic and Health Surveys published in the 10-year period 1988–99, the prevalence of low birth weight in sub-Saharan Africa ranges from 11% to 52%. Between 30% and 40% of children suffered from stunting due to chronic undernutrition, and 10% suffered from emaciation or wasting due to acute undernutrition. Half of the children aged under five years were iron deficient and a quarter were deficient in vitamin A. Between 4% and 40% of women of child-bearing age were underweight. The highest prevalence of undernutrition in adults was found among displaced people, including refugees.

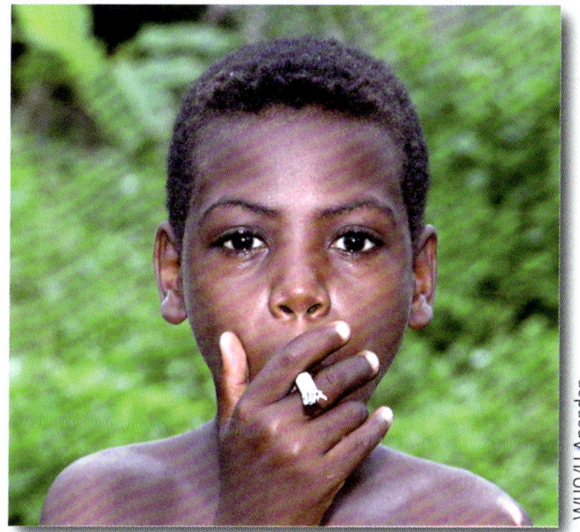

Young smokers are at risk throughout the Region.

| Single causes | Number of deaths | Rank |
|---|---|---|
| HIV/AIDS | 155 859 | 1 |
| *Ischaemic heart disease*[a] | *32 919* | 2 |
| *Homicide/violence* | *32 485* | 3 |
| *Stroke* | *32 114* | 4 |
| Tuberculosis | 29 553 | 5 |
| Lower respiratory infections | 22 097 | 6 |
| *Road traffic accidents* | *18 446* | 7 |
| Diarrhoeal diseases | 15 910 | 8 |
| *Hypertensive heart disease* | *14 233* | 9 |
| *Diabetes melitus* | *13 157* | 10 |
| *COPD*[b] | *12 473* | 11 |
| *Low birth weight* | *11 876* | 12 |
| Nephritis /nephrosis | 7 225 | 13 |
| *Trachea/bronchi/lung cancer* | *7 173* | 14 |
| *Asthma* | *6 987* | 15 |
| *Suicide* | *6 370* | 16 |
| Septicaemia | 6 047 | 17 |
| *Oesophageal cancer* | *5 803* | 18 |
| *Cirrhosis of liver* | *5 672* | 19 |
| Protein–energy malnutrition | 5 511 | 20 |

Source: *South African Health Survey 2000.*
[a] Text in italic indicates noncommunicable disease.
[b] Chronic obstructive pulmonary disease.

Surveys carried out in Nigeria show that the situation there is not really improving. In 1990, 43% of children under five years old were found to be stunted or short for their age. A repeat study in 2003 found that 38% of children were stunted, 19% were severely stunted, almost one in every 10 children was wasted and almost one in three children was underweight with 9% being severely underweight.

Early childhood undernutrition may be a risk factor for noncommunicable diseases in adulthood, particularly when coupled with lifestyle changes such as high consumption of sugars, fats and reduced physical activity. The African Region has seen an alarming increase in obesity since the early 1990s. The trend towards an unhealthy diet rich in saturated fat, sugar and salt and poor in fruit and vegetables means that in some countries, such as South Africa and Kenya, children are overweight but malnourished because they are receiving more than enough calories but not enough necessary nutrients to grow into healthy adults.

In South Africa, according to a survey undertaken in 1998, 29% of men and 56% of women were overweight. Almost one in 10 men and three in 10 women were obese with the general tendency towards being overweight increasing with age. Urban men and women were more likely to be obese than rural men and women. The proportion with a body mass index (BMI) greater than 30 reached 46% in women aged 45–64.

Obesity is a major risk factor for type-2 diabetes, which is increasing rapidly in the Region. In wealthier African countries such as Mauritius and Seychelles almost a quarter of middle-aged people are affected.

## Cancer

Cancer is the second leading cause of morbidity and mortality due to noncommunicable diseases. Tobacco use is the single largest causative factor, accounting for about 30% of all cancers in developed countries and an increasing number in the developing world. Smoking causes 90% of lung cancer and is a major risk factor for at least 11 other types of cancer as well as causing heart disease, stroke and chronic lung diseases such as bronchitis and emphysema. In Africa, there were 200 000 tobacco-related deaths in 2000. The prevalence of tobacco use was 29% in males and 7% in females in 2000. The Global Youth Tobacco Survey showed that smoking in 13–15-year-olds ranged from 13% in Kenya to 33% in Uganda.

Dietary factors account for around 20% of the burden of cancer in developing countries. Being overweight or obese is a serious risk factor for cancer, particularly for cancers of the stomach, colon, breast, uterus and kidney. Diets high in fruit and vegetables may reduce various types of cancer, while high consumption of preserved and/or red meat increases cancer risk. Eating a regular diet of highly salted foods doubles the risk of stomach cancer.

Some cancers are linked to infectious diseases. If these diseases were prevented or identified early enough then the associated cancers would not develop. For example, primary liver cancer is one of the top three causes of cancer death in much of Africa, Asia and the Pacific Basin but is relatively rare in the West. The major risk factor is infection with hepatitis virus B or C. Another risk factor is exposure to aflatoxin: a toxic substance present in mouldy peanuts, wheat, soybeans, groundnuts, corn and rice. People who eat these contaminated foods over a long period of time are at increased risk of developing liver cancer. This problem is more common in Africa and Asia than in other parts of the world.

Human papillomavirus (HPV) causes cervical cancer and is the fifth-leading cause of cancer death among females worldwide with some 239 000 deaths a year. About 68 000 cases of cervical cancer are reported each year in Africa. Cervical cancer offers a unique public health opportunity. Unlike most other cancers it is cost-effective to screen for precursor lesions and then treat them before they develop into cancer. The highest-risk lesions are most common among women in their thirties and forties, with the cancer that develops when the lesions are left untreated being most common among women in their forties and fifties. Countries that have a well managed cervical cancer screening service can achieve dramatic results in terms of treatment and prevention. For example, the age-standardized incidence for cervical cancer is 68.6 cases per 100 000 women in the United Republic of Tanzania compared with 7.7 cases per 100 000 women in North America.

## Injuries, violence and disabilities

Injury is a leading cause of death and disability in the African Region, particularly in those aged 5–29 years. Three of the top five causes of death for this age group are injury related. Armed conflict is a frequent occurrence in many African countries and is a major cause of ill-health and mortality. Five of the world's 10 most serious conflicts during the 1990s took place in the African Region. In addition to the deaths and injuries occurring on the battlefield, there are health consequences resulting from the displacement of populations, the breakdown of health and social services and the heightened risk of disease transmission. Even in countries that have not experienced armed conflicts there is a heavy toll from firearm injuries and other types of interpersonal violence which can lead to physical disability. This presents a special challenge for rehabilitation and contributes to poverty in the affected communities (see Box 4.1). Drowning is a leading cause of death in children. Burns are another common injury, especially for people with epilepsy who may fall into cooking fires when they have a fit. Because of inadequate care for the injured, all these conditions lead to more deaths and more severe disabilities than would be the case if trauma care systems and rehabilitation services were more developed (see Table 4.2).

Road traffic deaths in the African Region are 40% higher than in all other low- and middle-income countries and 50% higher than the world average. The epidemic of road traffic injuries in developing countries is still in its early stages but it threatens to grow exponentially with the rapid increase in the number of vehicles. Some countries, including Algeria, Benin, Kenya and Rwanda, are taking

## Rehabilitation for landmine victims in Angola

"I thought my life was over. I wanted to die," said Jose Antonio, as he recalls the day he stepped on an anti-personnel mine while fighting on the front line during Angola's civil war. The blast ripped off much of his left leg.

After recovering from his above-knee amputation Jose moved to Luanda, Angola's capital, for better medical care. There, he heard about the Centro Neves Bendinha, a rehabilitation centre for amputees, run by the provincial health authority and supported by the International Committee of the Red Cross (ICRC).

"I've been very lucky," said the father of seven, as he waded through a sand pit and climbed nimbly up and down steps, testing his new artificial limb. "For years after the accident I was nervous. I would jump at loud noises and was scared to leave the house. But my wife persuaded me I needed a job. Our family was growing and we were all relying too heavily on her. I could walk, so there was no reason not to work. I just needed courage."

Now spray-painting cars for a living, Jose believes that work stopped him from feeling sorry for himself. "Of course, I can't do all the things I used to do, but I'm alive, I have a job so I feel useful, and I have a good woman who made me see that there was more to life than me and my leg," he laughed.

An estimated six million landmines — a legacy of the country's brutal 27-year conflict — are littered around Angola's countryside. They have left a trail of physical destruction and one in every 415 Angolans disabled, according to UNICEF.

When available, rehabilitation services tend to be located in cities and provincial centres and are often inaccessible for people from rural areas. Beneficiaries of the few services available, like Jose, can lead productive lives. But the lack of post-trauma support services and life-skills training is hampering the integration of landmine victims into society. Many amputees think they are only fit to beg on the street.

"Physical rehabilitation is just one piece of the puzzle. Assistance to landmine survivors is much more complex," said Tracy Brown, country representative of the Viet Nam Veterans of America Foundation (VVAF), a nongovernmental organization that runs rehabilitation programmes for landmine survivors in eastern Angola.

Brown argues that post-trauma support and life-skills training are critical to social reintegration through training opportunities and employment. But they are expensive. Materials and assembly of an average limb already cost between US$ 300 and US$ 800, but that leaps to some US$ 2000 when post-trauma rehabilitation services are included.

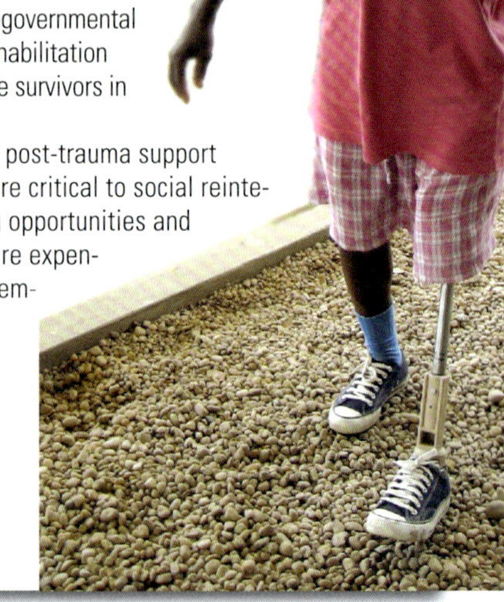


Jose Antonio tests his new leg at the Centro Neves Bendinha.

steps to reduce crashes involving pedestrians, cyclists, and passengers on public transportation (see Box 4.2).

Uganda has an annual road traffic fatality level of 160 deaths per 10 000 vehicles, one of the highest in the Region. Road traffic collisions cost the Ugandan economy around US$ 101 million per year, which is 2.3% of the country's gross national product. Road crashes not only place a heavy burden on national and regional economies but also on households. A study in Kenya showed that more than 75% of road traffic casualties were economically active young adults, and that those most at risk of death were pedestrians and users of motorized two-wheelers, who accounted for 80% of the deaths.

The death toll is only the tip of the iceberg with 20–50 million people injured or disabled each year in road traffic crashes worldwide. Pedestrians and users of motorized two-wheelers, who tend to be from lower-income groups, are most at risk of injury and death on the roads.

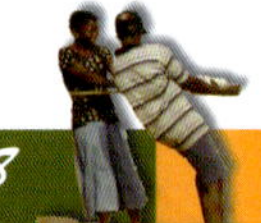

| Rank | 0–4 years | 5–14 years | 15–29 years | All ages |
|---|---|---|---|---|
| 1 | Malaria | Lower respiratory infections | HIV/AIDS | HIV/AIDS |
| 2 | Lower respiratory infections | HIV/AIDS | Tuberculosis | Malaria |
| 3 | Diarrhoeal diseases | Road traffic crashes | Violence | Lower respiratory infections |
| 4 | Perinatal conditions | Measles | Lower respiratory infections | Diarrhoeal diseases |
| 5 | HIV/AIDS | Trypanosomiasis | Road traffic crashes | Perinatal conditions |
| 6 | Measles | Fires | War | Cerebrovascular disease |
| 7 | Whooping cough | Drowning | Maternal haemorrhage | Tuberculosis |
| 8 | Protein-energy malnutrition | Tuberculosis | Abortion | Ischaemic heart disease |
| 9 | Tetanus | Malaria | Malaria | Measles |
| 10 | Congenital anomalies | Violence | Maternal sepsis | Road traffic crashes |
| 11 | Syphilis | Meningitis | Hypertensive disorders | Violence |
| 12 | Tuberculosis | Poisoning | Drowning | Whooping cough |
| 13 | Fires | Falls | Obstructed labour | Chronic obstructive pulmonary disease |
| 14 | Road traffic accidents | Upper respiratory infections | Syphilis | Protein–energy malnutrition |
| 15 | Vitamin A deficiency | Hepatitis B | Self-inflicted injuries | Nephritis and nephrosis |
| 16 | Anaemia | Epilepsy | Trypanosomiasis | Syphilis |
| 17 | Drowning | Protein-energy malnutrition | Epilepsy | War |
| 18 | Poisoning | Lymphomas, multiple myeloma | Poisoning | Tetanus |
| 19 | Endocrine disorders | Anaemia | Cerebrovascular disease | Diabetes mellitus |
| 20 | Meningitis | Leishmaniasis | Rheumatic heart disease | Drowning |

Source: *Global Burden of Disease 2002.*

Alcohol is an important factor in causing crashes. A study in South Africa found that around 29% of non-fatally injured drivers and over 47% of fatally injured drivers had been drinking. A later study found excess alcohol levels in over 52% of trauma patients involved in road crashes.

## Blindness

The major causes of blindness in the Region are cataract, trachoma, glaucoma, onchocerciasis and childhood blindness. The number of blind people in sub-Saharan Africa is expected to increase from about 9 million to 15 million by 2020 unless measures are taken to counter the problem. Some 80% of the causes of blindness are avoidable.

The most important cause of blindness in sub-Saharan Africa is cataract, which accounts for about 50% of blindness in this part of Africa. Trachoma is the most

## Making roads safer in Rwanda

Liliane Uwamahoro can still walk, but only with the help of crutches. She was one of six passengers in a public taxi who survived when it crashed in Rwanda's capital, Kigali, in 2002. Liliane lost her right leg, and has an artificial one. Eight fellow passengers lost their lives. She complains of pain in her left leg and still can't come to terms with the loss of her right leg. Liliane broke off her studies for three years and spent the first in hospital. Her family scraped their money together to pay for her treatment. This year she plans to return to college, but it won't be easy. "I have to do everything slowly now," she said.

Road traffic deaths in the African Region are 40% higher than all other low- and middle-income countries and 50% higher than the world average. Rwanda — a country of eight million people — is one of a growing number of African countries taking steps to combat this high mortality. Police spokesman Tony Kuramba said the number of traffic collisions reached unprecedented levels in 2002 and 2003. "We were doing a lot, but we realized that we had to double our efforts to bring discipline to the roads".

In 2003, Rwandan police launched a public awareness campaign. They told transport unions to make sure their staff were driving safely and used the media to reinforce the message that motorists and pedestrians must obey traffic regulations. As part of the campaign, primary and secondary schools started teaching road safety.

The number of people killed in road traffic collisions in the following year, 2004, fell by nearly a quarter compared with the previous year to 324 deaths, and the number of people injured on the roads fell by 10% to 3310, Kuramba said. "But we realize that losing over 3000 people in collisions … is still a big number," he said.

Under legislation passed since then, passengers who do not wear a seat belt and people on motorbikes or mopeds who do not wear a helmet face US$ 10 fine, one-fifth of a Rwandan civil servant's monthly salary. The number of traffic police in the capital has doubled to check for drunken or reckless driving, speeding and violations such as driving a vehicle with mechanical defects. Police posts have been created in rural provinces to monitor the highways leading to Kigali, where most crashes take place.

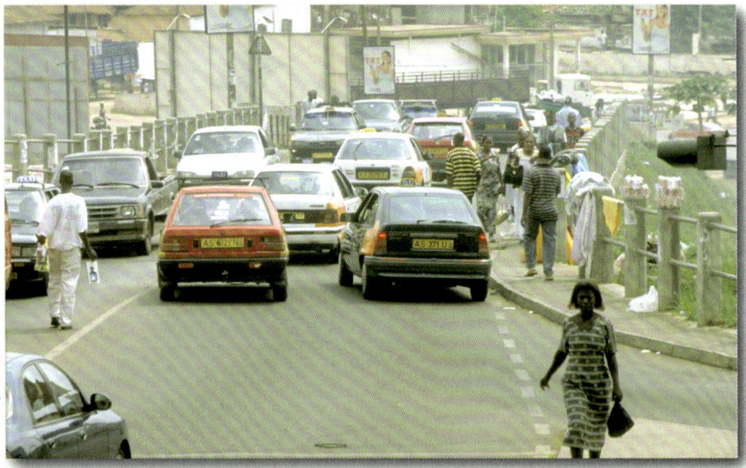

WHO/P.Virot

Road traffic injuries in developing countries threaten to grow exponentially with the rapid increase in the number of vehicles.

common infectious cause of blindness in the world, and is endemic in 48 countries, mostly in Africa. The Alliance for the Global Elimination of Trachoma by 2020 (GET 2020) adopted the SAFE strategy (**S**urgery for eyelids affected by trachoma, **A**ntibiotics, **F**acial cleanliness and **E**nvironmental improvement) as the means of achieving this goal, but most countries are still failing to ensure widespread implementation of this strategy.

In order to achieve sustainable control and elimination of trachoma, all four SAFE components must be implemented together. Likewise, all three essential components to the global initiative for elimination of avoidable blindness; disease control interventions, human resource development, and infrastructure development, must be addressed, and built upon the essential foundation of community participation.

Following the 1999 launch of the global initiative, VISION 2020: the Right to Sight, by WHO and key partners, several countries in the Region have stepped up blindness prevention and care efforts. The goal was to eliminate avoidable blindness worldwide by the year 2020. Yet at the beginning of 2005, only 22 of the 46 Member States in Africa had endorsed the global initiative, VISION 2020, by signing the Global Declaration of Support, and only 15 countries in the Region had formed a national committee for the prevention of blindness (NCPBL).

## Mental health problems

Mental health problems have been increasing throughout the African Region partly as a result of conflicts and post-conflict situations.

In 2002, mental disorders accounted for 5% of the total burden of disease in the Region. Moreover, despite a high burden of physical disease, mental disorders accounted for 19% of all disability in Africa. The burden of depression is particularly onerous, accounting for 5% of all disability.

In addition to conflicts, the increase in mental and neurological disorders is linked to the high prevalence of communicable diseases such as meningitis, cystircercosis, sleeping sickness (trypanosomiasis) and HIV/AIDS. The breakdown of traditional family structures and values is a further contributing factor since it can result in youth and adults who are poorly prepared to cope with life and who may turn to alcohol and illicit drugs. Indeed, reducing consumption of alcohol and illicit drugs has become a major challenge for the Region.

Poverty, exacerbated by difficult socioeconomic conditions, can lead to isolation and loneliness and, in turn, to depression, especially among vulnerable persons. There has been an increase of depression and acute psychotic disorders among adolescents, adults and the elderly. Without early diagnosis and appropriate care these conditions can become chronic.

Unfortunately, the financial and human resources in the African Region are insufficient to address adequately the burden of mental health disorders (see Table 4.3). The Region has fewer mental health professionals than other WHO regions. For example, the median number of psychiatrists per 100 000 people is only 0.04.

A similar trend is seen in the availability of psychiatric beds, whose median number per 10 000 population is 0.34. Also, only 56% of African countries have community-based mental health facilities and only 37% of countries in the Region have mental health programmes for children, while only 15% have programmes for the elderly.

People trying to access mental health care are also thwarted by its cost. In 18 countries in the Region the most common method of financing treatment involves out-of-pocket payments. Similarly, only 20 of these countries provide disability benefits. As a result most individuals with mental disorders in the African Region do not receive any medical treatment at all despite the fact that effective therapies exist for many of these conditions.

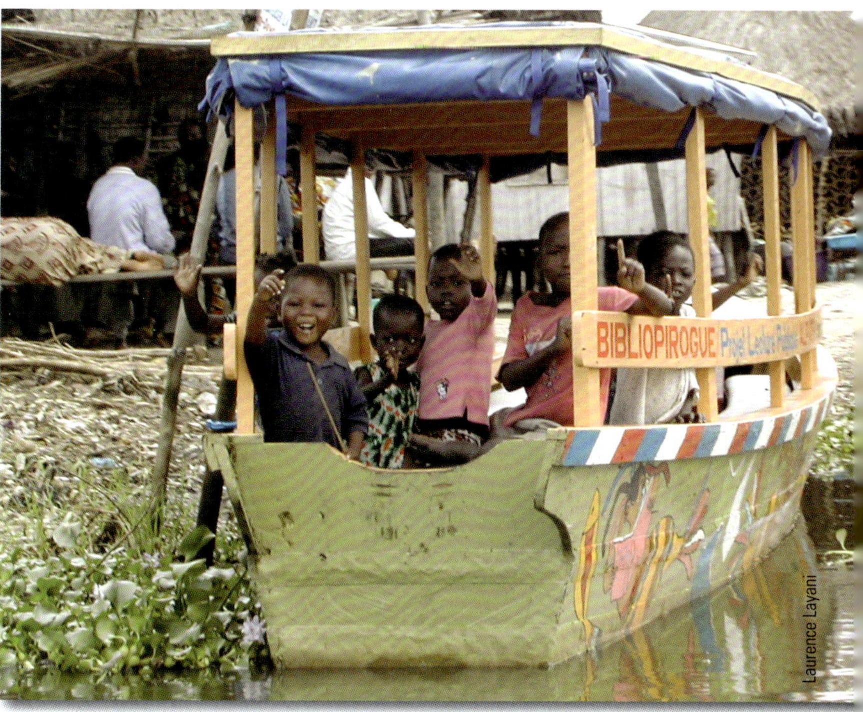

Laurence Layani

Healthy children can become healthy adults.

## Genetic diseases

The most prevalent genetic diseases in Africa are ones that alter the population's susceptibility to malaria. The main ones are: sickle cell, thalassaemia, elliptocytosis and glucose-6-phosphate dehydrogenase (G6PDH) deficiency. Sickle cell disease causes great suffering, frequent absenteeism in school and is a cause of premature death among children affected by it. Although there is no cure for the disease, a lot can be done in terms of management and prevention of symptoms. Unfortunately, even the more basic interventions, such as intravenous fluids and pain killers, are not always available to the majority of affected children in the Region.

**Mental health resources in selected countries in the African Region**

| Resources | Angola | Cameroon | Ethiopia | Mali | South Africa |
|---|---|---|---|---|---|
| Presence of mental health policy | Absent | Present | Present | Present | Present |
| Presence of substance abuse policy | Present | Present | Absent | Present | Present |
| Specific budget for mental health as a proportion of total health budget | Not available | 0.1% | Not available | 0.02% | 2.7% |
| Presence of treatment for severe mental disorders in primary health care | Absent | Absent | Present | Present | Present |
| Number of psychiatric beds/10 000 population | 0.13 | 0.08 | 0.07 | 0.2 | 4.5 |
| Number of psychiatrists/100 000 population | 0.07 | 0.03 | 0.02 | 0.06 | 1.2 |

Source: Project Atlas: A project of the Department of Mental Health and Substance Dependence, WHO, Geneva.

Much more could be done to screen children in Africa for these genetic abnormalities, prevent the complications of severe disease, educate the families of patients and provide advice on family planning for affected adults.

## Oral diseases

The African Region faces a number of serious oral diseases including noma, oral cancer, oral manifestations of HIV/AIDS and maxillofacial trauma. Dental caries and periodontal diseases are increasing in many African countries due to change of diet with growing consumption of sugars, increasing tobacco use and the high prevalence of oral manifestations of HIV/AIDS. Access to oral health services is limited in most African countries and oral health problems are left untreated or teeth are extracted because of pain and discomfort. Tooth loss and impaired oral function are therefore expected to increase. Oral cancer is closely related to the use of tobacco and excessive consumption of alcohol. The prevalence of oral cancer is particularly high among men. According to WHO estimates, oral and pharynx cancer represent the tenth leading cause of cancer in terms of incidence globally

Since many oral diseases have the same modifiable risk factors as cardiovascular disease, diabetes and cancer, a common risk factors approach has been developed by oral health programmes in the Region.

Noma — a gangrenous disorder that destroys the soft and hard tissues of the mouth and face — has been termed "the face of poverty" as it affects people in the very poorest parts of Africa. It mainly afflicts children aged under six years, with 70–90% of children with noma dying, while the survivors are disfigured for life, unable to eat, speak or breathe normally. An estimated 140 000 children contract noma each year, many of these live in the Sahelian region. The exact cause of noma remains unknown though it is believed to be bacterial. It has been linked to a combination of factors: malnutrition,

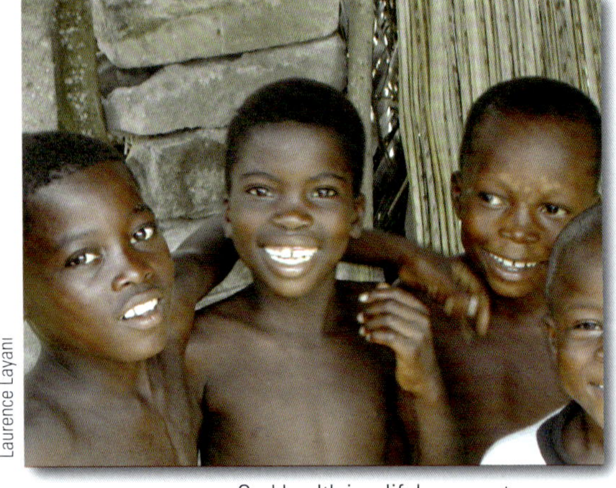
Oral health is a lifelong asset.

compromised immune system, poor oral hygiene and infection with several bacteria. If noma is recognized early enough treatment with antibiotics and nutritional support can halt the progression of the disease. However, the emphasis should be on prevention rather than treatment.

# Efforts to tackle the problems

Governments, donor agencies and research institutions in the African Region have sadly neglected the growing burden of noncommunicable diseases, although many of the causes are preventable. In contrast, cardiovascular diseases are now in decline in the industrialized countries. This decline is largely a result of the successes of primary prevention and, to a lesser extent, treatment. Many of the successful strategies that have worked in richer countries can, however, be just as effective in their poorer counterparts. In this context, ministers of health in the Region have adopted a number of strategies to address noncommunicable diseases, such as those on Noncommunicable Diseases in 2000, Health Promotion in 2001 and Mental Health in 1999.

# Legislation and marketing

One of the most effective measures that governments can take is to control the marketing of tobacco, alcohol, and salty, sugary and fatty foods. The modest amount of progress made in controlling the tobacco industry in recent years shows what can be achieved.

South Africa, for example, has some of the most stringent anti-tobacco legislation anywhere in the world and as a result the prevalence of smoking across most groups is declining. In 1994, the government imposed a tax increase on tobacco products amounting to 50% of the retail price. This action, combined with overall price increases, has doubled the price of tobacco products over the past decade. Along with other tobacco control interventions, tax increases have contributed to a 33% reduction in tobacco consumption. A survey carried out in October 1996 in South Africa showed that 34% of adults smoked. However, by 1998, following implementation of the Tobacco Products Control Act, only 24% of adults reported being current smokers. Significantly, fewer children are starting to smoke. In 1999, 18.5% of schoolchildren reported first smoking cigarettes before the age of 10 but this proportion had dropped to 16.2% in 2002.

The WHO Framework Convention on Tobacco Control has been signed by 39 of the 46 Member States of the African Region. By early 2006, 23 of those 39 African countries had ratified it. The next step is for these governments to pass appropriate anti-tobacco legislation.

The most effective intervention is a combination of tobacco taxation, comprehensive bans on advertising and dissemination of health information on the dangers of smoking. All of these strategies can be affordable and cost-effective in the Region.

*One of the most effective measures that governments can take is to control the marketing of tobacco, alcohol, and salty, sugary and fatty foods. The modest amount of progress made in controlling the tobacco industry in recent years shows what can be achieved.*

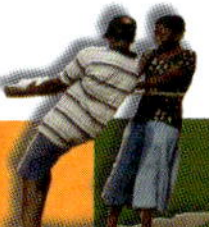

# Mental health legislation

Ghana is developing a new mental health law with the help of WHO that is expected to be a model for African countries. The idea is to provide a high standard of mental health care by protecting vulnerable groups and the rights of people with mental illness (see Box 4.3). This law also includes provisions to regulate the activities of traditional healers, to whom people with mental conditions often turn.

## Promoting healthy diets and lifestyles

Government-led action at the population level is needed to regulate marketing of unhealthy foods and to promote healthy lifestyles. One success story is a national healthy lifestyle intervention programme carried out in Mauritius between 1987 and 1992. The programme included extensive use of the mass media, community health promotion activities and, probably most importantly, legislation to change the composition of cooking oil from largely palm oil — which is high in saturated fatty acids — to soya bean oil. After five years there was a reduction in the prevalence of high blood pressure in men, from 15% to 12.1%, and the mean population total serum cholesterol concentration fell appreciably from 5.5 mmol/l to 4.7 mmol/l. Increased leisure exercise and decreased smoking and alcohol consumption were also seen.



### Ghana is drafting a new mental health law

Mr A. 67, has spent 40 years at the Accra Psychiatric Hospital, more than half his life. "We have many such in-patients whose families refuse to accept them back into their fold," said Ethel Lartey, Deputy Director of Nursing Services. "They have made this place their home".

While industrialized countries have been shifting from institutionalized mental health care to a care-in-the-community approach, many developing countries still keep patients with mental disorders in institutions. Shunned by their families and stigmatized by society, patients like Mr A. are still the luckier ones. Psychiatric services are in short supply and Ghanaians who suffer from depression, trauma, schizophrenia or the effects of substance abuse often seek help from unregulated religious or traditional practitioners.

At a religious healing camp in Ghana, some patients are constrained in chains. After four days 17-year-old Ms B. was still waiting to start treatment with "the Prophet". Meanwhile, her sister used severe coercive methods to stop Ms B. from stripping herself naked.

Under a new mental health law which Ghana is drafting in consultation with WHO's Department of Mental Health and Substance Abuse and the WHO Regional Office for Africa, such camps will have to be registered and supervised by working committees headed by a psychiatrist. Patients are to be treated with respect for their human rights and they should, when possible, remain integrated in the community while receiving care from psychiatric units attached to general hospitals. The law, which replaces a 1972 law, is expected to be passed in the next two years. It has gained the support of doctors, nurses and traditional healers and could serve as a model for other African countries wishing to develop progressive mental health laws that respect international human rights standards.

Dr Samuel Allotey, the psychiatrist in charge of Pantang Hospital outside the capital, said the current law only covers institutional care: "The current law … does not make provision for community psychiatric programmes. It does not cover traditional and spiritual healers and does not emphasize the rights of mental patients". One of the country's 16 psychiatrists in the country of 20 million people, Dr Allotey said that the new law will provide for the establishment of a National Mental Health Advisory Board and visiting committees that would have oversight and regulatory responsibilities of ensuring the rights of patients.

As far as alcohol consumption and its many negative public health consequences are concerned, the Regional Strategy for Mental Health 2000–10 and resolutions adopted by the World Health Assembly in May 2005 — notably resolution WHA58.26 on public health problems caused by harmful use of alcohol — show the way for governments to take appropriate measures.

The WHO Global Strategy on Diet, Physical Activity and Health, published in 2004, also provides guidelines for governments.

One obvious course of action is to regulate the amount of salt and sugar in foods, particularly those heavily marketed towards young people. Improved labelling of foods can also be beneficial.

For example, the Nigerian Heart Foundation has been successful in raising awareness about healthy eating habits and has recently started an initiative to label foods with a heart-friendly logo. Fortification of staple foods with micronutrients such as vitamin A is another key strategy.

## Low-cost management programmes

As well as action at the population level, strategies need to be developed for individuals at high risk such as setting up a recall system for patients who already have diabetes and hypertension. This can be achieved even in resource-poor settings such as rural South Africa, where a nurse-led noncommunicable disease management programme for hypertension, diabetes, asthma and epilepsy has been established within the primary health-care system for an overall population of around 200 000 people. This disease management programme includes use of clinic-held treatment cards and registries; diagnostic and management protocols; self-management support services, and regular, planned follow-up with a clinic nurse. Using this programme, nurses were able to achieve good disease control among most of the patient population: 68% of patients with hypertension; 82% of those with diabetes, and 84% of those with asthma.

## Closer collaboration

Collaboration between governments and nongovernmental organizations is vitally important. A global campaign for epilepsy, a joint initiative between WHO and leading nongovernmental organizations to raise awareness and develop national programmes on epilepsy, is being conducted in several countries, such as the Republic of the Congo, Senegal and Zimbabwe. The community-based approach to rehabilitating people with epilepsy that has been adopted in Togo is also interesting (see Box 4.4).

## Traditional health practitioners

The debate about conventional versus traditional medicine is often cast in "either/ or" terms. But in the mental health field many African communities and even some

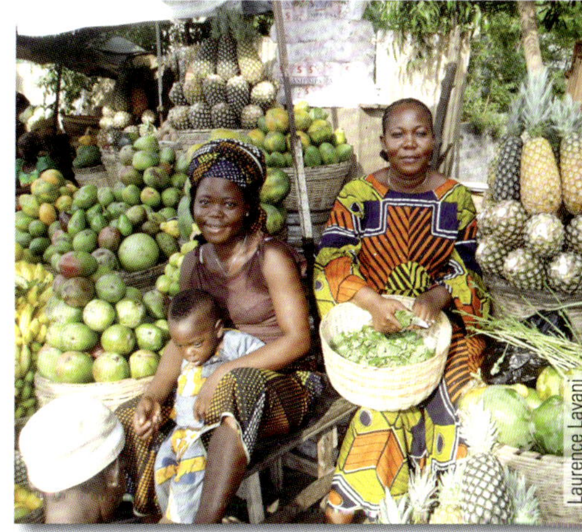

Fruit and vegetables are vital components of a healthy diet.





## Togolese people with epilepsy reintegrated into community

Sotoba district in northern Togo has worked hard to prevent people with epilepsy from becoming marginalized by society. Its approach to rehabilitation of these people is an example of good practice for intersectoral collaboration to integrate people living with epilepsy back into society. The Togolese Association against Epilepsy, community workers and members of the national mental health programme set up a programme in the district to provide essential care for people living with epilepsy. These people, who were mainly living on the streets, were given medication and psychosocial care as well as support for the families. After 18 months of such care social integration was possible in 35 adult cases. About 180 children and adolescents were monitored and around 60% of them were found to be seizure free.

specialists are happy for conventional and traditional health practitioners to treat patients at the same time. Mental health resources are limited and many Africans have little choice but to turn to traditional health practitioners.

Traditional health practitioners are highly respected in many communities because they share the same beliefs and perceptions on health care as members of those communities. African traditional healers are often the first point of care for people who are bereaved. These healers may guide people through rituals to help reduce their fear and depression. In some cases, however, clients with mental health problems are treated cruelly and physically mistreated by these practitioners.

More studies are needed into the potentially harmful effects of traditional approaches to mental health, and into how these approaches compare with practices such as psychotherapy. A number of African governments allow traditional health practitioners to register formally. Box 4.3 describes how healers in Ghana will soon be required to register under a mental health law that was drafted in 2005.

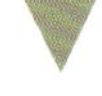



# The challenges

## Scarcity of resources

Money is a major constraint. Member States of the African Region have so many pressing issues, such as HIV/AIDS and tuberculosis, that swallow up limited health budgets and so it is easy to see why noncommunicable diseases are overlooked. But there is a ready source of new funds available if governments place a special tax on tobacco products and use the proceeds for disease prevention programmes. In South Africa, for example, government revenue from tobacco taxes has more than doubled in the last 10 years.

Not all interventions are costly. For example, giving aspirin to people with chest pain would prevent a quarter of the deaths associated with heart attacks and is more cost-effective on a population basis than interventions such as revascularization procedures. However, aspirin is strikingly underused when indicated. A study of diabetic patients in the United Republic of Tanzania found that 71.9% had high blood pressure (systolic pressure $\geq 140$ mmHg or diastolic pressure $\geq 90$ mmHg) and 12.2% were obese. All the other patients had at least one other indication for taking aspirin but only 39% were taking it regularly.

The lack of infrastructure in many parts of the African Region is a stumbling block. In many areas health care tends to be provided by nurses working in isolated clinics with limited access to drugs and equipment. First-class hospitals with hi-tech equipment do exist — the first heart transplant operation took place in South Africa — but often only a small number of wealthier citizens benefit. Certainly, more research is needed to examine what is feasible in low-resource settings.

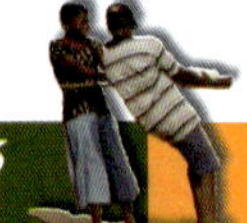

Setting up a traditional cervical cancer screening service, for example, can be costly. However, visual approaches using acetic acid or Lugol's iodine to identify suspicious precancerous cervical lesions are promising low-cost screening techniques.

Three centres have been set up to assess alternative approaches to screening and treatment of precancerous cervical lesions: in Guinea, Angola and the United Republic of Tanzania. As a result a screening programme has been put in place in 14 countries. More than 25 000 women have been screened and successfully treated for precancerous and cancerous cervical lesions over the last five years.

## Inadequate awareness and commitment

Inadequate awareness is a big problem. For example, many political leaders in the African Region are not fully aware of the magnitude and severity of road traffic injuries and that this is indeed a public health issue. A number of interventions can reduce road traffic crashes and minimize injuries. For example, setting and enforcing speed limits and seat-belt laws, requiring helmets to be worn on bicycles and motorbikes and setting and enforcing blood alcohol concentration limits. Using speed bumps and rumble strips to slow down traffic at crash-prone locations has proved highly successful in Ghana where fatality per 10 000 vehicles is about 30–40 times higher than in high-income countries. During the 16-month period between January 2000 and April 2001 when these measures were introduced, traffic collisions were reduced by 35%, fatalities by 55% and serious injuries by 76%.

There have been a number of WHO initiatives to raise awareness. For example the noncommunicable diseases strategy for the African Region, which was passed by the WHO Regional Committee for Africa in September 2000, aims to highlight the high and growing burden of noncommunicable diseases and galvanize governments into action.

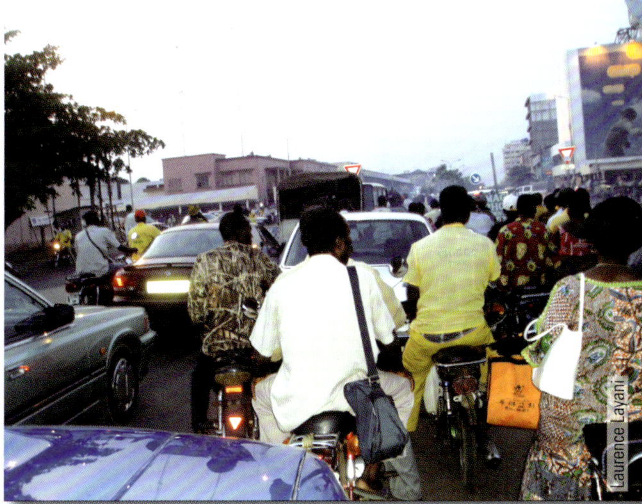

Helmet laws can reduce deaths.

## Limited data

The limited data on noncommunicable diseases in Africa and shortage of surveillance systems are important challenges. Surveillance systems play a key role in informing prevention and control programmes. The implementation of STEPS — a surveillance method based on risk factor approach — in Algeria, Eritrea, Cameroon and the Republic of the Congo shows that this method is feasible and affordable. A further six countries were being technically and financially supported to conduct STEPS surveys in 2005 (see Table 4.4).

Table 4.4



| Resource level | Population appproaches | | Individual high-risk approach |
| | National level | Community level | |
| --- | --- | --- | --- |
| Step 1:<br>Core | WHO Framework Convention on Tobacco Control (FCTC) is ratified in the country.<br><br>Tobacco control legislation consistent with the elements of the FCTC is enacted and enforced.<br><br>A national nutrition and physical activity policy consistent with the Global Strategy is developed and endorsed at Cabinet level; sustained multisectoral action is evident to reduce fat intake, reduce salt (with attention to iodized salt where appropriate), and promote fruit and vegetable consumption.<br><br>Health impact assessment of public policy is carried out (for example: transport, urban planning, taxation and pollution). | Local infrastructure plans include the provision and maintenance of accessible and safe sites for physical activity (such as parks and pedestrian-only areas).<br><br>Health-promoting community projects include participatory actions to cope with the environmental factors that predispose to risk of noncommunicable diseases: inactivity, unhealthy diet, tobacco use, alcohol use, etc.<br><br>Active health promotion programmes focusing on noncommunicable diseases are implemented in different settings: villages, schools and workplaces. | Context-specific management guidelines for noncommunicable diseases have been adopted and are used at all health-care levels.<br><br>A sustainable, accessible and affordable supply of appropriate medication is assured for priority noncommunicable diseases.<br><br>A system exists for the consistent, high quality application of clinical guidelines and for the clinical audit of services offered.<br><br>A system for recall of patients with diabetes and hypertension is in operation. |
| Step 2:<br>Expanded | Tobacco legislation provides for incremental increases in tax on tobacco, and a proportion of the revenue is earmarked for health promotion.<br><br>Food standards legislation is enacted and enforced; it includes nutrition labelling.<br><br>Sustained and well-designed national programmes (counter-advertising) are in place to promote non-smoking lifestyles. | Sustained, well-designed programmes are in place to promote:<br><br>• tobacco-free lifestyles, e.g. smoke-free public places, smoke-free sports;<br><br>• healthy diets, e.g. low-cost, low-fat foods, fresh fruit and vegetables;<br><br>• physical activity, e.g. "movement" in different domains (occupational and leisure). | Systems are in place for selective and targeted prevention aimed at high-risk populations, based on absolute levels of risk. |
| Step 3:<br>Optimal | Country standards are established that regulate marketing of unhealthy food to children.<br><br>Capacity for health research is built within countries by encouraging studies on noncommunicable diseases. | Recreational and fitness centres are available for community use. | Opportunistic screening, case-finding and management programmes are implemented.<br><br>Support groups are fostered for tobacco cessation and overweight reduction.<br><br>Appropriate diagnostic and therapeutic interventions are implemented. |

Source: *The world health report 2003*, Geneva: World Health Organization; 2003.

# Conclusion: Africa can learn from others' experience

Despite all the obstacles, a unique opportunity exists for governments in the African Region to produce and implement bold policies that can have large health benefits. The greatest gains would be in some of the poorest nations, where perhaps 10 more healthy life years might be achievable at relatively low cost. In order to achieve these gains, governments need to shift their main public health focus from a minority of high-risk individuals to include preventative measures that can be applied to the whole population. A coherent government-led strategy including legislation, regulation, protection of human rights, and education of the public is needed. It is imperative that the various government departments such as health, transport and education work together to ensure comprehensive interventions. In addition, collaboration between government, nongovernmental organizations, the media and others should be encouraged and expanded. *The world health report 2003* recommended a stepwise framework for the prevention and control of noncommunicable disease. Focusing on increased taxes on tobacco, legislation to reduce salt levels and stronger health safety and promotion alone would produce impressive results. Many developed countries are only now realizing the value of health promotion strategies, such as tobacco control. African countries have the opportunity to learn from the mistakes made in developed countries and to act early before the growing "epidemic" of noncommunicable disease gets out of control. ∎

> *Despite all the obstacles, a unique opportunity exists for governments in the African Region to produce and implement bold policies that can have large health benefits.*

## Bibliography

- Atlas: country profiles of mental health resources. Geneva: World Health Organization; 2001. Available from: http://whqlibdoc.who.int/hq/2001/WHO_NMH_MSD_MDP_01.3_P1.pdf

- Barker DJP, Osmond C, Winter PD, Margetts B, Simmonds SJ et al. Weight gain in infancy and death from ischaemic heart disease. *Lancet* 1989,2:577–80.

- Beaglehole R, Yach D. Globalisation and the prevention and control of non-communicable disease: the neglected chronic diseases of adults. *Lancet* 2003;362:903-8.

- Bradshaw D, Groenewald P, Laubscher R, Nannan N, Nojilana B, Norman R, et al. *Initial estimates from the South African National Burden of Disease Study, 2000.* Pretoria: South Research Council 2003. Available from: http://www.mrc.ac.za/bod/bod.htm

- Cappuccio FP, Micah FB, Emmett L, Kerry SM, Antwi S, Martin-Peprah R, et al. Prevalence, detection, management, and control of hypertension in Ashanti, West Africa. *Hypertension* 2004;43:1017-22.

- Coleman R, Gill G, Wilkinson D. Noncommunicable disease management in resource-poor settings: a primary care model from rural South Africa. *Bulletin of the World Health Organization* 1998;76:633-40.

- Department of Health, Republic of South Africa and Measure DHS+. *South Africa Demographic and Health Survey 1998: Full Report.* Pretoria: Medical Research Council; 2002.

- Dowse GK, Gareeboo H, Alberti KG, Zimmet P, Tuomilehto J, Purran A, et al. Changes in population cholesterol concentrations and other cardiovascular risk factor levels after five years of the non-communicable disease intervention programme in Mauritius. Mauritius Non-communicable Disease Study Group. *BMJ* 1995;311:1255-9.

- Eriksson GJ, Forsén T, Osmond, C, Barker DJP et al. Early growth and coronary heart disease in later life: longitudinal study. *BMJ*, 2001;322:949–53.

- Foster A. Vision 2020: The Cataract Challenge. *Community Eye Health* 2000;13:17-9.

- Guindon GE, Boisclair D. *Past, current and future trends in tobacco use.* Washington, DC: The International Bank for Reconstruction and Development/The World Bank; 2003. Economics of Tobacco Control Paper No 6. Available from: http://www1.worldbank.org/tobacco/pdf/Guindon-Past,%20current-%20whole.pdfhttp://www.measuredhs.com/

- Kolawole BA, Adebayo RA, Aloba OO. An assessment of aspirin use in a Nigerian diabetes outpatient clinic. *Nigerian journal of medicine: journal of the National Association of Resident Doctors of Nigeria* 2004;13:405-6.

- Magnus P, Beaglehole R. The real contribution of the major risk factors to the coronary epidemics: time to end the "only-50%" myth. *Archives of internal medicine* 2001;161:2657-60.

- Mahy M, Gupta N. *Trends and differentials in adolescent reproductive behavior in sub-Saharan Africa.* Calverton (MA): ORC Macro; 2002. DHS Analytical Studies No. 3.

- Murray CJ, King G, Lopez AD, Tomijima N, Krug EG. Armed conflict as a public health problem. BMJ 2002;324:346-9.

- *Nigeria Demographic and Health Survey 1990.* Lagos: Federal Office of Statistics and Colombia (MA): IRD/Macro International, Inc; 1992. Available from: http://www.measuredhs.com/

- *Nigeria Demographic and Health Survey 2003.* Lagos; National Population Commission, Federal Republic of Nigeria and Calverton (MA): ORC Macro; 2004. Available from: http://www.measuredhs.com/pubs/pdf/FR148/00FrontMatter.pdf

- Odero W, Khayesi M, Heda PM.Road traffic injuries in Kenya: magnitude, causes and status of intervention. *Injury Control and Safety Promotion* 2003;10:53-61.

- Peden M, Scurfield R, Sleet D, Mohan D, Hyder AA, Jarawan E, et al. World report on road traffic injury prevention. Geneva: World Health Organization; 2004.

- Peden M, van der Spuy J, Smith P, Bautz P. Substance abuse and trauma in Cape Town. *South African Medical Journal* 2000;90:251-5.

- Peden MM, Knottenbelt JD, van der Spuy J, Oodit R, Scholtz HJ, Stokol JM. Injured pedestrians in Cape Town — the role of alcohol. *South African Medical Journal* 1996;86:1103-5.

- *Status of infant and young child feeding in sub-Saharan Africa, situation analysis.* Brazzaville: WHO Regional Office for Africa; 2001.


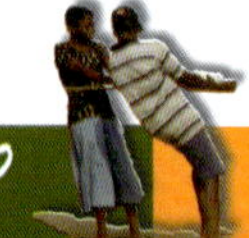

- Tsugane S, Sasazuki S, Kobayashi M, Sasaki S. Salt and salted food intake and subsequent risk of gastric cancer among middle-aged Japanese men and women. *British Journal of Cancer* 2004;90:128-34.

- Van Damme PA; Sokoto noma-team 19, September 2002. Noma. *Lancet Infectious Diseases* 2004;4:73.

- Walker RW, McLarty DG, Kitange HM, Whiting D, Masuki G, Mtasiwa DM, et al. Stroke mortality in urban and rural Tanzania. Adult Morbidity and Mortality Project. *Lancet* 2000;355:1684-7.

- WHO Regional Office for Africa, Noncommunicable Diseases: A Strategy  for the African Region, AFR/RC50/10, 2000.

- WHO Regional Office for Africa, Health Promotion: A Strategy for the African Region, AFR/RC51/12 REV1, 2001.

- WHO Regional Office for Africa, Mental Health: A strategy for Mental Health, AF/RC49/9, 1999.

- *The world health report 2001. Mental health: new understanding, new hope.* Geneva: World Health Organization; 2001. Available from: http://www.who.int/whr/2001/en/index.html

- *The world health report 2002: reducing risks, promoting healthy life.* Geneva: World Health Organization; 2002. Available from: http://www.who.int/whr/2002/en/index.html

- *The world health report 2003: shaping the future.* Geneva: World Health Organization; 2003. Available from: http://www.who.int/whr/2003/en/index.html

- *The world health report 2004: changing history.* Geneva: World Health Organization; 2004.

- *World report on violence and health.* Geneva: World Health Organization; 2002. Available from: http://whqlibdoc.who.int/hq/2002/9241545615.pdf

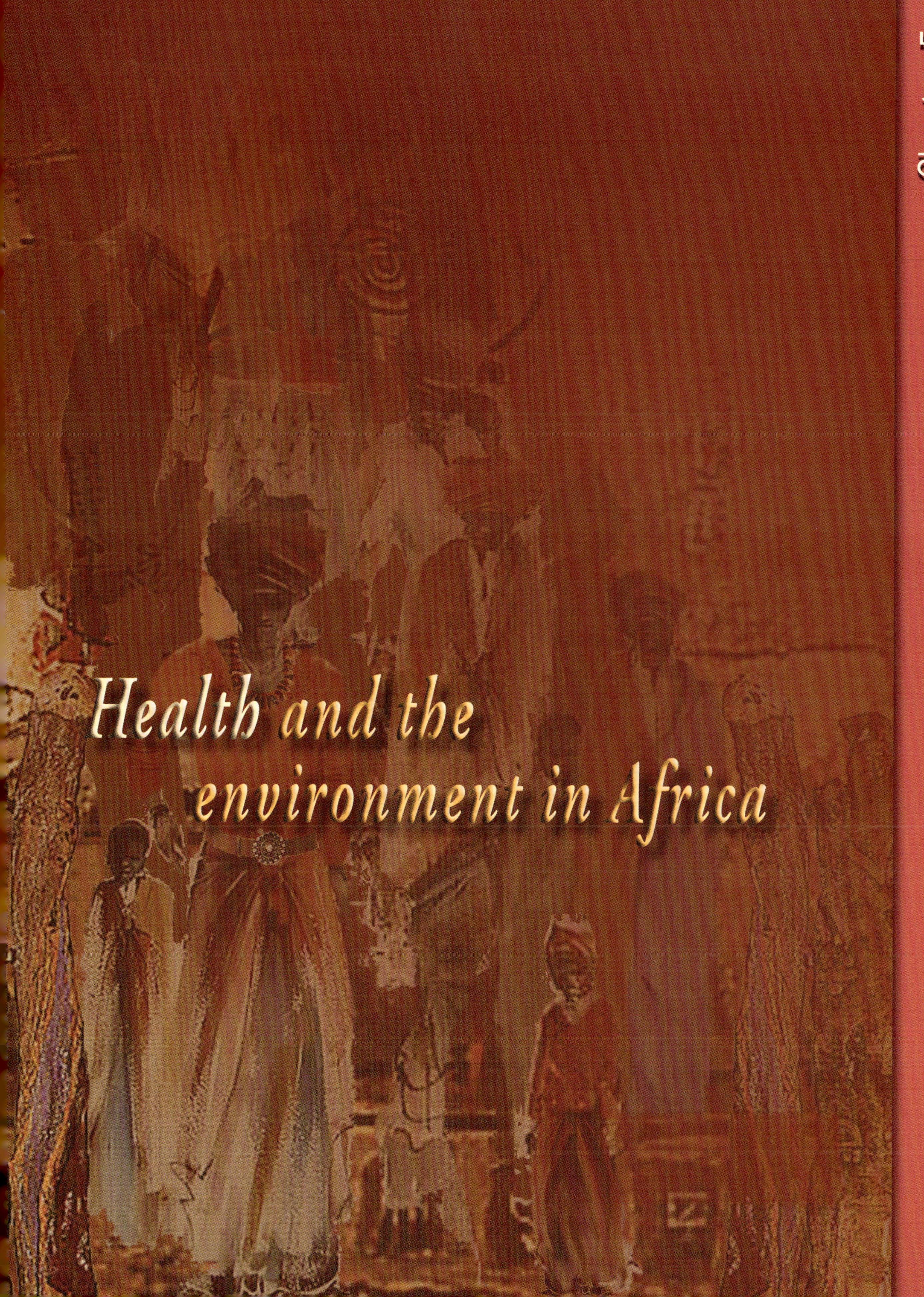



# Health and the environment in Africa

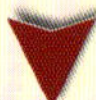

# Key messages

- Rapid urbanization poses major environmental health risks
- Widespread poverty limits ability to address environmental problems
- Inadequate access to safe water and sanitation exposes people to disease
- Emergencies cause a deterioration in the environment and in the health of people affected

# Solutions

- Scale up sustainable, low-cost solutions for water and sanitation
- Countries and international organizations need to work more closely together to prevent and resolve conflict
- Scale up food safety and hygiene education
- Closer cooperation between government ministries and other sectors to make the environment more healthy

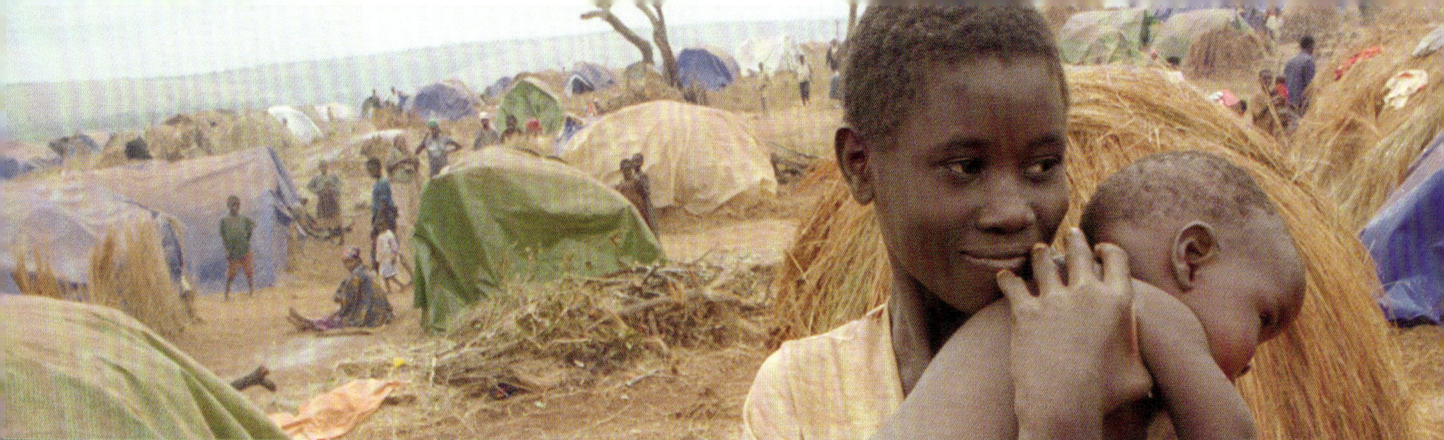

# Health *and the environment in Africa*

## Environmental health risks in Africa

People living in the African Region face a number of environmental health risks. High levels of air pollution, both within and outside the home, unsafe water supplies, inadequate sanitation and unhygienically prepared food are widespread in many parts of the Region. Rapid urbanization has left millions of people living in informal settlements lacking basic services — in the kind of environments that easily foster disease and high levels of stress and violence. In some parts of the Region, these day-to-day environmental threats are exacerbated by armed conflict and natural disasters. Apart from their direct impact, such events have an effect on the environment of people beyond the immediately affected area.

One of the main factors that determine environmental conditions and ill-health is the huge and seemingly intractable issue of poverty. Poverty limits people's ability to address the environmental factors that cause ill-health.

Urbanization can mean more affluence but also more pollution and different environmental risk factors compared to those faced by people living in rural communities. Clean water and sanitation facilities and functioning health systems, including immunization programmes and effective health education, need to be provided for people in areas that have undergone rapid and unplanned urbanization. Electrical power networks need to be constructed for these people to replace open fires. All of this requires money.

There are also a number of emerging environmental risks to health in the African Region such as ecosystem degradation and climate change. These are likely to increase the impact of current risks related to water availability, food producing ecosystems or changes in patterns of diseases, such as malaria.

Global efforts aimed at achieving the Millennium Development Goals (MDG) — especially MDG I to halve the number of people living in extreme poverty — could help to improve standards of living in the African Region. WHO and other agencies are working to make the environment in African countries more healthy and to reduce factors that predispose people to poverty.

# Challenges in the environment

## Water and sanitation

Access to a safe water supply and proper sanitation are essential parts of a healthy environment (see Fig. 5.1). Without safe water for drinking and for use in food preparation, populations are vulnerable to an array of waterborne diseases including cholera, typhoid and other diarrhoeal infections as well as to parasites, such as guinea worm and schistosomes.

The UNICEF/WHO Joint Monitoring Programme for Water and Sanitation found that within developing regions in 2002 the percentage of the population of sub-Saharan Africa with access to a safe water supply was 58%, with only the Pacific region having a lower rate. Coverage was low despite a concerted global effort. There have been two international drinking-water decades. The first was from 1981 to 1990, the second was launched in 2005. Global efforts have helped provide more than a billion people with safe water, producing a global coverage of access to drinking-water of 83%. But while access to safe water has improved, coverage for sanitation remains low. Only 58% of the world's population has access to adequate sanitation facilities, but sub-Saharan Africa has the lowest proportion of all, at just 36%. These figures show that the coverage of programmes to provide water and sanitation is too low and that they need to reach many more people.

Hundreds of thousands of Africans, particularly children, die every year from diseases caused by microorganisms, certain chemicals in the water supply, or diseases caused by poor sanitation. Poor water and sanitation also bring with them a host of non-fatal but debilitating diseases as well as severe problems of environmental degradation that have a further impact on health.

However, great strides have been made in the last 10 years in developing low-cost solutions and sustainable community-management approaches, such as the participatory hygiene and sanitation transformation (PHAST) approach, ecological sanitation and the AFRICA 2000 initiative to increase water supply and sanitation coverage in Africa. The PHAST approach involves community participation, which makes such projects more likely to be maintained and continued into the future.

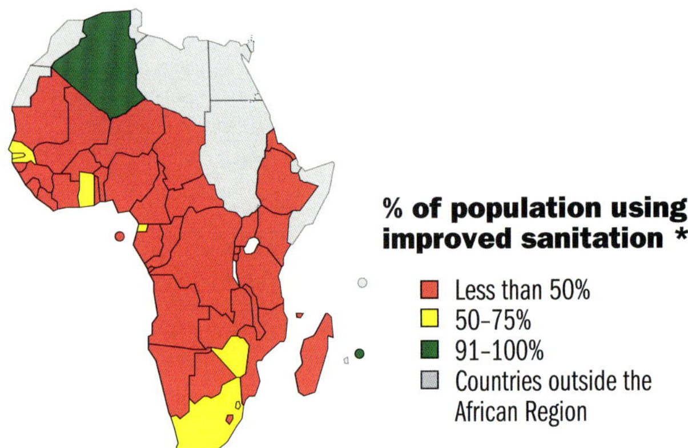

**Fig. 5.1**

Sanitation coverage in the African Region



Source: Based on: *Meeting the MDG drinking-water and sanitation target: a mid-term assessment of progress.* Geneva; World Health Organization: New York; UNICEF; 2004, Fig.7, p.12.

* No countries in the African Region were included in the 76–90% category.

Management of both solid and liquid waste is another environmental health problem in the African Region. Uncontrolled dumping attracts salvaging, vermin and vectors of diseases. Many communities inhabit old dump-sites, exposing themselves to a range of toxic risks and burns from explosions of built-up gases, plus risk of infections from the mixing of medical waste with other types of waste. Regular waste collection is far from adequate in urban areas. Waste dumped into storm drains, creeks, lagoons and other waterways also creates serious environmental problems that can turn into disasters.

## Pollution and industrial waste

Air pollution is one of the most serious environmental problems in the African Region and a major threat to public health, especially in urban areas (see Table 5.1). As cities grow, more vehicles, industries, homes and power stations are contributing to the pollution load.

Children are more susceptible to the adverse effects of indoor air pollution than adults. Indoor air pollution has a direct impact on people's health. Most people living in rural areas, informal settlements and city slums in the African Region rely on traditional fuels such as crop residues and firewood for cooking and heating. These low-quality fuels — combined with inefficient stoves and poor ventilation — create high levels of pollutants inside the home, often many times greater than outdoor air pollution levels. Urban air pollution contributes to illnesses, such as lung cancer, heart disease, asthma and bronchitis.

Cities may face many environmental problems, but rural areas have their problems too. There is less provision of waste disposal in rural areas than in urban areas. Indoor air pollution in traditional mud huts has been linked to acute respiratory infections, but in recent years some rural communities have found innovative ways to tackle the problem, such as the installation of smoke hoods in Kenya (see Box 5.1).

Chemical pollution is another environmental source of damage to health in the African Region. Exposure to certain chemicals can cause effects ranging from acute intoxication to birth defects and cancer. Hazardous practices in agriculture or public-health use of certain chemicals have had profound repercussions on health. The use of DDT is a particular problem. Banned in much of the world because it remains in the soil long after it has been applied and can travel great distances, this pesticide is used in some parts of Africa in the absence of cheaper alternatives and because of its effective role in vector control. DDT is only used at particular times of the year in



| | DALYs* | Mortality |
|---|---|---|
| Attributable | 12 318 000 | 392 000 |
| % of total in the Region | 3.4 | 3.5 |

* Please see glossary for explanation of DALYs
Source: *World health report 2002*

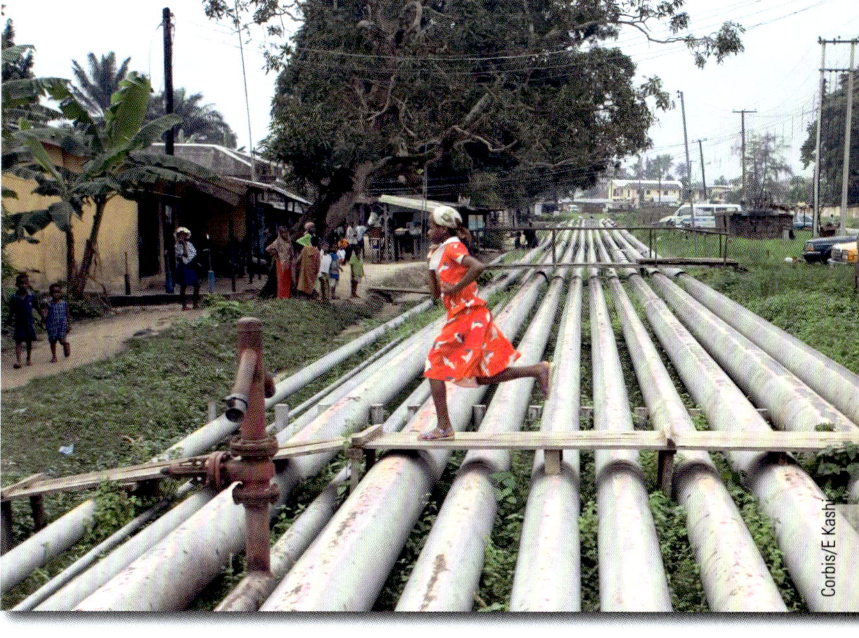

Children play on oil pipelines in Okrika, Nigeria.

## Clearing the air with smoke hoods in Kenya

Happiness Lemuliet, 37, is delighted with the new smoke extractor that has been installed in her traditional hut. "This thing has changed my life," says Lemuliet, a mother of six from Kenya's Maasai community in Kajiado, a rural district near the capital, Nairobi. "My children can now study in the evening, and they don't get colds and coughs as often as they used to."

The hood clears at least 80% of indoor smoke, dramatically lowering health risks, according to Intermediate Technology Development Group (ITDG), the nongovernmental organization which developed it.

In Kajiado, where an initial 25 homesteads were involved in the pilot project, the smoke extraction system consists of a fireplace base, a smoke hood and a lightweight chimney to take smoke out of the house. The smoke hood is a simple frame made of sheet metal that is installed above the cooking fire, drawing smoke towards the chimney. It can easily be dismantled and transported on animals to the next homestead, and costs from US$ 20 to US$ 70. The Maasai community were closely involved in developing the ventilation systems, as the smoke hoods, fireplace bases and chimneys were constructed locally using old water drums, scrap metal and anthill soils.

Adaptability and low cost are essential in communities where more than half the people live on less than US$ 1 a day and rely on biomass — especially firewood, charcoal, dry dung and crop waste — for heating and cooking. In urban areas, the rising cost of wood is driving people to burn plastic, which emits even more dangerous by-products.

The result is that indoor environments in many of the country's households are highly polluted. Traditional hut designs, such as the Maasai's windowless mud-and-dung shelters, compound the problem through poor ventilation.

"Our research in Kajiado shows that the indoor environment in a traditional Maasai hut has particulate levels up to 100 times those accepted internationally," Dr Jacob Kithinji, a consultant to the ITDG project and lecturer at the University of Nairobi's Department of Chemistry says. "In western Kenya, where hut design is circular with a thatched roof, particulate levels are usually about 20 times higher than the international standard — still very dangerous levels."

"Children from poorly ventilated households have an especially difficult time coping with domestic chores and school work," says Justin Nyaga, the Kenyan manager of ITDG's indoor smoke programme. "These children have a high incidence of coughs, upper respiratory infections and eye irritation."

"In Kajiado, the smoke hoods have made a good impact," says Nyaga. "The houses are cleaner and children are able to study."

"The intervention should be participatory in all aspects," says Nyaga. "It should take account of culture and hut design, local sensibilities, available resources and the traditional knowledge base, as well as sustainability and cost-effectiveness."

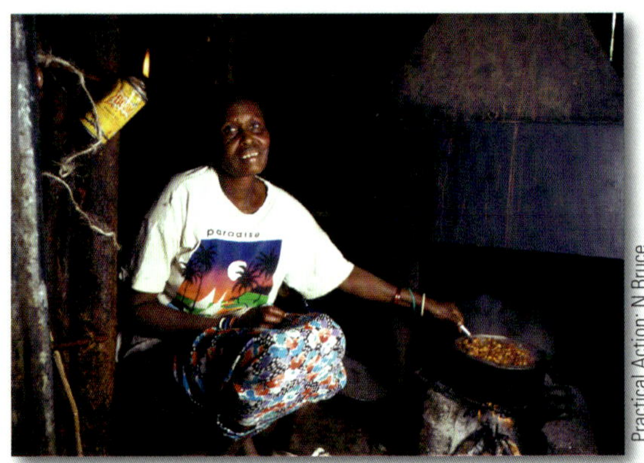

Woman cooking on a fire under a smoke hood in Kajiado, Kenya.

Africa when there are lots of mosquitoes, or for vector control in exceptional circumstances. For example, when a refugee population arrives in a malaria-endemic area, the use of DDT is sometimes necessary to protect the refugees, who — coming from an area where malaria is not endemic — are particularly vulnerable to the disease.

The accumulation of chemical waste is also becoming a serious problem, and one which communities are facing as urban growth has brought residential areas close to previously isolated chemical plants, and towns have been built over former waste disposal sites. The long-term effect of exposure to compounds such as polychlorinated biphenyls, potent pesticides, accelerators and plasticizers has yet to be studied and quantified. In addition to industrial waste, there are problems associated with health-care waste from medical facilities which pose a risk to human health. This is because such waste is often contaminated with infectious agents, such as HIV and the hepatitis B virus. Efforts to improve the situation have included the adoption of low-cost incinerators and other technologies.

Many countries in the African Region also have yet to enact regulations to control the levels of lead in fuels used for road vehicles. Particularly in urban areas, dispersed lead emissions from vehicles that run on leaded gasoline, as well as industrial emissions from smelters and battery recycling plants, contribute to poor air quality.

## Urbanization

From being an overwhelmingly rural part of the world just 20 years ago, Africa is urbanizing rapidly and its population is well on the way to becoming primarily an urban one. The annual average urban growth rate in Africa is 3.6%, one-third higher than in Asia and more than two-thirds higher than in Latin America. Currently 37% of Africans live in cities, but by 2030 this proportion is expected to reach 53%.

Rapidly expanding cities are often characterized by slum-dwelling, inadequate water and sanitation services and wastewater problems. Currently, 72% of city-dwellers in sub-Saharan Africa live in slums. The lack of effective waste disposal services is becoming a major problem. Lagos, Africa's largest city with an estimated population of 15 million people, is trying to crack down on illegal waste dumping with mixed results (see Box 5.2).

Informal urban settlements without adequate sanitation, water, transport or health services make very unhealthy environments. Microbes flourish and infectious diseases become epidemic. The overcrowding that always accompanies rapid



## Tackling mountains of waste in Lagos

Taofeek Raheem earns his living by working as a household refuse collector in Lagos. He fills his cart with household waste collected for a fee, and then rummages through this waste in the hope of finding something he can sell. Once he has finished, he pushes the waste to a legal dump site. Taofeek is registered to take waste to this dump site, but the problem is that many cart pushers are not registered and dump waste illegally in the city.

Lagos has been beset with the difficulties of clearing over 10 000 tonnes of solid waste generated daily. The city's population has grown from 5.7 million people in 1991 to an estimated 15 million in 2005. Many new arrivals, often unskilled youths like Taofeek, turn to the streets for shelter and to the dumps for a livelihood.

During this rapid expansion, city officials have experimented with every conceivable ploy to rid the streets of the mounds of refuse that often squeeze pedestrian and road traffic routes into little more than narrow channels, including private sector participation (PSP), the use of highway managers and the registration of neighbourhood refuse cart pushers like Taofeek.

Gbolahan Sulaiman, spokesman for Lagos Waste Management Authority, says that indiscriminate dumping is an added complication: "It costs more to evacuate loose waste than bagged refuse". Sulaiman blames the illegal operators for the dumping of refuse in the Lagoon, on the strip of land in the middle of the road and on the side of motorways.

Despite several strategies adopted to address the menace, mountains of refuse still litter the streets, public places, markets and bus stops, with the side or middle of highways becoming the unofficial communal dumpsites in most neighbourhoods. In many areas, a heavy pall of smoke emanating from these dunghills settles permanently over the surrounding areas.

Professor Jide Alo, an environmentalist from the University of Lagos, says the state waste management authority is genuinely overwhelmed by the volume of refuse generated in the city. He believes that until the environmental concept known as the "polluter pays principle" is effectively implemented and various agencies working on refuse collection are empowered with funds, the problem will persist.

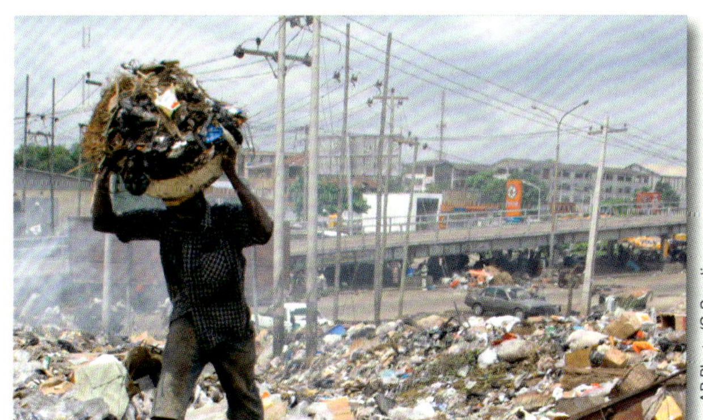

Making a living from waste in Lagos, Nigeria.

urbanization contributes to a host of social and behavioural problems including disintegration of families, homelessness, crime, violence, drug use and sexual abuse, and each of these problems spawns its own set of health risks to the people living within these settlements.

The WHO Regional Office for Africa is working with a number of countries to help tackle the negative environmental consequences of urbanization as part of the Healthy Cities project. So far, Cameroon, the Central African Republic, Ethiopia, Kenya, Mozambique, Namibia, Niger, the Republic of the Congo, Togo, Zambia and Zimbabwe have developed plans to address the poor environments in their cities that are caused by inadequate water and sanitation, illegal refuse dumps and unsafe handling of food.

## Food safety

The shift in population throughout the African Region from rural communities to largely informal urban settlements has brought a fundamental change in eating habits. Whereas in the rural setting food is usually prepared and served in the home, poorer city-dwellers frequently have neither the facilities nor space to store and prepare food nor the time and resources to gather ingredients and ensure that preparation is adequate. As a result, the use of street food vendors and the consumption of ready-to-eat food have soared.

Hygiene arrangements among vendors of cheap ready-to-eat food are often very poor in most developing countries (see Box 5.3). Adequate running water, toilets and washing facilities are rare, many vendors fail to disinfect surfaces or wash their hands, food is not usually protected from insects and refrigeration is seldom available. Poor food-handling increases the transmission of microorganisms including *Campylobacter* spp., *Salmonella* spp., the hepatitis A virus and *Escherichia coli* (*E. coli*). Practices such as using the same tools for cutting all ingredients, sharing tools with other vendors and using the same water both for washing ingredients and for dishwashing all add to the risk of food becoming contaminated.

Inadequate refrigeration and storage increase the incidence of food poisoning. Contamination with pesticides, mycotoxins, other naturally occurring toxins, industrial chemicals and heavy metals is an ongoing problem, as is the use of antibiotics in animal husbandry, which brings with it the risk of transferring antibiotic-resistant pathogens. The use of sewage sludge and animal manure as agricultural fertilizer is another source of food contamination.

Poor handling and preparation of staple foods are of concern in both urban and rural communities, especially when traditional food preparation technologies, such as fermentation, are used. For example, konzo, a disease that causes paralysis, occurs in rural Africa as a result of insufficiently processed cassava, a food staple in many African countries. There are also concerns about the safety of some of the products received as food aid.

Because of the informal, fragmented nature of much of the food-supply chain in the Region, ensuring food safety is difficult. Outbreaks of disease are often well




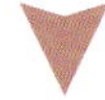

## Making street foods safer in Ghana

Street food vendors are important in the African Region. They feed millions of people every day. But studies in Ghana show that street food has often been prepared in an unhygienic way, sparking concerns over the health risks.

Nine-year-old Setorwu eats breakfast at home before leaving for school. For his lunch, his parents give him 2000 *cedis* (US$ 0.25) to buy lunch from the street food vendor. His father, Christian, a public servant, does not eat breakfast at home. His only meal at home on weekdays is dinner. Both Setorwu and his father patronize street food vendors. Many Ghanaians like Setorwu and his father rely on street vendors for many of their meals.

These vendors play a key role in providing as many as three meals a day for schoolchildren, workers, families, travellers, migrants and itinerant traders in Ghana. And they are everywhere: from the street corners, where the food is sold on tables, to the women who go from house-to-house carrying food in baskets on their heads to local canteens known as "chop bars". Food vendors also operate at work places and construction sites where they are popular, as they open credit lines for workers. Their menus range from beverages such as tea and coffee to porridge and more substantial meals.

But Ghana's health authorities have been warning for some time that some street food may be unsafe and calling for more control over the ingredients that go into street food and over the way this food is handled, prepared and stored. Poor food-handling increases the transmission of microorganisms including *Campylobacter* spp., *Salmonella* spp., hepatitis A virus and *E. coli*.

There are training programmes for food handlers and consumers on safe food-handling and personal hygiene. Ghana has adopted the hazard analysis critical control point (HACCP), an internationally established system, which predicts for preventive action the points in the food chain where contamination could occur.

But although Ghana has food safety regulations and has adopted the HACCP system, officials there say these are not being implemented rigorously enough. A survey conducted among street vendors in the capital, Accra, shows that 18% of them would associate diarrhoea with germs but none was aware that dirty hands were a risk factor for diarrhoea.

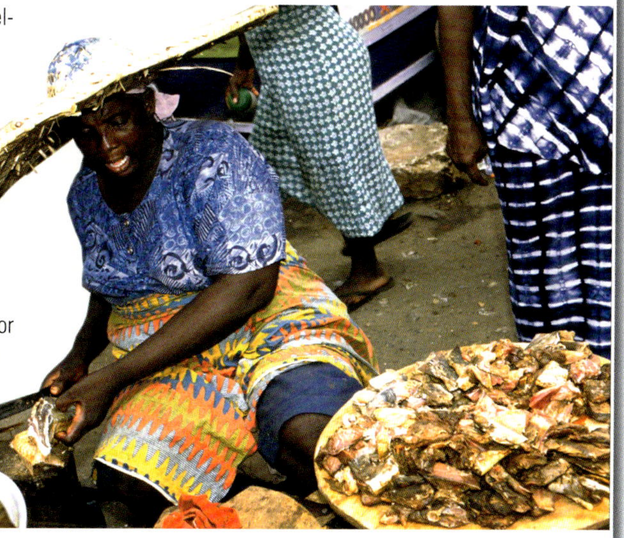

WHO/ P. Virot

Street food vendors often make do with minimal equipment

advanced before they come to the attention of health authorities. In Kenya in 2004, for example, an outbreak of acute aflatoxicosis due to consumption of contaminated maize led to 317 reported cases and 125 reported deaths. The heavy toll of death and disease associated with such outbreaks could be prevented by effective surveillance and monitoring systems. During this outbreak, laboratories were improved to test for food aflatoxins and other mycotoxins, and surveys were carried out to identify predisposing factors and to assess the magnitude of the problem. The laboratory tests allowed contaminated maize to be removed from the food supply system and from households, destroyed and replaced with "clean" food.

## Emergency situations

The African Region continues to struggle under the severest onslaught of man-made disasters and disasters associated with natural hazard. In January 2006, of 46 countries worldwide that WHO's Health Action in Crisis unit listed as experiencing a crisis, 25 were in the African Region. In 2006, Southern Africa and the Horn of Africa faced the "triple threat" of food shortage, increasing HIV/AIDS prevalence and natural hazards, while the Great Lakes region and West Africa faced complex humanitarian emergencies. The impact on the environment in countries affected by these crises — and to some extent on their neighbours' environment — is immense.

Civilians are more likely to suffer the most as a result of illness caused by communicable diseases, untreated chronic conditions, reproductive ill-health or violence when there is no rule of law. There are also crises or emergency situations that develop slowly and insidiously — such as those caused by HIV/AIDS — and these can have a profound and long-term impact on society.

In health terms, the direct effects of war, civil conflict, floods, droughts, famine and infectious disease are formidable. These factors reduce the resilience of people and of health systems, and they are quickly compounded when shelter, water, nutrition, security, sanitation and disease control are inadequate. The primary threat to people's health is posed by common illnesses because these are made even more dangerous by the crisis conditions. The most vulnerable people are the first to suffer and die in crisis situations.



### Healing post-conflict societies by healing peoples' minds

Mental health is often neglected in the places it is needed most. There is a peace, of sorts, in Liberia. Former combatants have faced each other across a cabinet table and an election has been held. Psychiatrists say international donors fail to realize that re-establishing a mental health system in a country like Liberia is of vital importance and can contribute to a stable society that is more able to develop socially and economically.

WHO consultant Danish psychiatrist Dr Søren Buus Jensen assessed post-conflict mental health needs in Sierra Leone to neighbouring Liberia. He says he could have reduced his report on Liberia to four words: "Needs: immense. Resources: none". He says that people with mental illness are some of the most marginalized members of society and providing care for them is not just a public health but also a human rights issue. "They have their voices in their heads and no voices speaking on their behalf," Buus Jensen says.

In Sierra Leone, the country's only psychiatrist Dr Edward Nahim agrees: "Sierra Leone is a post-conflict and a low-income country. Therefore mental health should be the number one priority, but unfortunately it is completely neglected".

The prevalence of mild and moderate common mental disorders in any given general population is 10%, while that of severe mental health problems, such as psychosis or severe depression, typically affect 2–3% of any given population but can increase to 3–4% after a disaster. For the traumatized populations of post-conflict states, the mental health needs are even greater.

When he arrived in Liberia in 2004 the consultant said that "not one patient was in treatment" and the country's only psychiatric hospital had long been destroyed. He argues that unless people with mental disturbances in fragile societies are treated, there is little hope of ending the cycle of violence that hampers social and economic development.

"It doesn't take a lot of psychotic patients to terrorize a village. If we don't do anything there is no chance to create a healing environment where justice and democracy might grow. We get a lot of sympathy, but no money. We can't pay a salary to anyone, we can't set up a pilot project to show what is possible."

Common preventable and treatable illnesses such as diarrhoea, malaria, measles, malnutrition and respiratory tract infections claim a disproportionate number of lives, while diseases such as meningitis and cholera can quickly flare into epidemics, exacerbated by endemic malnutrition and malfunctioning health systems. The conditions leading to epidemics are caused mostly by secondary effects and not by the primary hazard, except in the case of flooding, which can cause an increase in waterborne and vector-borne diseases. Disasters can result in the rupture of water mains and sewerage systems or the interruption of electricity supplies required to pump water.

In addition, in post-conflict situations mental health problems require specialized treatment (see Box 5.4).

Sudden, large-scale movements of people between and within countries often produce emergency conditions. Dramatic loss of livelihoods and increased spending due to emergencies can place people in a precarious situation. Epidemic diseases, such as cholera, can easily overwhelm the capacity of an under-resourced health service, triggering an urgent need for support.

The length of time that people spend in temporary unassisted settlements is an important determinant of the risk of disease transmission. The prolonged mass settlement of refugees in temporary shelters with only minimal provision of essential services is typical of a situation that can cause outbreaks of infectious diseases.

In the Democratic Republic of the Congo, an estimated 3.3 million people died as a result of the war between 1998 and 2002, according to the International Rescue Committee (IRC) study on mortality in the Democratic Republic of the Congo. Dubbed Africa's "first world war" because at least six nations were involved, the conflict was characterized by extreme violence, mass population displacements, widespread rape, and a collapse of public health services. The outcome has been a humanitarian disaster, unmatched by any other in recent decades.

Crises are often characterized by a high level of sexual violence against women and young children. WHO published guidelines with UNHCR for health workers on best practice in the care and treatment of victims of sexual violence in 2004. WHO ran projects in the Democratic Republic of the Congo and in Liberia from 2004 to December 2005 to address the health and psychological effects of sexual violence. These provided specialized training for health workers, counselling centres and medical supplies. As part of the projects, lawmakers received advice on drafting legislation on sexual violence and training was provided for community health leaders to fight sexual violence.

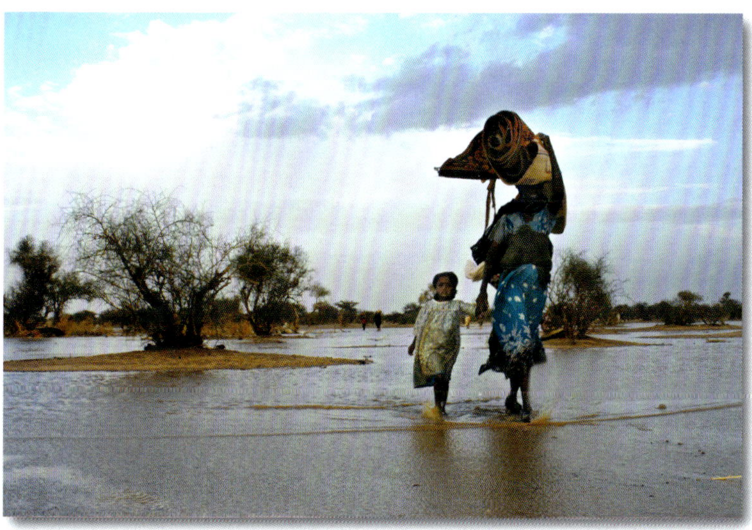

A refugee family carrying their belongings out of reach of the water when the first heavy rains near Bahai, Chad, flooded the seasonal riverbed.

As many as two million people have been displaced after two decades of conflict in northern Uganda. A study of internally displaced people in three districts in northern Uganda showed that in the first six months of 2005 a cumulative excess mortality of 25 694 persons was calculated. Malaria and HIV/AIDS were the two top causes of death reported by people surveyed, while violence was found to be the third most frequent cause of death. The crude mortality rate and under-five mortality in two of the districts were four times the overall levels in non-crises areas of sub-Saharan Africa.

Thousands of farmers lost their crops during an invasion of locusts in West Africa from April to December 2004 leading to food shortages across the region. In parts of some countries, including Burkina Faso, Chad, Mali, Mauritania, Niger and Senegal, the price of food — especially millet — doubled.

Angola's recent history also demonstrates the links between crisis situations and outbreaks of infectious disease. In April 1999, Angola suffered one of the largest polio outbreaks ever recorded in Africa. The outbreak came after 30 years of war and destruction of health services, massive population displacement that had resulted in overcrowding, poor sanitation and inadequate water supply — an ideal environment for the spread of the poliovirus. In March 2005, an outbreak of Marburg haemorrhagic fever in Angola led to 329 deaths, making it the most deadly outbreak of Marburg fever to date. There is no cure or vaccine for Marburg. Neither the source of the outbreak nor the reservoir has been identified to date.

WHO and other UN agencies have many roles to play in crises. One is to evaluate past and current social protection programmes that target vulnerable people. Another is to support countries in the recovery process. WHO is providing this support to Angola, Burundi, the Central African Republic, Côte d'Ivoire , the Democratic Republic of the Congo, Eritrea, Ethiopia, Liberia, Mozambique, Niger and southern African countries among others. This type of assistance represents a shift in focus, from saving lives to restoring livelihoods. Experience shows that it is possible to transform disaster into an opportunity to develop the health sector.

# Tackling poverty and environmental risks

## Poverty reduction

Determined efforts to make the environment in the African Region healthier are frequently hampered by the nature of the underlying problems, not least of which is poverty. The challenges of tackling poverty are considerable, but there are tried and tested solutions that are achieving results and need to be scaled up. One initiative is WHO's strategy on poverty and health in the African Region. Its core idea is that health is vital for poverty reduction, economic growth and human development. The strategy aims to promote health system reform that provides poor people with access to basic health services and to advise non-health sectors on how to factor heath issues into policies and practices. The strategy also seeks to shift the focus of health systems away from the dominance of a curative approach to more health prevention and promotion.

## Conflict prevention and management

The conflict-based emergencies that have been so widespread in the African Region bring with them a multifaceted set of problems for the environment. As with poverty, these emergencies can only be tackled by a large and sustained international effort, or by countries solving conflicts in a peaceful way.

That means improving the management of government incomes from natural resources, using aid in a better way to tackle the causes of conflict, implementing international agreements on how to control the conflict resources that fuel or finance hostilities, and controlling the trade in small arms.

International and African organizations can help prevent and resolve conflict when tensions cannot be managed at the national level through effective early warn- ing, mediation and peacekeeping. Coordination and funding of post-conflict peace- building and development must be improved to prevent states that emerge from violent conflict from sliding back into it.

WHO's African Regional emergency and humanitarian strategy urges Member States to develop or strengthen their capacity to manage emergencies. The recom- mended methods are focusing on country or areas vulnerable to emergencies through emphasis on prevention, preparedness and readiness, and capacity-building. Other recommended methods are training staff and strengthening institutional capacities, including early-warning systems, and allocation of appropriate resources to create — where this does not already exist — a National Emergency Fund. Countries are also urged to integrate emergency and humanitarian programmes and activities into their national health development plans. Also countries are encouraged to strengthen community involvement in emergency preparedness and response, and to identify, classify and map potential sources of emergencies. Effective and well- prepared relief efforts can transform the most daunting of crises. As a result of this strategy, several countries have improved their capacity for emergency prepared- ness and response.

In emergency situations, whether due to human or natural causes, insufficient resources and preparation render many governments in the Region incapable of miti- gating the impact on the environment. Humanitarian organizations are often required to underwrite and administer health interventions in emergencies. But reliance on outside help inevitably delays the arrival of assistance and increases the period of risk for the affected population.

Along with other agencies, WHO has also responded by taking a more proactive role in helping countries to prepare for the health impact of emergencies and put- ting systems in place to alleviate health problems caused by crises as quickly as possible.

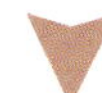

*A key to an effective response to emergencies in the African Region is improving coordination and technical support between the people and governments receiving relief as well as the organizations providing it.*

WHO's emergency and humanitarian strategy for the African Region, launched in 1997, contains a series of measures countries can take to be better prepared for emergencies. WHO is helping Member States to assess health risks and vulnerability, build technical support for response and improve coordination during crises. WHO has developed a minimum health package for emergencies, guidelines for action and other tools for technical support. WHO also helps countries to rebuild destroyed health systems after a natural disaster or armed conflict.

A key to an effective response to emergencies in the African Region is improving coordination and technical support between the people and governments receiving relief as well as the organizations providing it. Crises such as the famine in Ethiopia and Eritrea and the conflicts in the Central African Republic, the Democratic Republic of the Congo, Liberia and other West African countries have had an impact on the environment well beyond the borders of any one country, and coordinated action by governments in the Region and international agencies is crucial to controlling that impact.

## Sustainable, low-cost solutions: water and sanitation

The crucial area of water and sanitation is one where progress has been made, even if it is slower than hoped. The last 10 years have seen the development of low-cost solutions and sustainable community-management approaches to this central problem. Decentralizing responsibility and ownership and providing a choice of service levels to communities have proven to be particularly effective in improving access to safe water.

Community-management programmes run by WHO and other agencies have shown results. For example, schemes using the PHAST demand-responsive approach for water and sanitation as well as ecological sanitation projects. The AFRICA 2000 water and sanitation programme has also galvanized efforts to improve safe water supplies and sanitation in the African Region.

Several countries in the Africa Region have adopted WHO's healthy settings approach, which focuses on making cities, schools, villages and food markets healthier and which is based on the idea that health depends on a supportive environment as well as good health services. By adopting the healthy settings approach, these countries are addressing complex urban health problems in a holistic way for the first time.

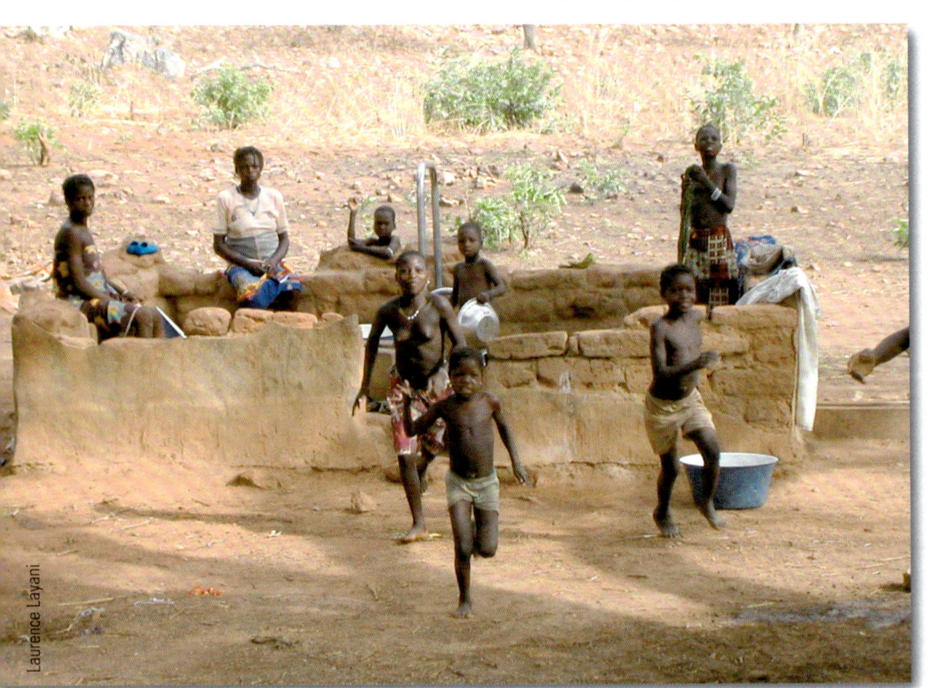



Fresh water is an invaluable resource.

The tools and expertise needed to run cost-effective programmes for improved water supplies and sanitation facilities are now readily available, and as awareness of those tools spreads so too should solid results, in turn, making the environment more healthy to live in.

One example of an environmentally friendly solution to water-supply problems, and of the kind of creative thinking that holds the key to solving the problems in this area, is the play pump: a merry-go-round that also functions as a pump, allowing children to pump water for their communities while they play.

Water supplies sometimes harbour diseases. One way of tackling waterborne disease is through environmental control. For example, public health workers in Malawi are controlling snail populations that carry schistosome parasites in rivers and lakes to reduce transmission of schistosomiasis (see Box 5.5).



## Environmental control of schistosomiasis in Malawi

Around 85% of the estimated 200 million people globally who suffer from schistosomiasis and the 600 million people at risk of contracting the disease live in Africa. Africa is now the focus of considerable international and national efforts to lessen the ravages caused by this infection.

Most of this effort is going into locating sufferers and providing them with treatment, but in Malawi, promising research is being conducted into controlling populations of snails that transmit the parasites responsible for schistosomiasis, also known as bilharziasis, in humans.

The country's Bilharzia Control Programme coordinator Samuel Jemu said environmental control was as important as identification, treatment, nutrition and sanitation to tackle schistosomes and other intestinal parasites.

His teams give priority to finding what they call "infection hot spots". These are the snail-rich environments where snails are passing parasites to water and where the parasites may be picked up by people collecting water, washing, fishing or playing.

"We look at the habitat and see if it is good for the snail," Jemu said. "We try to mobilize communities in those areas to make sure they clear the waterways," Mr Jemu said. "The water can then move a little faster and that way no transmission can take place. We also build footbridges so people have less contact with the water in those areas."

In the past pesticides were used to control snail populations but this practice was abandoned because of the disastrous environmental consequences, according to snail expert Dr Henry Madsen of DBL-Institute for Health Research and Development (Danish Bilharziasis Laboratory).

Peter Furu, Senior Adviser at the institute who was involved in setting up and evaluating the trial programmes in 28 villages on Nankumba Peninsula, leading to conference papers in 1998 and 1999, said the project was "innovative in its implementation because it was a health project integrated in a biodiversity conservation project in Lake Malawi".

A full evaluation could not be completed after Danish aid to Malawi was reduced in 2001, scientists said. The research linked schistosome transmission and snail numbers to the declining populations of mollusc-eating fish: Lake Malawi's celebrated cichlids.

Madsen said even if more fish turns out to mean fewer snails, it will not provide a complete answer to the schistosomiasis problem in Malawi or anywhere else. Where funds are limited and cost-effective drugs are available, it makes sense to treat people as the first priority. "However, I do believe that once prevalence has been reduced there will be a great need for environmental control to get rid of the disease," Madsen said.

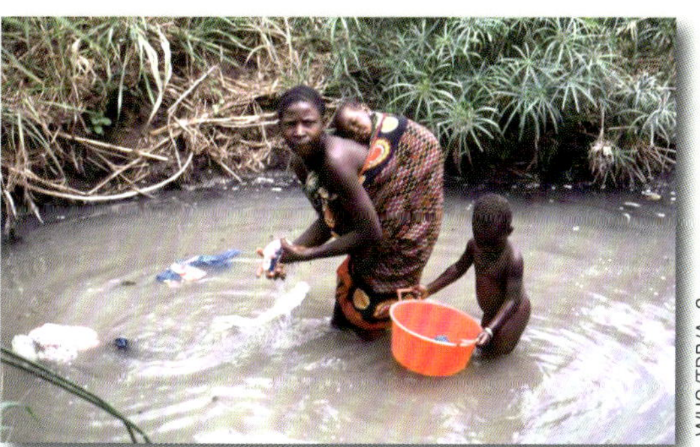

WHO/TDR/A. Crump

Unavoidable contact with snail-infested water puts many people at risk of contracting schistosomiasis.

# Making food safer: a shared responsibility

Improving food preparation and storage can reduce the health risks of unsafe food. Targeting hygiene practices at a localized level, monitoring the level of hygiene and disease transmission and educating food handlers have yielded good results.

Through the integrated disease surveillance strategy developed by the WHO Regional Office for Africa in 1999, all countries in the Region are now providing data on cholera, typhoid and infections due to *Salmonella* spp., *Shigella* spp. and other microorganisms. A major constraint is the lack of well trained technical staff, but this lack is being addressed. Training of such staff in foodborne disease surveillance and microbiological monitoring has been going on in 10 francophone countries since 2002. There are plans to cover the rest of the countries in the Region in the future.

In the francophone countries of the African Region, there is also an ongoing project to monitor antibiotic resistance in *Salmonella hadar* as a result of the Global Salm-Surv workshops, an international *Salmonella* surveillance programme initiated in 2000. Other research activities include microbiological monitoring of food from production to consumption as well as imported food products such as infant formula.



## MDG 7 on water and sanitation

One of the targets of MDG 7, which is concerned mainly with environmental sustainability, is to halve the number of people who do not have sustainable access to safe drinking-water and basic sanitation by 2015. This target requires coverage of 75% of the population by improved water sources. In sub-Saharan Africa, that proportion only rose from 49% to 58% between 1990 and 2002, well short of the progress needed to reach the 2015 target.

In the area of sanitation, the target is 66% coverage by improved services by 2015, but here sub-Saharan Africa is even further from the goal. From 32% in 1990, coverage had risen to only 36% by 2002. To be on track, it should have reached 49% by that time. There are some bright spots, however, such as Cameroon, where coverage was only 21% in 1990 but had reached 48% by 2002; Senegal, where coverage rose from 35% to 52%; and Ghana, rising from 43% to 58%, but progress in general is far too slow.

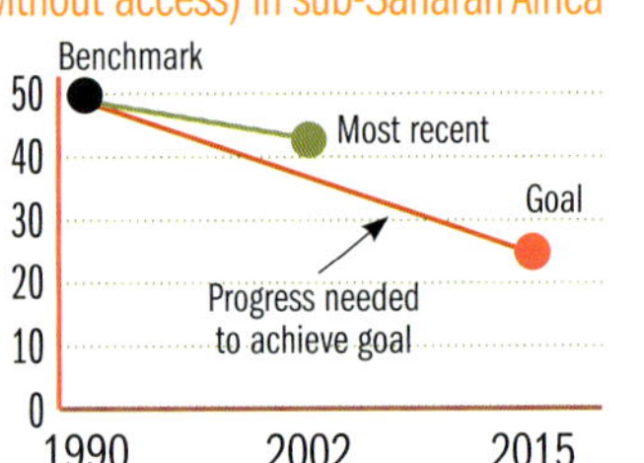


Source: WHO/UNICEF Joint Monitoring Programme for Water Supply and Sanitation – Water for life: make it happen. 2005.

Benin and the Republic of the Congo have been working to strengthen surveillance and microbiological monitoring of foods.  The Global Environment Monitoring System/Food Contamination Monitoring and Assessment Programme (GEMS/FOOD) has been introduced in about 10 francophone African countries through the Third International Total Diet Study Workshop held in May 2004.  A project on the chemical contaminants in food, in the form of a total diet study — these are the primary sources of information on the levels of various chemical contaminants and nutrients in the diet — is planned in Cameroon.

The rising incidence of foodborne disease and the emergence of new microbial threats to the food-chain prompted the WHO Regional Committee to make food safety a priority area of work in 2003. The establishment of the Codex Trust Fund in the same year has allowed many countries in the Region to commit themselves to implementing international food safety standards.

The food safety resolution endorsed by the Regional Committee for Africa in 2003 calls on Member States to develop or update food safety policies and legislation based on scientific risk assessment and prevention along the entire food-chain. The idea is to harmonize national food safety regulations with international food standards and guidelines, including those set out by the Codex Alimentarius Commission. Under the 2003 resolution, Member States are also encouraged to integrate food safety in the curricula from primary school level to higher learning institutions; to incorporate food safety education and information into training programmes for food handlers at all levels — consumers, producers, and farmers; to provide functional laboratory facilities with adequate resources as part of national surveillance systems; and to ensure national, subregional and regional coordination and networking.

Botswana, Ghana, and the United Republic of Tanzania have adopted the hazard analysis of critical control points (HACCP), an internationally established system of food safety management. This system anticipates points in the food chain where contamination could occur and promotes voluntary controls to prevent them.

Activities are also under way in Burkina Faso, Guinea-Bissau and Kenya to assess the quality and safety of street foods, to educate food handlers and consumers on safe food-handling and personal hygiene, and to train food control inspectors. The concept of healthy food markets has been applied in a number of countries, including Mozambique, the Republic of the Congo and the United Republic of Tanzania, to improve the safety of food sold in markets. The WHO *Five keys for safer food* poster, Bringing food safety home, is being implemented in Botswana, Mozambique and the Republic of the Congo to educate schoolchildren on food hygiene.

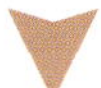

# Conclusion: Tracking progress

People in the African Region are faced with a wide range of health risks, many of which are of environmental origin. There are high levels of air pollution, both within and outside the home, unsafe water supplies, inadequate sanitation and unhygienically prepared food in most communities in the Region. The Region is also characterized by disparity in health outcomes. The result is poverty, poor transportation, inadequate housing, poor access to services, especially clean water and sanitation (see Box 5.6), and stress due to poor social and environmental conditions. Emergencies caused by man-made and natural disasters often result in huge displacement of populations, which in turn may trigger a deterioration in living conditions and in the immediate environment.

WHO has been working with its partners in the African Region to improve the health of the people by applying tried and tested solutions. For example, the PHAST approach has been applied to tackle problems with water supply and sanitation. By taking a healthy settings approach, much is being done to improve sanitation in cities and improve food safety in food markets. Improving food hygiene in the food industry has largely been achieved through the application of HACCP, while the WHO *Five keys for safer food* helps to provide consumer education and has been particularly useful for educating school children.

WHO has implemented a number of strategies in the African Region to help Member States make their environments more healthy, notably WHO's 2002 Strategy on Environment and Health, which stresses the development and implementation of environmental health policies in the health sector. The strategy also seeks to encourage communities to improve their knowledge and awareness of the crucial link between the environment and health.

Other strategies include: Poverty and Health: A strategy for the African Region; Microeconomics and Health: the Way Forward in the African Region; Emergency and Humanitarian Strategy in the African Region, and others on Food Safety and Occupational Health. All these strategies provide clear directives on how to alleviate poverty and reduce contamination of the environment.

These strategies draw on a wealth of knowledge on how to enable the poor to get the food and health care they need. There is plenty of evidence on how to make sure food is safe at every point from the farm to the table, and to ensure safety in the workplace. Methods for preventing and managing emergencies are also known. Member States, WHO and partners should work more closely together to apply these tried and tested methods and knowledge to make the environment more healthy and reduce the burden of diseases of environmental origin in the African Region. ■

*Member States, WHO and partners should work more closely together to apply these tried and tested methods and knowledge to make the environment more healthy.*

## Bibliography

- *Africa Statement – Water and Sanitation Africa Initiative. Africa Consultative Forum, Abidjan, 17–20 November 1998.* Geneva: Water

- *African Ministerial Conference on Housing and Urban Development, 2005.* Available from: http://www.housing.gov.za/amchud/top.html

- *AIDS epidemic update December 2004.* Geneva: Joint United Nations Programme on HIV/AIDS; 2004. Available from: http://www.unaids.org/wad2004/EPlupdate2004_html_en/epi04_00_en.htm

- Azziz-Baumgartner E, Lindblade K, Gieseker K, Schurz Rogers H, Kieszak A, Njapau H, et al. Case-Control Study of an Acute Aflatoxicosis Outbreak, Kenya, 2004 *Environmental Health Perspectives* 2005;113:1779-83.

- Chitsulo L, Engels D, Montresor A, Savioli L. The global status of schistosomiasis and its control. *Acta tropica* 2000;77:41-51.

- *Clinical management of rape survivors: developing protocols for use with refugees and internally displaced persons.* World Health Organization, United Nations High Commissioner for Refugees; 2004. Available from: http://www.who.int/reproductive-health/publications/clinical_mngt_survivors_of_rape/clinical_mngt_survivors_of_rape.pdf

- Coghlan B, Brennan R, Ngoy P, Dofara D, Otto B, Clements M, et al. Mortality in the Democratic Republic of the Congo: a nationwide survey. *Lancet* 2006;367:44-51.

- *Environmental health in emergencies and disasters: a practical guide.* Geneva: World Health Organization; 2002. Available from: http://whqlibdoc.who.int/publications/9241545410.pdf

- *Food Safety and Health: Situation Analysis and Perspectives* (AFR/RC53/R5). Brazzaville: WHO Regional Office for Africa, Brazzaville, Republic of the Congo; September 2003.

- *Health and Environment: A Strategy for the African Region* (AFR/RC52/10). Brazzaville: WHO Regional Office for Africa, Brazzaville, Republic of the Congo; 2002.

- *Health and mortality survey among internally displaced persons in Gulu, Kitgum and Pader districts, Northern Uganda.* Study partnership: WHO, UNICEF, WFP, UNFPA and IRC under the auspices of the Ministry of Health of the Republic of Uganda, July 2005). Available from: http://66.102.9.104/search?q=cache:ZWu60LwAeWMJ:www.theirc.org/resources/N-20Uganda-20MOH-20Survey-20Report-20July-202005-20FINAL.pdf+health+and+mortality+survey+among+internally+displaced+persons+in+Gulu&hl=en

- IASC (Inter Agency Standing Committee) *Early Warning-Early Action Report for the IASC WG (3rd Quarter - 2005).* Available from: http://www.humanitarianinfo.org/iasc/

- *Meeting the MDG drinking water and sanitation target.* New York and Geneva: UNICEF and World Health Organization; 2004. Available from: http://www.who.int/water_sanitation_health/monitoring/jmp04.pdf

- Mensah P, Yeboah-Manu D, Owusu-Darko K, Ablordey A. Street foods in Accra, Ghana: how safe are they? *Bulletin of the World Health Organization* 2002;80:546-54.

- Occupation Health and Safety in the African region: Situation Analysis and Perspectives (AFR/RC54/10) WHO Regional Office for Africa, Brazzaville, Republic of the Congo; September 2004.

- *Our common interest: report of the Commission for Africa.* London; Commission for Africa; 2005.

- Outbreak of Poliomyelitis – Angola 1999, *MMWR*, 1999;48:327-9

- Poverty and health: a strategy for the African Region (AFR/RC52/11). WHO Regional Office for Africa, Brazzaville, Republic of the Congo 2003.

- *Regional strategy for emergency and humanitarian action, Report of the Regional Director,* AFR/RC47/7. Brazzaville: World Health Organization, Regional Office for Africa; Brazzaville, Republic of the Congo; 1997. Available from http://www.afro.who.int/hac/pdf/strategieregional.pdf

- *Strengthening the coordination of emergency humanitarian assistance of the United Nations; report of the Secretary General.* Draft from June 2005.

■ Supply and Sanitation Collaborative Council. Available from: http://www.wsscc.org/dataweb.cfm?edit_id=164&CFID=827742&CFTOKEN=59731633

■ *Technical Guidelines for Integrated Disease Surveillance and Response in the African Region.* Brazzaville: WHO Regional Office for Africa, Brazzaville, Republic of the Congo and Centers for Disease Control and Prevention Atlanta, Georgia, USA; 2001.

■ *The world health report 2005: make every mother and child count.* Geneva: World Health Organization; 2005.

■ T. Tylleskär. *The association between cassava and the paralytic disease konzo.* ISHS Acta Horticulturae 375: International Workshop on Cassava Safety. http://www.actahort.org/books/375/375_33.htm

■ Van Ommeren M, Saxena S, Saraceno B. Aid after disasters. *BMJ* 2005;330:1160-1.

■ WHO/UNICEF Joint Monitoring Programme for Water Supply and Sanitation. *Water for life: make it happen.* Geneva: UNICEF/World Health Organization; 2005.

■ *World urbanization prospects: the 2003 revision.* New York: United Nations; 2004.

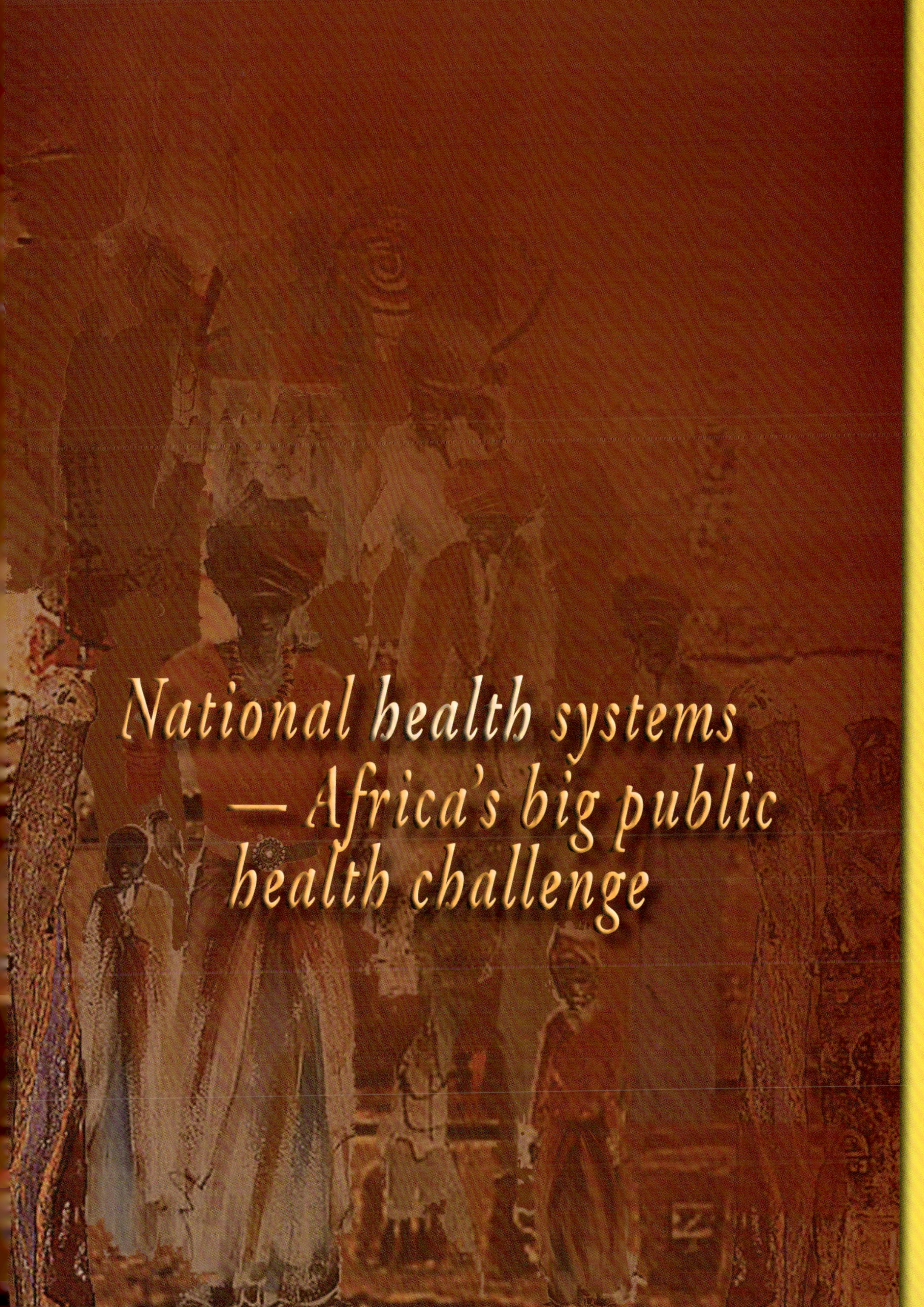



# National health systems — Africa's big public health challenge

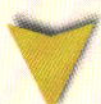

# *Key messages*

- Health-care delivery is hampered by shortage of health workers and inadequate infrastructure
- Out-of-pocket payments for health care drag people into cycle of poverty and ill-health
- Better health information needed to gauge appropriate public health response
- Half the population in parts of the Region have no access to medicines

# *Solutions*

- African governments and their partners should allocate more funds for health systems
- Subsidized health care and social health insurance schemes are needed
- Sector-wide approach would allow for effective coordination of domestic and external resources
- Strong health systems would be an effective platform for delivering all essential health care

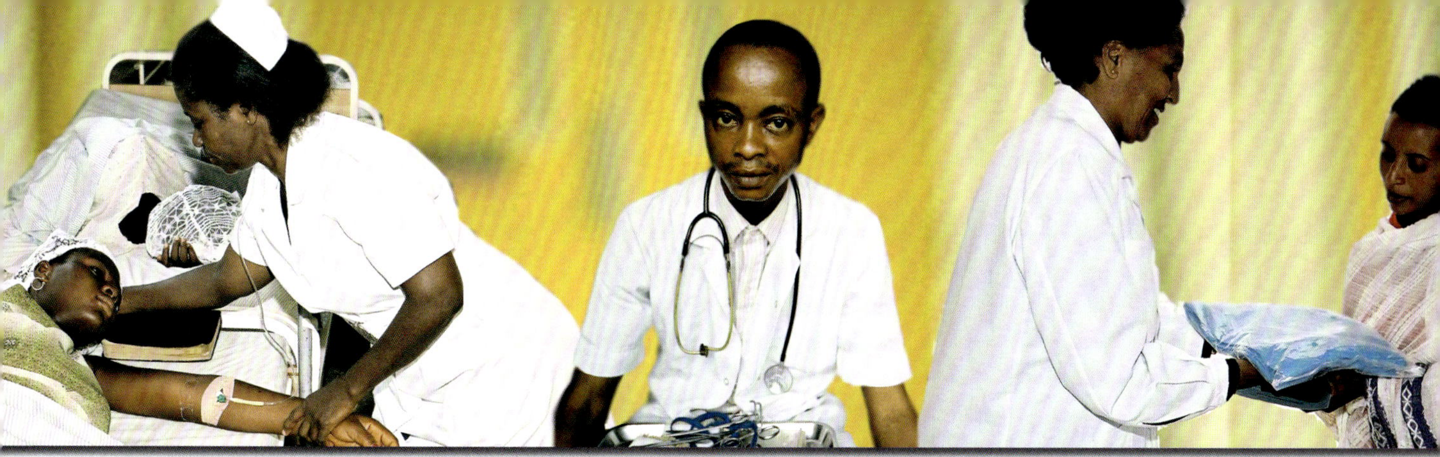

# National *health* systems — Africa's big public health challenge

**M**ost countries in the African Region have carried out health sector reforms to improve their health service delivery. Despite these efforts, health systems in many countries of the African Region are weak and not fully functional. The major constraint on governments is inadequate financial and human resources. Inevitably these governments welcome international support for their efforts to control diseases and alleviate suffering. Some "vertical" or single-disease programmes, provided and funded by external donors, have achieved dramatic results; for example, smallpox eradication and progress in the control of polio, guinea-worm disease, onchocerciasis and measles. However, vertical programmes tend not to address a major underlying cause of ill-health: weak health systems (see Box 6.1). This chapter is about Africa's big public health challenge — strengthening these weak and dysfunctional health systems.

People get sick and die in many cases because the systems for disease prevention and control are not in place or — if they are — they do not function properly. Some may argue that building health systems in Africa is prohibitively expensive. But a groundbreaking experiment in the United Republic of Tanzania proved the contrary: that it is possible to strengthen health systems at little additional cost with spectacular public health improvements. It has yet to be seen whether these gains can be sustained in the two Tanzanian districts where the experiment was carried out and whether the same approach can be applied successfully in other Tanzanian districts or in other countries in the Region. The experiment, however, shows that improved health systems performance can lead to progress in disease control.

# Building and reinforcing health systems

In countries where many of the basic ingredients of a health system — skilled health workers, information and knowledge, funds, infrastructure, as well as essential medicines and medical equipment — are either absent or limited, the outlook can be bleak.

Many people living in the African Region, particularly those in rural areas, often have to travel long distances to receive basic health care. Once they reach a hospital or clinic, they may only receive health care if they pay for it out of their own pockets. Inevitably, many people forego treatment because they cannot afford it, while those who pay may find the costs ruinous and the quality of services limited. Either way, people face impoverishment through incapacitating illness or catastrophic expenditures. Some countries, including Ghana, Kenya, Nigeria and Zambia, are developing national social health insurance schemes to help people cover their health costs.

One long-term solution to these problems, which are common in the African Region, lies in further health sector reform, calling for increased financing and more effective use of funds combined with better governance and improved access to affordable interventions that are known to work. A key element of this reform is to establish health districts as the basis for health service delivery. Once established as such, health districts across the Region need be made fully functional so that they can deliver essential health-care services to people in an appropriate, affordable and effective manner.

## Public and private health-care provision

The private sector plays an important role in the provision of health care in Africa. This is partly because governments have been unable to provide basic health care for a population who — in the absence of state-subsidized health care — has no choice but to seek alternatives. Private providers complement the public sector, stepping in where the state fails to provide essential services. But the private sector suffers from a lack of regulation and it may discriminate against people who cannot afford its services. The private sector includes nongovernmental and charitable agencies that provide free or subsidized care. In some countries, the private sector provides a significant proportion of the health care that is available, whether subsidized or fee-based.

As medical goods and services flow between public, commercial, philanthropic, traditional and informal providers, the distinction between private and public health sectors is becoming increasingly blurred. Some doctors charge fees for services that are supposed to be free in the public sector. Some drugs and medical equipment



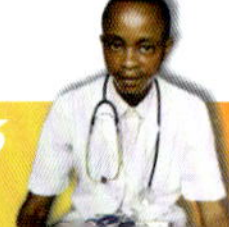

purchased for public hospitals are sold on the black market. Some health workers earn so little they have two jobs — one in the private and one in the public sector — to make ends meet. Yet both sectors are needed. The private sector tends to allow more competition, flexibility and innovation, while the public sector is responsible for ensuring more equitable access to essential health care.

## Scaling up health systems

Scaling up health systems means increasing human resources, improving infrastructure and training, and working on all fronts to make quality health-care services more widely available. No region needs to scale up its health systems more than Africa. Improved health systems are the only coherent solution to the scale of public health problems confronting the African Region. In the absence of functioning health systems, HIV/AIDS has taken hold and spread rapidly to create one of the biggest public health problems in history. Today, the HIV/AIDS pandemic has reversed hard-won gains in life expectancy. This reversal is a telling indictment of the inadequacy of health systems to cope with the enormous burden of the pandemic.

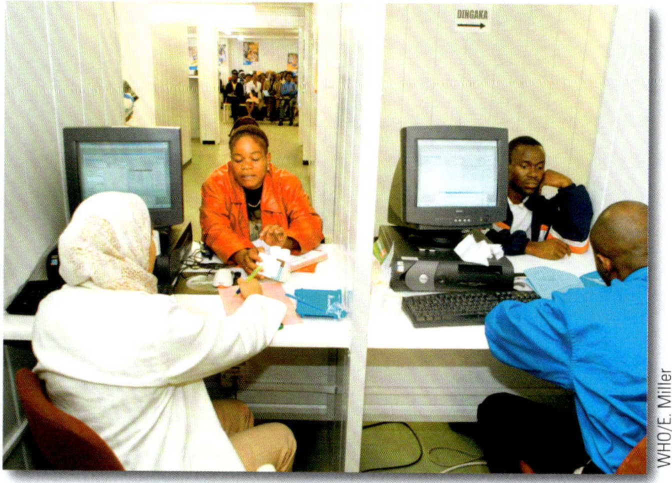


WHO/E. Miller

People visit big HIV/AIDS clinic in Gaborone, Botswana, in order to receive antiretroviral (ARV) treatment.

There are affordable and effective interventions to counteract the diseases that are taking away the lives of people in Africa, but the health workforce has dwindled so much — partly as a result of the HIV/AIDS pandemic — that there is often no one left to deliver them. Health-care delivery in the Region is often piecemeal, with some tried and tested interventions provided free of charge in small-scale projects in one clinic or hospital. These projects need to be scaled up first to health district level and then to the whole country. But scaling up is more easily said than done.

There are increasing efforts to help countries in the African Region achieve the health-related Millennium Development Goals (MDGs), such as the "3 by 5" initiative to deliver HIV/AIDS treatment, the Global Fund to fight AIDS, Tuberculosis and Malaria and the US president's Emergency Plan for AIDS Relief. The challenge is to muster enough funding for countries to build and reinforce their health systems as the overall conduit not just to fight HIV/AIDS but for all disease control and treatment efforts.

## Vertical programmes

By any measure of health systems function — immunization coverage, skilled birth attendance, malnutrition, and maternal and child mortality — the African Region is in poor shape. The challenge is to expand access to and coverage of basic health services, although efforts have been made in this regard (see Box 6.2). Specific programmes focusing on particular health conditions have been implemented as vertical or single-disease programmes, with varying success.

## Delivering health care to isolated communities

For the last 11 years, the Phelophepa health-care train has been bringing health care and education to communities across South Africa.

The train stops mainly in isolated farming areas, where the railway stations often have no platform and there isn't a hospital for 100 km. About 42% of South Africa's population of 44.8 million live in rural areas like these.

But Phelophepa, which means "good clean health" in the Sotho and Tswana languages, also brings health care to towns, such as Malmesbury in the Eastern Cape, where many people are too poor to pay for health services that are available. The response is overwhelming.

"I work until about 8 pm but sometimes there are still people waiting to be seen. Some of them sleep on the platform because they don't want to lose their place. It's heartbreaking," said optometrist Emma Rapoo, 27, one of train's staff members who are mainly final-year and post-graduate medical students.

Phelophepa started as an eye clinic in 1994 and has since expanded to 16 wagons housing a primary care centre, dental clinic, counselling team and education unit. They are limited, however, to conditions and illnesses that can be treated on the spot. If a patient appears with symptoms of a serious disease, such as malaria, cancer, HIV/AIDS or tuberculosis that requires long-term treatment that person will be referred to the nearest clinic or hospital.

The train does try to address these needs, however, by training local community volunteers in home-based health care, which may include the DOTS strategy for tuberculosis or basic AIDS care. These volunteers are then placed under a local coordinator from the department of health, usually a nurse in the area.

To date, the train has provided health care to 500 000 people and health screening and education to a further 800 000 people.

Every year, Phelophepa stops for a week at a time at one of 36 destinations in four of the country's nine provinces. Train Manager Lillian Cingo says that, by providing education, "hopefully" it also leaves something behind to sustain the community "to the extent that some people will no longer need its services when it returns".

Phelophepa's marketing team works closely with communities months in advance to discuss their needs and identify patients who cannot afford the US$ 0.50–1.00 fee.

The project requires planning and coordination. Its annual operating costs are about US$ 4.0 million, 60% of which is provided by the Transnet Foundation and the rest by corporate and other private donors. Organizers plan to build a second train in the next two years, for which they are raising US$ 6million. Dr Cingo's dream is to extend the health train's route into the rest of Africa. Further information can be obtained from the following web site: http://www.mhc.org.za/

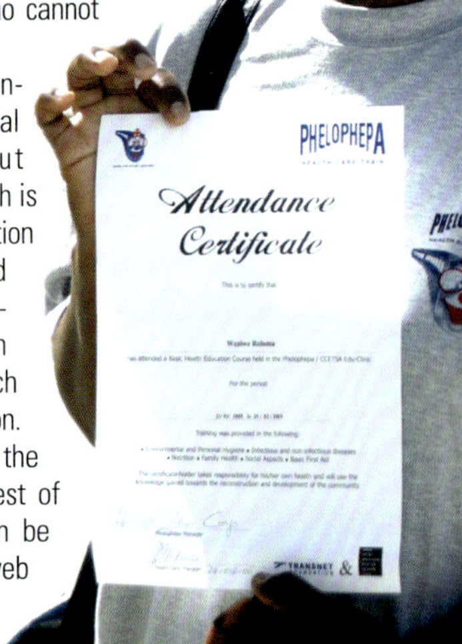

Weziwe Rholowa, from Grahamstown, South Africa, attended a five-day training course in basic health run by Phelophepa staff.

These programmes tend to focus on one disease or one target group. They may achieve great success in these terms, but they cannot be expected to address the population's health needs as a whole. This vertical approach to public health care can result, for example, in lost opportunities for delivering more comprehensive care to isolated communities. Lack of coordination between vertical programmes can lead to duplication of effort, poaching of skilled staff from essential health-care services as well as unsustainable and short-term services.

Individual programmes that focus on one area or disease of interest, such as HIV/AIDS or malaria, inevitably fail to provide people with the full range of the basic health services they need.

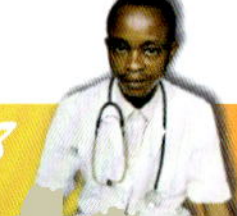

Another problem with single-disease programmes is that they are short-term. Often when they cease operating, recipients seek the same services from their local health system, which may have deteriorated in the meantime. As a result of the failure to build and reinforce health systems, while providing vertical programmes, and the failure to coordinate such programmes, many people in Africa have no reliable health care at all.

## Sector-wide approach

One way to improve the coordination of donor, government and other funding for health-care programmes is to adopt a sector-wide approach (SWAP). This approach means that all significant funding agencies support a shared policy and strategy that applies to the whole health sector, i.e., that is sector-wide. The approach allows governments to agree on health policies and strategic plans, and on where resources should be allocated, with donors and other development partners. By adopting a sector-wide approach, funding and other development partners commit themselves to greater reliance on government financial management and accountability systems. Ghana, Mozambique, Uganda, the United Republic of Tanzania and Zambia are just some of the countries in the African Region that have adopted a sector-wide approach in recent years.

Identifying the key constraints to scaling up health systems was a key factor when the MDGs were formulated. The 1990 baseline picture of health systems function in the African Region underscores just how far there is to go in terms of achieving these goals.

In 1998, countries in the African Region agreed to review their national health policies and strategies and to monitor their progress towards the goal of health for all. This pledge, made in a Regional Committee resolution, covers all facets of health systems, from district services, hospitals, health research and information systems to financing, essential technology, blood safety, essential and traditional medicines, and human resources. The resolution also includes goals to give district health systems more of a community focus, and to provide an essential package of care and to broaden access to this care.

Almost all countries in the African Region have taken different approaches to developing national health policy. Only a few, however, have recently developed or reviewed these policies, with WHO support, to make their health-care services stronger, more efficient and more widely available. For example, Burundi, the Central African Republic, Mauritania, Gabon and the United Republic of Tanzania did such reviews in 2004.

A great deal of work has yet to be done across much of the Region in terms of developing national health policy, a key step towards taking a sector-wide approach. In 2004, WHO increased the number of staff working in the Region to help countries build up and reinforce their health systems. WHO's Regional Office for Africa has also produced technical guidelines to help Member States draw up their own national health policies and development plans.

Many countries, however, face key constraints for improving the health services that are available to their people, such as rapid turnover of staff in key positions; lack

of continuity in policy; lack of resources; poor management of available resources; and poor implementation.

# Health information systems

Governments need reliable evidence based on population health data to develop a public health policy that responds to the needs of the people in their country. These data are vital for planning public health programmes and for monitoring and evaluating progress made by these programmes. Furthermore, population health data can be used to ascertain whether the burden of disease has changed and whether resource allocation needs to be adjusted. This approach enables a government to be more accountable in the way it spends public money on health care.

Such a system provides basic, timely information on a number of factors: how many people die and of what causes; what are the chief causes of disease; who is treating patients; how many people can access care; how much does it cost; what treatment outcomes are; and where the gaps in coverage are shifting. Patient registration, keeping medical records and running an appointment system not only make it possible to manage patients but also enable health authorities to collect data that can be collated and used to set priorities.

Despite limited resources Eritrea, the Gambia, Niger and the United Republic of Tanzania have managed to develop information system policies, national health indicators and integrated data collection forms over the last decade. Some countries in the African Region have also developed and maintained user-friendly databases that are models of efficient health data collection from the level of primary care to the ministry of health. However, efforts in the Region to use information technology effectively have been hampered by the lack of computer hardware; poor internet connections; inadequate system maintenance; the lack of sustainable energy sources; and a shortage of adequately trained personnel. In addition, countries often use different definitions, sources and methods for collecting data, rendering international comparisons difficult. There is, however, increasing support for unified methods of providing improved population health data which can be converted into evidence or knowledge for policy-making, such as Multiple Indicator Cluster Surveys (MICS), and demographic and health surveys (DHS) (see Fig. 6.1).

Most countries in the African Region do not have a health information system that is capable of collecting, storing, analysing, using and reporting these types of data.

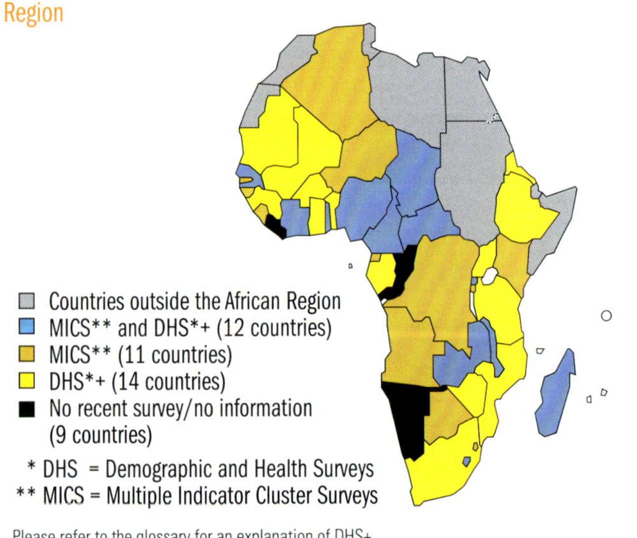

Fig. 6.1

Types of household surveys that have been conducted in the African Region



Please refer to the glossary for an explanation of DHS+
Source: WHO Regional Office for Africa.

That means that governments and global agencies have to compensate for the lack of information by employing other methods, such as mathematical models to predict possible trends and best-guess scenarios based on estimates or extrapolations. Sometimes these methods provide the only available source of information, but they are clearly inadequate. A lack of reliable population health information can result in misdirected funds or the failure on the part of donors to renew aid in spite of continuing need.

In response to the inadequacies of national health information systems in the African Region, global initiatives such as the Health Metrics Network (HMN) have started to help countries improve and align their health information systems, including the quality of vital registration, which is a crucial prerequisite to a more responsive and appropriate use of health systems resources. By April 2006, 25 countries had applied for funds and help as part of the HMN in the African Region and 19 of those applications had been approved.

## Vital registration

The critical baseline for judging a population's health is derived from the registration of births and deaths, but these vital events go unrecorded for the vast majority of people in Africa. Less than 10% of deaths are registered in the African Region and even when deaths are registered, often the causes are either not attributed reliably or not reported at all. This low coverage plus the fact that decision-makers are forced to work with presumed causes of death can result in wide margins of error.

Only a few of the 46 countries in WHO's African Region have some form of vital registration data and only one country has complete current vital registration data, while others have reported incomplete data — including no mortality data collected since 1990 — and some have never reported such data (see Fig. 6.2).

There are, however, alternatives to vital registration. Verbal autopsy is the reporting of the circumstances surrounding a death by interviewing relatives or others who are familiar with the death but who have no medical expertise. Sample registration — another method — tries to capture the causes of mortality of a defined portion of the population. Also, sentinel demographic surveillance involves monitoring a representative group for the vital events of interest.

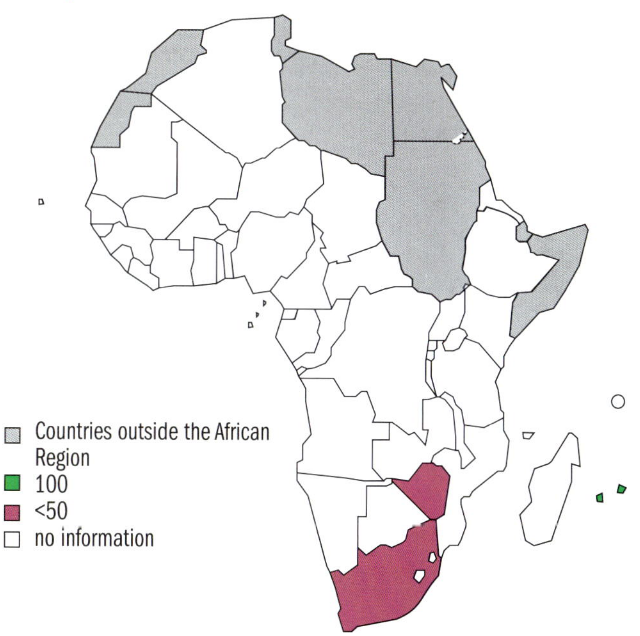

Fig 6.2

Coverage of death registration: mortality data (1995 onwards), by cause, available to WHO



Source: Mathers CD, Ma Fat D, Inoue M, Rao C, Lopez AD. Counting the dead and what they died of: an assessment of the global status of cause of death data. *Bulletin of the World Health Organization* 2005;83:171-7

## Getting the numbers right

For health information systems to measure how effectively a health system is working, it is important to get reliable data. Some data — immunization coverage, health-care facility attendance and antenatal care coverage — may be generated by the routine health information system. Other data, especially on long-term indicators such as maternal and child mortality, life expectancy and fertility rates of a given population, may require other sources of data. These other sources include population censuses, and demographic and health surveys. Such data, however, are not sensitive to short-term changes in health service provision, nor are they specific enough to distinguish the impact of a change in policy from other factors, such as civil unrest or natural disasters, which are common in the African Region. On the other hand, disease-specific interventions aimed at preventing and controlling diseases require reliable data to show changes in incidence of the disease in question. However, gathering reliable incidence data is dependent upon research capacity and/or valid reporting systems, both of which are among the first casualties when health systems decline.

The quality of data is often not given adequate attention and yet it is crucial for deriving reliable information from that data. There are various methods for checking data quality, including health facility patient/client satisfaction surveys, supervisory visits and community surveys. The data obtained from these surveys allow for cross-checking and validation of data obtained routinely. In addition, these data would complement those routinely collected.

Some countries in the Region have developed tools to monitor key indicators of health system performance. The Health Systems Trust, a nongovernmental organization in South Africa, established the District Health Barometer. The aim of this tool is to compare the health data in the country's 53 districts and make the information accessible to the public, thereby improving transparency and accountability. It shows how districts are performing relative to one another and relative to their province and the national average. It is designed to help managers identify gaps and deficits in data collection, so that they can improve the quality of the health indicators they use in decision-making.

Despite some countries' efforts to strengthen their national information systems, much remains to be done. WHO and its partners are providing support to Member States in the African Region to implement priority interventions to strengthen na-

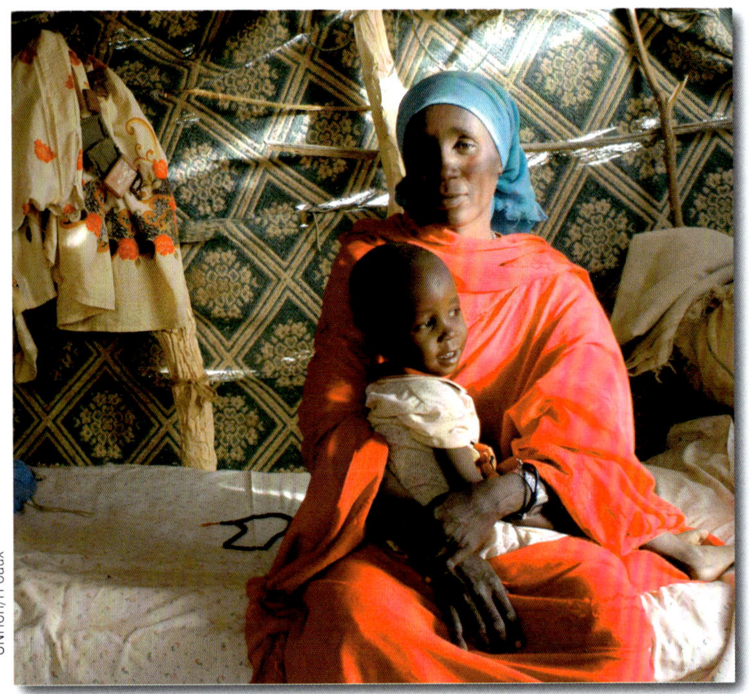



Sudanese refugees from the Darfur region of Sudan. Mother and son in their shelter in Iridimi. They were due to move to a proper tent in the camp. Iridimi, Eastern Chad.

tional health information systems. WHO has helped Kenya, Rwanda, Uganda and Zambia to compile inventories of their health facilities, human resources and health interventions — plotting them on maps in a process known as service availability mapping. These maps show the coverage of health services and give a clear picture of current facilities and staff, and help to identify gaps in services more easily.

# Essential medicines

In some parts of the African Region, over half of the population do not have access to essential medicines and are unable to benefit from proven treatment for common diseases.

Thirty Member States now have national medicine polices (Fig. 6.3), including traditional medicine. These policies have been drawn up with WHO's help to improve equitable access to quality medicine at affordable prices and to promote their rational use. That is an encouraging increase from three countries in 1991. Full implementation of these policies, however, is hampered by many factors, including: the shortage of skilled workers; insufficient funding; poor planning and management; and conflict and poverty. These factors are crucial to the long-term improvement of the pharmaceutical sector in the countries of the African Region.

Medicines account for the second-largest share of the health budget after salaries in countries in the African Region. Government resources allocated to medicines are insufficient to provide for the whole population. There is a need to improve the efficiency of the medicines supply system, including rational selection, procurement, effective distribution and use. Furthermore, prices for new medicines for the most prevalent diseases — HIV/AIDS, tuberculosis and malaria — are often high.

**Fig 6.3**

Member States with official national medicine policies, WHO African Region

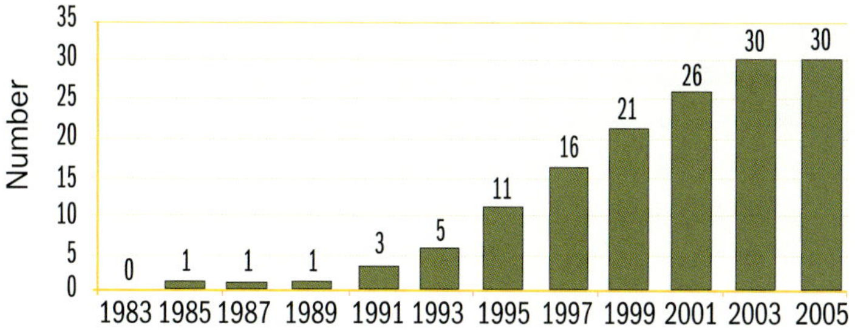

Source: WHO/AFRO/EDM

## Improving access

According to WHO's Medicines Strategy, equitable access to essential medicines can only be ensured by meeting several criteria: rational selection and use; affordable prices; adequate and sustainable financing; and reliable supply systems.

WHO has helped several countries in the African Region carry out medicine price surveys in 2004. The surveys in Algeria, Chad, Ethiopia, Ghana, Kenya, Mali, Nigeria, South Africa, Uganda, the United Republic of Tanzania and Zimbabwe found that prices of similar medicines vary considerably and are often unaffordable. In many countries in the Region, medicine prices are not regulated; even in countries that have medicine pricing policies, these policies are not always enforced.

In the absence of affordable and good quality medicines, some people in the Region unwittingly resort to poor quality or cheap counterfeit medicines. It is illegal in all countries in the Region, but common practice in most, to sell pharmaceutical products on the street often, these medicines are counterfeit. In most cases these are more harmful than no medication at all. Only four countries in the Region have comprehensive medicine regulatory capacity. Inadequacies in this capacity can be ascertained by quality screening of commonly used medicines. For example, a 2002 WHO survey found that chloroquine and sulfadoxine–pyrimethamine for the treatment of malaria in Gabon, Ghana, Kenya, Mali, Mozambique and Zimbabwe failed standard quality tests. Moreover, samples of rifampicin and isoniazid, essential medicines for the treatment of tuberculosis, collected in Chad, Ethiopia, Ghana, Rwanda, Senegal, Uganda, and the United Republic of Tanzania in 2004 were found to be substandard when tested for quality.

Local production of traditional medicines is one solution to the lack of availability of essential medicines, but only when there is evidence to show that the medicines are safe and effective. The best example is provided by artemisinin derivatives for malaria. The plant *Artemisia annua* was introduced from China to the United Republic of Tanzania in 1990, where it is now cultivated commercially. The Tanzanian National Institute for Medical Research showed that rather than exporting the plant to Europe for processing, then re-importing the artemisinin-based medicines to Africa at US$ 6–7 per dose, domestic production could reduce costs to US$ 2 per dose (see Box 6.3).

Some countries in Africa are trying to foster innovation in traditional medicines as a long-term way of providing more affordable medicines to address public health needs. But to do this, countries need to build a research and development capacity, create gene banks and they need patent protection. For example, scientists in South Africa are conducting research to find a vaccine for HIV that addresses the country's specific health needs. The aim is to produce a vaccine for subtype C of the virus, which accounts for more than 90% of HIV infections in southern Africa. Most HIV vaccine research aims to develop a vaccine for virus subtype B, the dominant strain in the United States and Europe.

WHO has developed a number of policies and standards to help Member States address the problems with safety and quality, supply, management and rational use of essential medicines. The illicit trade in pharmaceuticals needs to be controlled, and the rights of pharmacists to sell generic medicines — which are cheaper than their patented originals — need to be upheld. Member States should collaborate to produce affordable essential medicines in the Region, and negotiate bulk purchases wherever possible to reduce medicine prices.

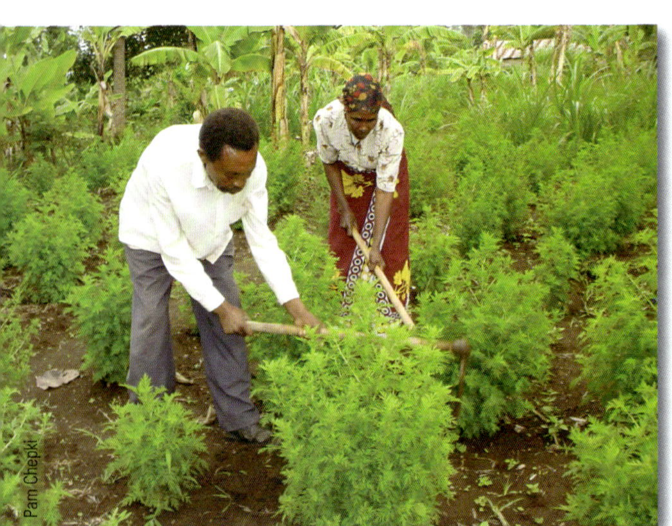


The Leserian family tending their valuable sweet wormwood crop in Arusha, the United Republic of Tanzania (see Box 6.3).

## Tanzanian farmers grow their own *Artemisia annua*

Cultivation of *Artemisia annua,* or sweet wormwood, in the United Republic of Tanzania is the first step to improving people's access to antimalarial medicines, and it has economic advantages too. Farmers in Arusha say that growing *Artemisia* is more profitable than growing vegetables and will raise their living standards.

Joseph Leserian uproots sweet wormwood seedlings from a nursery and transplants them to his main garden, taking care not to damage their roots. The 64-year-old hopes that the miniature plants will provide him with a better income than his vegetables. A bumpy unpaved road leads to his simple bungalow in Arusha, a poor area near Africa's tallest peak, Mount Kilimanjaro.

Until recently *Artemisia annua*, was grown mainly in China and Viet Nam. The plant is the source of artemisinin, which is the active ingredient in the most effective antimalarial medicines available today. These drugs — known as artemisinin-based combination therapies (ACTs) — are badly needed in Africa because malaria parasites have become resistant to former mainstays of antimalarial treatment, such as chloroquine. A global shortage of artemisinin, however, means that not all countries can obtain sufficient quantities of ACTs. That is where farmers like Leserian come in. *Artemisia* thrives in Tanzanian soil, which makes local production of artemisinin a viable commercial proposition. Now WHO is coordinating the efforts of a nongovernmental organization called TechnoServe and African Artemisia Ltd to produce the crop locally.

"We help farmers with cultivating, harvesting and selling their crop. We hope that by producing artemisinin in East Africa, we are helping to provide an African solution to an African problem," said TechnoServe's project director, Michael Baddeley.

Leserian was the first of 300 farmers in Arusha to start cultivating the plant in February 2004. His three-quarter hectare plot — part of his two-hectare farm — now boasts leafy well tended *Artemisia* shrubs. An optimistic Leserian says he switched from growing tomatoes and potatoes to cultivation of *Artemisia annua* after being convinced that the new venture could change his life. He points out that the *Artemisia* shrubs are easier to tend than vegetables, and easier to sell. "We had to struggle and to sell our vegetables, unlike *Artemisia,* sweet wormwood, which has a ready market". African Artemisia Ltd will purchase the crop: extract the artemisinin and sell it to international pharmaceutical companies. Farmers will be paid for the weight and quality of the crop; Tsh500 (US$ 0.5) per kilogram of leaves, with a bonus for higher artemisisin content. Each hectare is expected to produce an average of two tonnes of *Artemisia.*

"Once I sell the crop and venture into other projects … I shall improve the living standards of my family," Leserian said.

## Blood safety

Ensuring that blood supplies are safe is one example of the challenges health systems face in Africa. Blood transfusions save many lives each year, but many people also die when blood supplies are inadequate or unsafe. Women and children are particularly affected. Women receive transfusions to replace blood lost during pregnancy and delivery. Children often need transfusions because they are prone to life-threatening anaemia caused by the all-too-common problems of severe malnutrition and malaria. An unsafe blood supply can be worse than no blood supply, as the long-term risk of being infected with and dying from HIV/AIDS or viral hepatitis B or C can outweigh the risks of dying from anaemia in the short term.

In 1994, WHO's Regional Committee for Africa noted with concern that only 10 of the 46 Member States could guarantee the safety of blood transfusion in their hospitals. Countries were urged to enact blood safety policies and improve hospital transfusion services. Yet by 1999, only 14 countries had a national blood transfusion policy, and even these were not always fully implemented. Haphazard practices exposed many patients and health-care staff to potentially fatal risks. The rest of the countries in the Region have since developed a national blood policy, but due to lack of funds, inadequate infrastructure and shortage of skilled personnel, implementation has been slow.

The way blood banks are run and transfusions are handled are problems. The source of the blood is another. The safest blood source is from regular, unpaid, voluntary donors, as their blood is the least likely to be infected with HIV or the hepatitis viruses. In the absence of adequate supplies, patients are asked to find a family member who will donate blood for their transfusion or an unrelated person who will replace the units of blood taken from the hospital's short supplies. Cases of paid donations have been reported by a few countries.

In 1999, only Botswana, Côte d'Ivoire, Namibia, Rwanda, South Africa and Zimbabwe were collecting 100% of blood supplies from voluntary non-remunerated donors. Four additional countries, Benin, Burundi, Swaziland and Togo, have reported using this source exclusively. In 2002, only half of the entire blood supply in the Region came from unpaid donors, while about 44% came from family or replacement donors and 4% from paid donors. However, it is often hard to tell how much of so-called family or replacement donations have been purchased. In the early years of the HIV/AIDS epidemic some paediatric cases of HIV/AIDS were caused by transfusion with contaminated blood. Well organized blood donation programmes in Côte d'Ivoire, South Africa and Zimbabwe have shown that it is possible to find a population of willing, unpaid blood donors with uninfected blood, even in areas with a high prevalence of HIV.

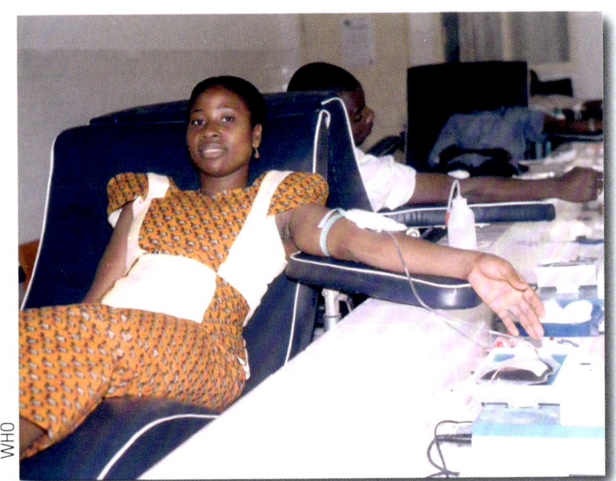
Healthy blood donors are a vital resource.

Selecting donors is the first step to ensure a safe blood supply. Screening the blood is the second. Despite progress made in HIV screening — 99.9% of blood is screened compared with 75% in 1999 — less than 60% of the African Region's blood supply is currently screened specifically for the four major transfusion-transmissible infections (HIV, viral hepatitis B and C, and syphilis). Reliable blood screening is impossible without high quality reagents and test kits, properly trained and skilled staff, and regular quality assurance. Twenty countries in the African Region still struggle with irregular or incomplete supplies of reagents and test kits, with the result that patients are given transfusions with potentially infected blood. This is doubly tragic when patients who could have survived without a blood transfusion are given one and when, on top of that, those patients die from an infection transmitted through blood that they did not need in the first place.

Despite WHO courses — 200 quality managers were trained between 2000 and 2003 — national blood quality systems have since been established fully in only 12 countries, and partially in 15 countries. Twelve countries in the Region currently have no quality assurance of blood transfusions.

Ensuring a safe blood supply is a long and costly exercise, but countries in the African Region are making progress in improving transfusion practices. More funds are needed to train staff, build and equip blood transfusion services, purchase reagents and implement quality assurance programmes. Patients in need should have equitable access to safe blood, and HIV should not be transmitted through blood transfusions. The medical indications for transfusion also need to be critically examined to make sure that patients are only given blood when there is no viable alternative treatment.

# Human resources: a continent in crisis

A major gathering of experts in human resources for health in Addis Ababa, Ethiopia, in January 2002 put the African Region's health workforce crisis firmly on the international agenda. Delegates at the meeting reported alarming figures; for example, 50% of doctors in Namibia were expatriates, and medical doctor vacancy rates in the public sector in 1998 were reported to be 43% in Ghana and 36% in Malawi. Nurse vacancy rates in the public sector in Lesotho were reported to be 48% in 1998. The meeting heard that for 15 years there had been no public recruitment of health personnel in Cameroon, while Ghana, Zambia and Zimbabwe estimated losses of 15–40% of employees in the public sector every year. This underscores the instability of the health workforce and the lengths some countries must go to fill vacancies (see Box 6.4).

Many factors have contributed to the growing shortage of health workers across the Region — Africa's human resources for health crisis. A high disease burden means that more health workers are needed to take care of the sick. Another factor is the loss of many health-care workers due to death, migration and poor conditions of service. Human resources for health policies and plans have not been able to address the increasing demands of health service delivery, while weak or stagnant health system infrastructures have not adapted to population growth. The devastating impact of the HIV/AIDS pandemic has drastically cut large swathes of the health workforce in some African countries and made working conditions more intolerable in the health sector. But even before the HIV/AIDS pandemic, the human resources for health sector — a key element of a well functioning health system — was already badly neglected. Until recently, scant attention was paid to the remuneration, deployment and continuing education of health staff in Africa. To draw more attention to the problem, WHO devoted the *World health report 2006* and World Health Day 2006 to this issue. Increased awareness at national and global level is only the first step to fixing the problem.

A WHO survey, published in 2004 of trends in Cameroon, Ghana, Senegal, South Africa, Uganda and Zimbabwe over the period 1991–2000, found that although the absolute numbers of health professionals had increased, the overall doctor: population ratio had fallen. Health workers migrate within countries from rural to urban practices, from the public to the private sector, and between countries, in search of better working conditions, higher salaries, and opportunities for training and recognition. It is difficult to gather reliable data on the scale of this migration.

## Malawi's health sector "brain drain"

The growing shortage of doctors and nurses across parts of the African Region is one of the greatest obstacles to tackling the heavy burden of disease, particularly in countries with a high prevalence of HIV/AIDS. Malawi is one of the Region's worst hit countries. It is often said that more Malawian doctors work in the English city of Manchester than in the whole of Malawi. But there is more than just anecdotal evidence to suggest the drift.

"We have a critical shortage of nurses. We need 10 to 12 nurses to a ward. At the moment we have about five to a ward of 70 or 80 patients," said Chief Nursing Officer Fannie Kachale at Kamuzu Central Hospital, one of Malawi's largest state referral hospitals. The hospital in the capital Lilongwe needs 532 nurses to be fully staffed, but in March 2005 had only 188. More than half the nurses' posts were vacant. Many had left to work in Malawi's private sector or the United Kingdom, attracted by better pay and work conditions.

At Kamuzu Central, work conditions are grim and staff, who divide their time between this and another hospital, are barely able to cope. Wards are overflowing as patients spill out on to the verandah and most patients have relatives helping to look after them. Their conditions are serious, ranging from tuberculosis to pneumonia, often related to HIV/AIDS.

Dr Damsom Kathyola, the director of the hospital, said the shortage of nursing staff was "a crisis, which, if not reversed, could lead to the collapse of the entire health delivery system in Malawi". Development agencies have started to respond to the crisis. The UK Department for International Development doubled its development aid to Malawi in 2005 to US$ 176 million (£100 million) over the following six years. Just over half will be spent on human resources for health.

The idea is not only to train double the number of nurses and doctors currently being trained in Malawi but once they start working to offer them higher salaries and additional incentives to stay in Malawi. The aid would also cover the costs of paying nurses and doctors from other countries to fill gaps, while the Malawians are being trained.

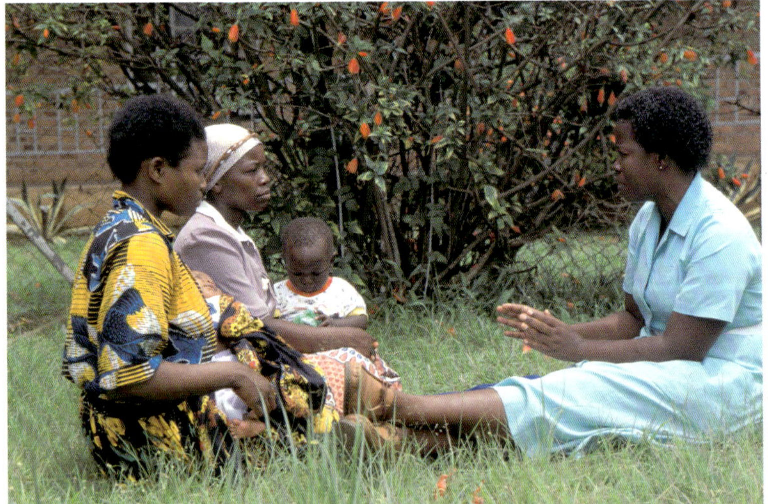

Panos/ G Pirozzi

Nurse talking to mothers about childcare at a rural health clinic in Malawi.

However, regulatory bodies in developed countries have data on health workers registered to work in their countries. While this information is inevitably partial, it provides an overview of foreign-trained health workers in developed countries. Table 6.1 shows the number of doctors and nurses from African countries working in developed countries. They represent more than 30% of the stock of doctors in the source countries. Rough estimates can also be made based on the numbers of requests for certificates of good standing from national licensing bodies as well as from the number of expatriate doctors employed to fill in the gaps and the number of vacant posts.

Table 6.1

Outflow of health workers from 16 African countries, 1993–2002

| Country | No. of health workers reported migrated | Main destination |
|---|---|---|
| Burundi | 127 | Belgium, Benin, France, Rwanda |
| Cameroon | 82 | Canada, Central African Republic, France, Namibia, Senegal, UK, USA |
| Central African Republic | 176 | Cameroon, Côte d'Ivoire, France, Senegal |
| Côte d'Ivoire | 641 | Canada, France |
| Democratic Republic of the Congo | 337 | Canada, Côte d'Ivoire, France, Senegal, USA, Zambia |
| Gabon | 128 | Canada, France |
| Gambia | 233 | UK, USA |
| Ghana | 1169 | Gabon, Saudi Arabia, South Africa, UK, USA |
| Kenya | 1734 | Saudi Arabia, UK, USA, Zambia |
| Madagascar | 341 | France, Zambia |
| Malawi | 484 | UK, USA |
| Mali | 93 | Cameroon, Canada, Côte d'Ivoire, France, USA, Zambia |
| Nigeria | 213 | France, Gambia, Kenya, Namibia, UK, USA, Zambia |
| Sao Tome and Principe | 103 | Gabon, Namibia, Portugal |
| United Republic of Tanzania | 446 | Botswana, Comoros, Equatorial Guinea, Kenya, Mauritania, Namibia, UK, United Arab Emirates, Zimbabwe, USA |
| Zambia | 974 | Botswana, UK, USA |
| **Total** | **7281** | |

Source: *Survey on migration of health workers in the African Region.* Brazzaville: WHO Regional Office for Africa; 2003.

Hospital development needs to complement other levels of the health system, and improve referral patterns while ensuring that poor people have access to services. Hospitals also need to develop their role in the provision of medical care to include more specialized training and to promote research and the use of information systems.

## Approaches to filling the gap

To address growing shortages of health workers, some countries are testing models where certain tasks are re-assigned from highly qualified health workers to less qualified staff under further orientation and supervision. Botswana has tested community home-based care as a way of involving families and other members of the community in caring for people with HIV/AIDS (see Box 6.5). Likewise, Uganda has led the way in terms of training health workers to deliver simplified HIV/AIDS treatment. (see Box 6.6).

Like Uganda, the Eastern Cape region of South Africa has adopted simplified guidelines to deliver antiretroviral (ARV) treatment to people with HIV/AIDS. Researchers have called on the government to roll out the approach to the rest of the country by giving more nurses greater responsibility to dispense ARVs, permission to screen HIV-positive patients to determine whether they were eligible for treatment, and permission to monitor patients' adherence to medication. They argue that with adequate orientation and supervision, nurses can prescribe ARVs.

In rural Tanzanian districts, assistant medical officers often work as medical doctors, and those with specialist training are in charge of clinical disciplines such as the department of anaesthesiology and ophthalmology when no specialists are available in these disciplines. In Zanzibar, an island in the Indian Ocean, where the shortage of medical doctors is more serious, and in the mainland of the United Republic of Tanzania, assistant medical officers work as district medical officers.

International efforts are under way to address Africa's growing health workforce crisis. The World Health Assembly passed a resolution on migration and human resources for health in 2004 and the High Level Forum meeting to discuss progress towards the health-related Millennium Development Goals in 2004 also recognized human resources for health as vital for achieving the goals.

WHO and its partners are working closely with Member States in the African Region to find ways to motivate and retain their health workers. WHO has been helping countries develop and implement motivation and retention strategies with the support of development partners as part of these countries' national health plans. This support includes scaling up training — especially of mid-level cadres — to fill in staffing gaps. Various methods, including distance learning and continuing medical education can also help to achieve better staffing coverage.

Countries have tested different ways of preventing health workers from migrating. These include allowing health workers to engage in private practice while working in the public sector, raising salaries and improving working conditions.  These also include retaining certificates of graduates until they have returned to their country of origin, allowing communities in decentralized systems to directly recruit their



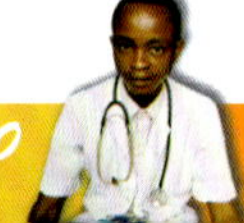

## Community home-based care in Botswana

Banyefudi Sampora is full of praise for the community home-based care (CHBC) programme, which has taught her how to look after her sick daughter at home and emerged as a powerful tool in Botswana's response to HIV/AIDS.

"These people have been like the second mother to my daughter, she eats well and gets medicine," said the 68-year-old grandmother referring to the community health workers who visit Sampora and her family every month.

Sampora has been taking care of her HIV-positive daughter since 2002 at her rural home at Mmopane village, 20 km north-west of Botswana's capital, Gaborone. She is the only breadwinner as her daughter is too ill to work. She also has to care for her daughter's four children who are still in school.

Sampora was given a basic education in HIV/AIDS. Community health workers explained how to care for her daughter, prevent transmission of the virus to other members of the family and monitor that her daughter is taking her medicine every day.

Every month they deliver a package to each home containing basic medical supplies and food. If her daughter gets an infection, the family must go to the village health post 2 km away.

Botswana has one of Africa's most developed health systems. But with the rapid spread of HIV/AIDS over the last decade that system is badly overstretched. The community home-based approach is a way of making scarce health resources go a long way and of delivering health care to patients in the comfort of their homes.

The village of 5000 was selected in 2002 by the Department of Nursing and Midwifery at the University of Botswana, a WHO Collaborating Centre, to develop CHBC teaching and learning material for the rest of English-speaking Africa. The department also created a day centre for patients, which gives the home-based caregivers time to get on with their own lives. Sampora tends a vegetable garden and sells her produce to support the family.

Director Dr Esther Seloilwe said the village was chosen because it is underdeveloped despite being close to the capital. It has a health post staffed by a nurse but no telephone, which makes referring patients to hospital very difficult.

"The Botswana family structure is ideal for the CHBC programme because the culture dictates that families support and care for the sick and the dying," said Seloilwe. "Home-based care has been in our tradition for years, it was just a case of us now placing the emphasis on caring for those with HIV/AIDS."

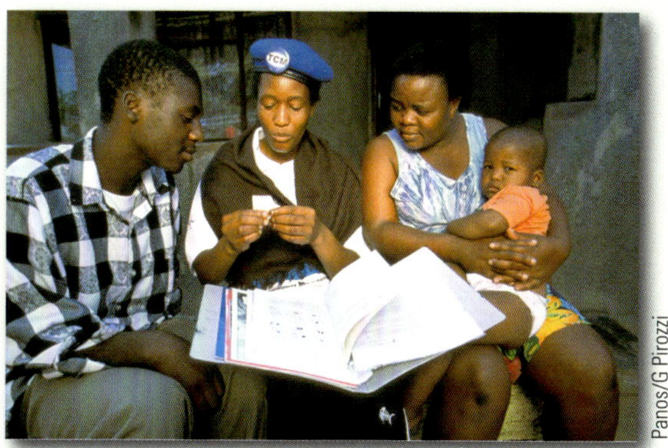

Mobile health educator teaching a family about HIV/AIDS.

health workers and pay them. While recognizing the right of individuals to migrate, governments can also use this to mutual benefit through, for example, bilateral exchanges of specialists.

# Health financing

African countries spent on average 5% of their gross domestic product (GDP) on health in 2003, 51% of which were expenditures by the government. The median share of government expenditure on health funded by external resources is 26%, with a wide range of countries' share of government expenditure on health funded by external resources, from less than 1% (e.g. Algeria) to over 75% (e.g. Rwanda). Expenditures on health by the private sector (households, nongovernmental organizations, private enterprises, insurance) on average made up 49% of total expenditure on health,

## Uganda leads the way in simplified AIDS care

Few countries in the African Region can afford the "gold standard" package of HIV/AIDS chronic care that is routinely provided in industrialized countries. Botswana, one of the Region's wealthiest countries, adopted this approach and by the end of 2004 it was the only African country to have reached the 50% treatment target level. But Uganda hopes that a new, simplified approach to delivering HIV/AIDS treatment will help it overcome the lack of cash and health workers and be just as effective as Botswana. So far Uganda has started delivering treatment to a third of the people who need it. It hopes this new approach will help it reach the rest over the next few years.

The idea is to train nurses to do some of the work of doctors and for lay health workers and community workers to carry out some nurses' tasks. Patients are prescribed combination pills to be taken twice daily, rather than several different medicines. As long as a doctor diagnoses a patient or endorses the diagnosis of a nurse, and as long as the doctor writes the prescription, the counselling and supervision of drug intake can be done by others.

"If you can make a good diagnosis, the counselling is good and the patient adheres to the drugs, I don't see how the level of qualification can be a problem," said Elizabeth Madraa, manager of Uganda's National AIDS Programme, adding that simplified treatment guidelines were key not only to delivering HIV/AIDS treatment but basic health care in general. "Unless we do things differently to address the human resource capacity gap, we shall never deliver even the basic health-care services, let alone ART (antiretroviral therapy)".

The approach called Integrated Management of Adult and Adolescent Illness (IMAI) is a health services delivery model characterized by simplified guidelines and training material. It is based on full involvement of nurses, lay health workers and — in the case of HIV/AIDS chronic care — HIV-positive patients who help to train health workers.

The approach has been inspired by successes elsewhere in Africa, Latin America and the former Soviet Union where relatives, friends or other community volunteers have been trained to help treat tuberculosis patients in poor settings.

One of the principles is community home-based care — which has already proved a success in Botswana (see Box 6.5) — to ease congestion in health facilities. If complications arise, the nurses and others who visit the patients at home can refer them to a doctor or a health facility.

More than 1400 health workers in Uganda have completed HIV training across the country. Ethiopia, the Eastern Cape Province of South Africa, Swaziland and Zambia have also started training health workers in this simplified approach. If successful, they could serve as a model for other low-income countries.

with households representing the largest share (80%). Fig. 6.4 shows a breakdown of expenditure on malaria in Ghana, illustrating the disproportionate burden on households.

The WHO Commission for Macroeconomics and Health estimated that a minimum expenditure of US$ 34 per person per year was required to provide an essential package of public health interventions in order to achieve both the relevant MDGs and the New Partnership for Africa's Development (NEPAD) targets. Thus, governments in the 35 Member States that are currently spending less than US$ 34 on health per capita per year will need to increase their budgetary allocations to reach the recommended minimum health spending (Fig. 6.5).

Heads of state of countries in Africa made a commitment in Abuja to allocate at least 15% of their annual budgets to the health sector. By the end of 2003, only one country's government had spent 15% or more of its national budget on health, including spending funded by external resources. The other 45 Member States in the African Region will need to take appropriate steps to honour the commitment made by their heads of state.

In 2005, the Abuja pledge to allocate 15% of their national budgets to health was reconfirmed by African heads of state in the Gaborone Declaration at the October 2005 session of the Conference of African ministers of health in Botswana.

WHO has devised a method called National Health Accounts, a system which 23 of the Region's 46 Member States have already used to track their health expenditure. This system can also be used to analyse the financial flows within national health systems to see where funds are adequate or in short supply. Health authorities can use this to allocate finances more effectively to improve the overall performance of health systems.

## Donor funding

Donor funding, on average, represented 16% of overall health-care spending in the African Region in 2003. In the Maputo Declaration, African heads of state urged donor countries to honour their pledge to allocate 0.7% of their gross national product as official aid to developing countries to boost funds for health and development.

There is little coordination between international donors, who tend to focus on different diseases in an unsystematic way. Donors may, for example, insist on using different drugs from one another. They may demand different delivery methods. They may fail to live up to their funding pledges, and they may provide funds over short time-frames. The UK's Commission for Africa called upon health development partners to harmonize and align their support with recipient countries' national health policies and strategic plans to make aid more effective.

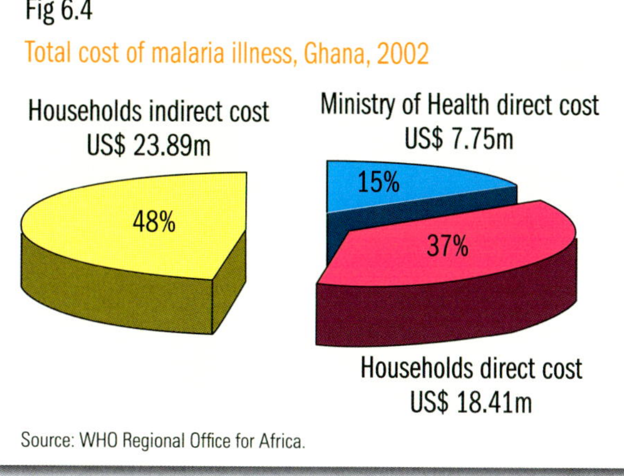



Where aid is ineffective, donors can be to blame as much as the recipient countries themselves. There is broad agreement — and this is one of the demands of the UK's Commission for Africa — that donor countries change their approach to funding, but there is less consensus on how.

Ideally, donors should all work to a single agreement drawn up by the government of each recipient country and they should be legally bound to pay as promised. They should pledge aid over a longer time frame to allow African governments to plan the use of those resources better. One way governments in the Region have started to improve coordination of external and domestic funds for health is by taking an intersectoral approach to streamline the efforts of all the sectors involved.

Health is determined by a number of factors that lie outside the health sector's direct influence, such as water, sanitation and other environmental factors as well as food availability, education, political and social environment. These social determinants of health can be addressed by strengthening inter-sectoral collaboration.

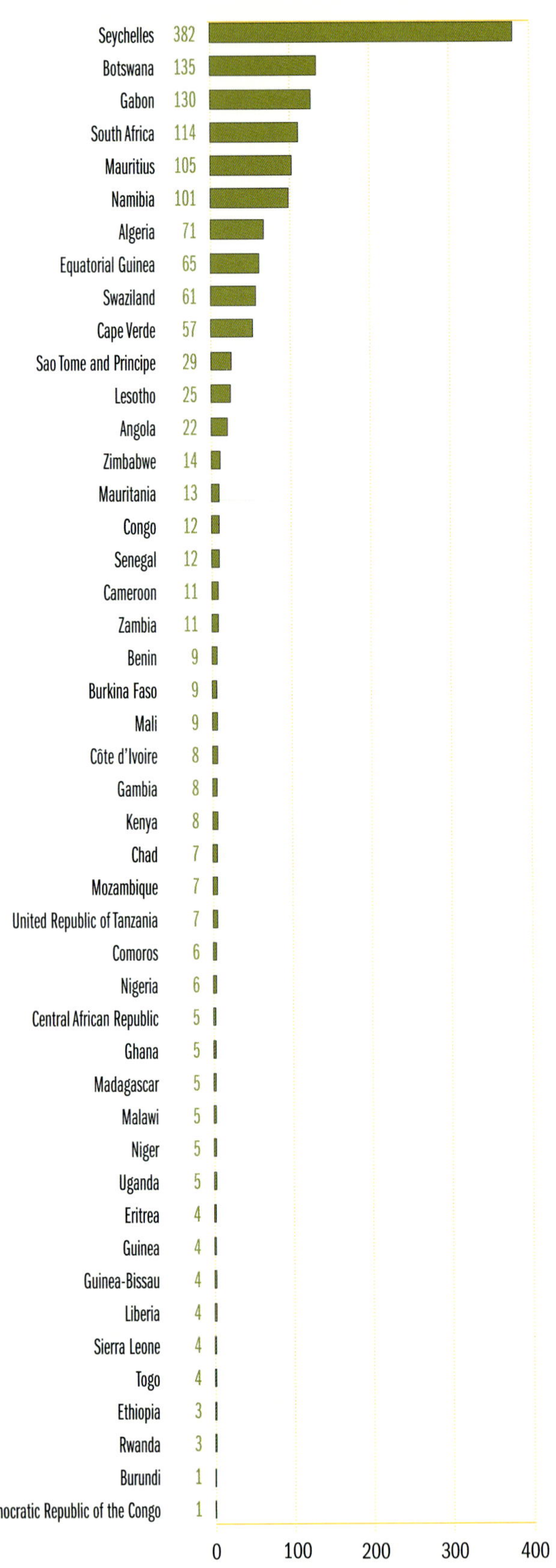



Source: WHO/ World Health Report, 2006.

## User fees

User fees charged by public facilities are often around 5% of total government recurrent health expenditure. However, analysis in the United Republic of Tanzania showed that the abolition of primary health care fees would cost only US$ 13 million per year. Rich nations should support poor countries to offset the financial loss arising from the removal of direct out-of-pocket payments for basic health care until governments in Africa can afford to take on these costs themselves. Basic health care should be subsidized for the poorest members of society. User fees may be entirely covered by alternative financing methods, but many providers prefer charging a minimal, symbolic fee to ensure that services are appreciated and not used unnecessarily.

There are many types of social protection schemes, such as social health insurance, voluntary-based insurance, cash transfers to carers, social pensions, and child-care grants. These can be of great benefit to many people, especially the most vulnerable: the elderly, the young and the disabled.

## Evidence for resource allocation

Once governments have collected and pooled from various sources their scant public revenues, policy-makers face the task of having to decide how to allocate them to buy health services. Often policy-makers do this with very little evidence to guide their choice of the many possible public health interventions. This lack of evidence sometimes results in decisions being made to invest in expensive interventions that benefit few people rather than in low-cost interventions which potentially benefit more people. To guide such priority-setting, WHO runs a project called Choosing Interventions that are Cost Effective — also known as WHO CHOICE — to help countries in this task. WHO has compiled databases, which can be found under http://www.who.int/choice/links/related_links/en/index.html of the evidence of cost-effectiveness on over 500 public health interventions addressing broad categories of problems: unsafe water, addictive drugs, sexual health, malnutrition, malaria, tuberculosis,

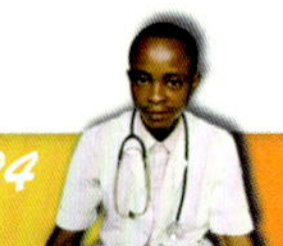

maternal and neonatal diseases, iron deficiency, unsafe injections, mental illness and blindness. Information on 200 interventions for cardiovascular diseases and cancer will be added to the databases.

Once resources have been allocated to pay for various health-care services, it is important to monitor the efficiency of the use of those resources. There is also growing evidence in the African Region that hospitals and health centres can attend to more patients if the resources available to them are better managed. Since hospitals and health centres consume a significant proportion of development and recurrent budgets of ministries of health, there is a need for vigilance in monitoring the use of those resources.

# Conclusion: Health systems – the key to better health

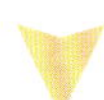

The countries of the African Region need to build and reinforce their health systems as a platform to provide a broad range of essential health-care services to their people. There is no "one-size fits all". These health systems must be tailored to the needs of each country, each region and each community — whether rural or urban, affluent or poor. Health systems must provide services that address key public health needs and these must be delivered in an effective and accountable way. There is an urgent need to establish accountable and transparent systems to monitor and evaluate health expenditure as health spending from public and private sources increases. Getting this right is one of Africa's big public health challenges.

Several key elements need to be in place for health systems to function properly: adequate human resources and infrastructure, reliable evidence on public health needs, as well as health financing systems. Governments, working together with all partners, need to make a deliberate effort to build and reinforce health systems to make them responsive to public health needs and to be more effective. Governments — in the African Region and elsewhere in the world — need also to be more involved in research into the health problems that affect their people most and engaged in the quest for sustainable public health solutions to those problems.

In view of the significant role being played by the private sector and civil society in health services delivery, it is imperative that governments strengthen their collaboration with them and also create the right regulatory and legal environment for the private sector and civil society to effectively play that role.

As we have seen, building, reinforcing and scaling up health system interventions are vital steps towards the goal of equitable health care in the spirit of the 1978 Declaration of Alma-Ata on primary health care to achieve the goal of health for all. There is widespread recognition among African governments and in the donor community that the African Region has little chance of achieving the health-related MDGs if it cannot strengthen and operate such systems effectively. Health systems have enormous untapped potential to contribute to economic and social development.

The challenge is to make governments more aware that health has a crucial role to play in the social and economic development of their countries. Health needs to be placed higher on the political agenda of countries in the Region and their leaders need to develop policies and strategies to strengthen their health systems. That means providing sufficient resources to make health systems work effectively and to sustain them into the future.

Governments in the Region and donors need to make health systems a top priority in national and international development agendas. This is vital for establishing integrated primary health care at district level and to strengthening the overall public health infrastructure. These vital health system elements require long-term political commitment and substantial additional funds. Those involved must also accept that results will be slow, but solid. The health systems that result would provide a much needed platform for delivering all the necessary services for the health of the people. ■

## Bibliography

- African Union: *Maputo declaration on Malaria, HIV/AIDS, Tuberculosis, and other related infectious diseases.* Addis Ababa; 2003.

- Asbu EZ, McIntyre D, Addison T. Hospital efficiency and productivity in three provinces of South Africa. *South African Journal of Economics,* 2001;69:336-58, .

- Awases M, Gbary A, Nyoni J, Chatora R. *Migration of health professionals in six countries: a synthesis report.* Brazzaville; WHO Regional Office for Africa; 2004

- Brown A. *Current issues in sector-wide approaches for health development. Mozambique case study.* Geneva: World Health Organization; 2000. WHO document WHO/GPE/00.4. Available from: http://whqlibdoc.who.int/hq/2000/WHO_GPE_00.4.pdf

- Brown A. *Current issues in sector-wide approaches for health development. Tanzania case study.* Geneva: World Health Organization; 2000. WHO document WHO/GPE/00.6. Available from: http://whqlibdoc.who.int/hq/2000/WHO_GPE_00.6.pdf

- Brown A. *Current issues in sector-wide approaches for health development. Uganda case study.* Geneva: World Health Organization: 2000. WHO document: WHO/GPE/00.3. Available from: http://whqlibdoc.who.int/hq/2000/WHO_GPE_00.3.pdf

- Chatora R. Health financing in the WHO African Region. *African Health Monitor.* 2006;5:13-6.

- Commission for Africa. *Our common interest: an argument.* London: Penguin Books; 2005.

- Documenting Best or "Promising" Practices In Human Resources For Health Development In The Who African Region.

- Evans D, Edejer TT. Choice: an aid to policy. *African Health Monitor.* 2005;5:27-9.

- Foster M, Brown A, Conway T. *Sector-wide approaches for health development: a review of experience.* Geneva; World Health Organization; 2000. WHO document WHO/GPE/00.1. Available from: http://whqlibdoc.who.int/hq/2000/WHO_GPE_00.1.pdf

- Freedman LP, Waldman RJ, de Pinho H, Wirth M E, Chowdhury AMR, Rosenfield A. Transforming health systems to improve the lives of women and children. *Lancet* 2005;365:997-1000.

- Guidelines for evaluating traditional medicines in WHO African Region. Regional Office for Africa. Brazzaville.

- Kirigia JM, Emrouznejad A, Sambo LG, Measurement of technical efficiency of public hospitals in Kenya: Using data envelopment analysis, *Journal of Medical Systems,* 2002;26:29-45.

- Kirigia JM, Emrouznejad A, Sambo LG, Munguti N and Liambila W. Using Data Envelopment Analysis to Measure the Technical Efficiency of Public Health Centers in Kenya. *Journal of Medical Systems,* 2004;28:155-66.

- Kirigia JM, Sambo LG, Scheel H. Technical efficiency of public clinics in Kwazulu-Natal province of South Africa, *East African Medical Journal,* 2001;78:S1-S13.

- Marmot, M. Social determinants of health inequalities. *Lancet* 2005;365:1099-104.

- Masiye F, Ndulo M, Roos P, Odegaard K. A comparative analysis of hospitals in Zambia: a pilot study on efficiency measurement and monitoring. Chapter 7, pp. 95-107. In: Seshamani V, Mwikisa CN, Odegaard K. *Zambias, Health Reforms Selected Papers 1995-2000.* Lund: Sweden; 2002.

- Mathers CD, Ma Fat D, Inoue M, Rao C, Lopez AD. Counting the dead and what they died from; an assessment of the global status of cause of death data. *Bulletin of the World Health Organization* 2005;83:171-7.

- New WHO Regional Director for Africa pledges to do better for Africa. *Bulletin of the World Health Organization* 2005;83:9.

- Organization of African Unity: *Abuja declaration on HIV/AIDS, tuberculosis and other related infectious diseases.* Addis Ababa; 2000.

- Osei D, d'Almeida S, George MO, Kirigia JM, Mensah AO, Kainyu LH. Technical efficiency of public district hospitals and health centres in Ghana: a pilot study. *Cost Effectiveness and Resource Allocation* 2005;3:9. Article URL: http://www.resource-allocation.com/content/2/1/9.

- Regional Committee for Africa  fifth session, International migration of health personnel: a challenge for health systems in developing countries. An information document. AFR/RC55/inf/Doc.2 2005.

- Renner A and Kirigia JM. Technical efficiency of health centres in Sierra Leone. *African Health Monitor.* 2005;5:39-42.

- *Report on the Consultative Meeting on Improving Collaboration between Health Professionals, Governments, and Other Stakeholders in Human Resources for Health Development, Addis Ababa, 29 January – 1 February 2002*. Brazzaville; WHO Regional Office for Africa: 2002. Available from: http://www.afro.who.int/hrd/consultative_meeting_report.pdf

- Tools for institutionalizing traditional medicine in health systems in WHO African Region. Regional Office for Africa. Brazzaville. http://www.prometra.org/Documents/ToolsforINstitutionalizingTraditionalMedicineinHealth.pdf

- WHO Regional Office for Africa (2004) Priority Interventions for Strengthening National Health Information Systems. WHO Regional Office for Africa (2004) AFR/RC54/12.

- Commission for Macroeconomics and Health Report. Geneva; World Health Organization 2001.

- *World health report 2004: Changing history.* Geneva; World Health Organization 2004.

- *World health report 2005: Make every mother and child count.* Geneva; World Health Organization 2005.

- *World Health Report 2006: Working together for health.* Geneva; World Health Organization 2006.

- *World development indicators 2004.* Washington, DC: World Bank; World Health Organization 2004.

- World Health Organization: Sustainable health financing, universal coverage and social health insurance. Geneva; WHO; 2005.

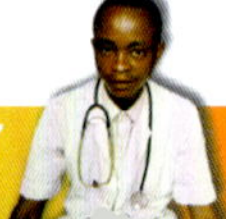

# Health statistics in the African Region

# African Region of the World Health Organization

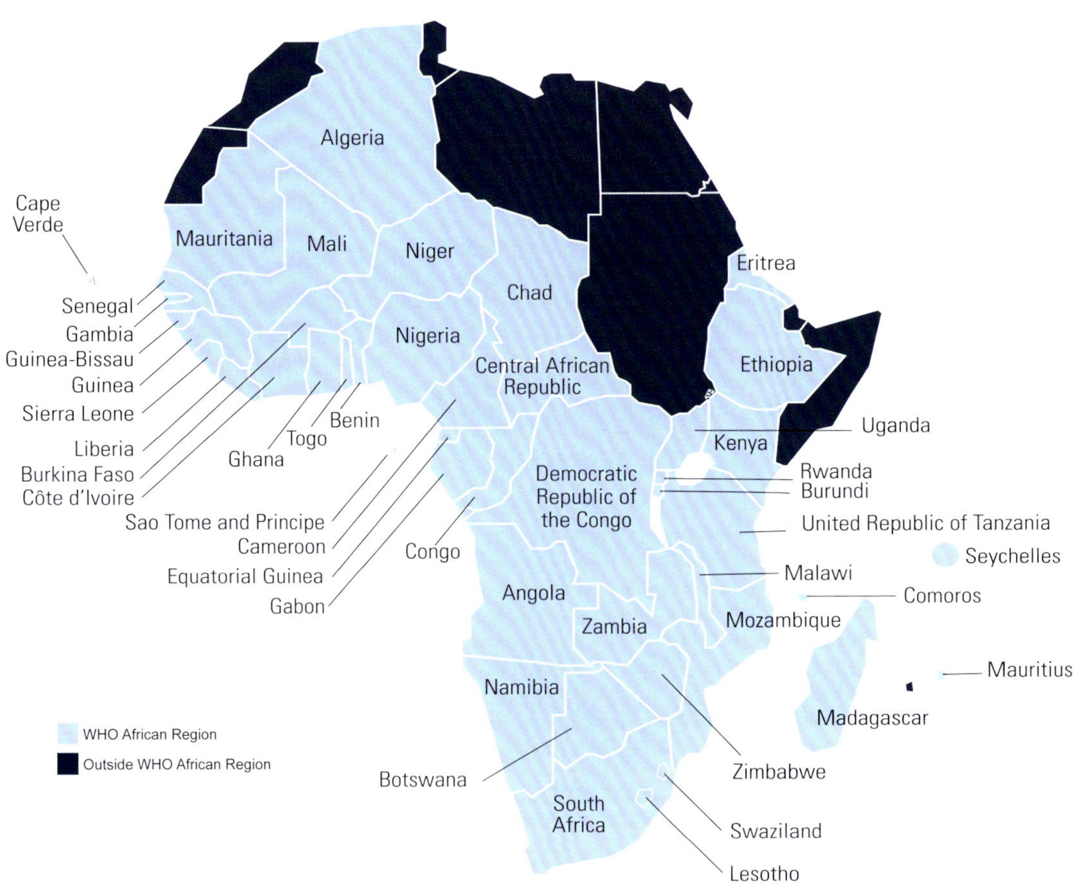


This report is about the 46 Member States of the African Region of the World Health Organization (WHO), as illustrated in this map. The African Regional Office of WHO is based in Brazzaville, the Republic of the Congo. When this report refers to "Africa", it is referring to the continent and islands as a whole. When the report refers to "the African Region" or "the Region", it is as defined by WHO.

It is important to note that the WHO African Region does not include all the countries on the African continent and the Region itself is not limited to all of sub-Saharan Africa.

Please note: the World Bank divides the continent into two regions: North Africa and sub-Saharan Africa, while UNICEF divides it into three regions: Eastern and South Africa, West and Central Africa, and the Middle East and North Africa.

# Introduction

These tables include some of the most recent statistics since 1997, based on health indicators from the African Region's 46 Member States. All of these tables have been selected from *World Health Statistics 2006*. In addition, historical data for some of these indicators have been reproduced from the *World health report 2006: Working together for health*. The statistical tables cover the following categories: mortality, morbidity, health service coverage, risk factors, health systems, inequities in health, and demographic and socioeconomic status.

*World Health Statistics 2006* includes an expanded set of statistics from all 192 WHO Member States, with a particular focus on equity between and within countries. It was collated from publications and databases of WHO's technical programmes and regional offices. The core set of indicators was selected on the basis of relevance for global health, availability and quality of data, and accuracy and comparability of estimates. The statistics for the indicators are based on an interactive process of data collection, compilation, quality assessment, and estimation between WHO technical programmes and its Member States. In this process, WHO strives to maximize accessibility, accuracy, comparability, and transparency of country health statistics.

In addition to national statistics, this publication presents statistics on the distribution of selected health outcomes and interventions within countries, disaggregated by gender, age, urban/rural setting, wealth/assets, and educational level. Such statistics are primarily derived from the analysis of household surveys and are only available for a limited number of countries. The number of countries reporting disaggregated data is expected to increase during the next few years.

The core indicators do not aim to capture all relevant aspects of health, but to provide a comprehensive summary of the current status of population health and health systems at country level: 1) mortality outcomes; 2) morbidity outcomes; 3) risk factors; 4) coverage of selected health interventions; 5) health systems; 6) inequalities in health; and 7) demographic and socioeconomic statistics.

All statistics have been cleared as WHO official figures in consultation with Member States, unless otherwise stated. The estimates published here should, however, still be regarded as the best estimates by WHO rather than the official view of Member States.

As demand for timely, reliable, and consistent information on key health statistics continues to increase, users need to be well informed on definitions, quality, and limitations of health statistics. More detailed information is available from the WHO Statistical Information System (WHOSIS) at: http://www.who.int/whosis.

| | Country | Population[a] | | | Total fertility rate[a] | Adolescent fertility proportion[b] | |
|---|---|---|---|---|---|---|---|
| | | number | annual growth rate | in urban areas | | | |
| | | (000) 2005 | (%) 1995–2004 | (%) 2005 | (per woman) 2004 | (%) | Year |
| 1 | Algeria | 32 854 | 1.4 | 60 | 2.5 | ... | |
| 2 | Angola | 15 941 | 2.3 | 37 | 6.7 | ... | |
| 3 | Benin | 8 439 | 2.8 | 46 | 5.7 | 9.3 | 1999 |
| 4 | Botswana | 1 765 | 0.9 | 53 | 3.1 | ... | |
| 5 | Burkina Faso | 13 228 | 2.7 | 19 | 6.6 | 10.1 | 2002 |
| 6 | Burundi | 7 548 | 1.7 | 11 | 6.8 | ... | |
| 7 | Cameroon | 16 322 | 1.9 | 53 | 4.5 | 13.9 | 2003 |
| 8 | Cape Verde | 507 | 2.1 | 58 | 3.6 | ... | |
| 9 | Central African Republic | 4 038 | 1.6 | 44 | 4.9 | ... | |
| 10 | Chad | 9 749 | 3.0 | 26 | 6.7 | 14.7 | 2003 |
| 11 | Comoros | 798 | 2.5 | 36 | 4.7 | ... | |
| 12 | Congo | 3 999 | 2.9 | 54 | 6.3 | ... | |
| 13 | Côte d'Ivoire | 18 154 | 1.9 | 46 | 4.9 | 12.3 | 1997 |
| 14 | Democratic Republic of the Congo | 57 549 | 2.2 | 33 | 6.7 | ... | |
| 15 | Equatorial Guinea | 504 | 2.1 | 50 | 5.9 | ... | |
| 16 | Eritrea | 4 401 | 3.2 | 21 | 5.4 | 8.1 | 2000 |
| 17 | Ethiopia | 77 431 | 2.3 | 16 | 5.7 | 9.4 | 1998 |
| 18 | Gabon | 1 384 | 2.0 | 85 | 3.9 | 16.9 | 1998 |
| 19 | Gambia | 1 517 | 2.9 | 26 | 4.6 | ... | |
| 20 | Ghana | 22 113 | 2.0 | 46 | 4.2 | 8.3 | 2002 |
| 21 | Guinea | 9 402 | 2.0 | 37 | 5.8 | 14.7 | 1997 |
| 22 | Guinea-Bissau | 1 586 | 2.6 | 36 | 7.1 | ... | |
| 23 | Kenya | 34 256 | 2.1 | 42 | 5.0 | 11.7 | 2002 |
| 24 | Lesotho | 1 795 | 0.6 | 18 | 3.5 | ... | |
| 25 | Liberia | 3 283 | 4.2 | 48 | 6.8 | ... | |
| 26 | Madagascar | 18 606 | 2.6 | 27 | 5.3 | 14.5 | 2002 |
| 27 | Malawi | 12 884 | 2.2 | 17 | 6.0 | 13.0 | 1998 |
| 28 | Mali | 13 518 | 2.6 | 34 | 6.8 | 13.7 | 2000 |
| 29 | Mauritania | 3 069 | 2.6 | 64 | 5.7 | 8.9 | 1999 |
| 30 | Mauritius | 1 245 | 0.9 | 44 | 2.0 | 9.6 | 2000 |
| 31 | Mozambique | 19 792 | 2.1 | 38 | 5.4 | 16.2 | 2002 |
| 32 | Namibia | 2 031 | 2.0 | 34 | 3.8 | 10.5 | 1999 |
| 33 | Niger | 13 957 | 3.1 | 23 | 7.8 | 14.5 | 1997 |
| 34 | Nigeria | 131 530 | 2.2 | 48 | 5.7 | 11.1 | 2002 |
| 35 | Rwanda | 9 038 | 5.0 | 22 | 5.6 | 4.6 | 1999 |
| 36 | Sao Tome and Principe | 157 | 1.8 | 38 | 3.9 | ... | |
| 37 | Senegal | 11 658 | 2.2 | 51 | 4.9 | ... | |
| 38 | Seychelles | 81 | 0.6 | 50 | 2.1 | ... | |
| 39 | Sierra Leone | 5 525 | 2.6 | 40 | 6.5 | ... | |
| 40 | South Africa | 47 432 | 1.2 | 58 | 2.8 | ... | |
| 41 | Swaziland | 1 032 | 0.8 | 24 | 3.8 | ... | |
| 42 | Togo | 6 145 | 2.9 | 36 | 5.2 | ... | |
| 43 | Uganda | 28 816 | 2.9 | 12 | 7.1 | 13.6 | 1999 |
| 44 | United Republic of Tanzania | 38 329 | 2.0 | 38 | 4.9 | 12.2 | 1998 |
| 45 | Zambia | 11 668 | 1.8 | 37 | 5.5 | 13.7 | 2000 |
| 46 | Zimbabwe | 13 010 | 0.9 | 36 | 3.4 | 13.3 | 1997 |
| | **Region** | | | | | | |
| | African Region | 738 083 | 2.2 | 38 | 5.3 | 11.7 | |

... Data not available or not applicable.

[a] World Population Prospects: The 2004 Revision. Population database. Population Division. Department of Economic and Social Affairs. United Nations Secretariat. (http://esa.un.org/unpp)

[b] Population Division. Department of Economic and Social Affairs. United Nations Secretariat.

[c] United Nations Educational, Scientific and Cultural Organization. (http://gmr.uis.unesco.org/selectindicators.aspx)

| Adult literacy rate[c] | Net primary school enrolment ratio[d] | | Gross national income per capita[e] | Population living below the poverty line[f] | |
|---|---|---|---|---|---|
| (%) 2000–2004 | Males (%) | Females (%) | (PPP Int.$) 2004 | (% with <$1 a day) | Year |
| | | 1998–2004 | | | |
| 69.8 | 96 | 94 | 6 260 | ... | |
| 66.8 | 66 | 57 | 2 030 | ... | |
| 33.6 | 69 | 47 | 1 120 | ... | |
| 78.9 | 79 | 83 | 8 920 | ... | |
| 12.8 | 42 | 31 | 1 220 | 44.9 | 1998 |
| 58.9 | 62 | 52 | 660 | 54.6 | 1998 |
| 67.9 | ... | ... | 2 090 | 17.1 | 2001 |
| 75.7 | 100 | 98 | 5 650 | ... | |
| 48.6 | ... | ... | 1 110 | ... | |
| 25.5 | 72 | 49 | 1 420 | ... | |
| 56.2 | 59 | 50 | 1 840 | ... | |
| 82.8 | 55 | 53 | 750 | ... | |
| 48.1 | 67 | 54 | 1 390 | 10.8 | 2002 |
| 65.3 | ... | ... | 680 | ... | |
| 84.2 | 91 | 78 | 7 400 | ... | |
| ... | 49 | 42 | 1 050 | ... | |
| 41.5 | 55 | 47 | 810 | 23.0 | 1999-00 |
| ... | 79 | 78 | 5 600 | ... | |
| ... | 79 | 78 | 1 900 | 59.3 | 1998 |
| 54.1 | 64 | 62 | 2 280 | 44.8 | 1998-99 |
| ... | 73 | 58 | 2 130 | ... | |
| ... | 53 | 37 | 690 | ... | |
| 73.6 | 66 | 66 | 1 050 | 22.8 | 1997 |
| 81.4 | 83 | 89 | 3 210 | ... | |
| 55.9 | 79 | 61 | ... | ... | |
| 70.6 | 78 | 79 | 830 | 61.0 | 2001 |
| 64.1 | ... | ... | 620 | 41.7 | 1997-98 |
| 19.0 | 50 | 39 | 980 | ... | |
| 51.2 | 68 | 67 | 2 050 | 25.9 | 2000 |
| 84.3 | 96 | 98 | 11 870 | ... | |
| 46.5 | 58 | 53 | 1 160 | ... | |
| 85.0 | 76 | 81 | 6 960 | ... | |
| 14.4 | 45 | 31 | 830 | ... | |
| 66.8 | 74 | 60 | 930 | 70.2 | 1997 |
| 64.0 | 85 | 88 | 1 300 | 51.7 | 1999-00 |
| ... | 100 | 94 | ... | ... | |
| 39.3 | 71 | 66 | 1 720 | ... | |
| 91.9 | 100 | 99 | 15 590 | ... | |
| 29.6 | ... | ... | 790 | ... | |
| 82.4 | 89 | 89 | 10 960 | 10.7 | 2000 |
| 79.2 | 75 | 75 | 4 970 | ... | |
| 53.0 | 99 | 83 | 1 690 | ... | |
| 68.9 | ... | ... | 1 520 | 84.9 | 1999 |
| 69.4 | 83 | 81 | 660 | ... | |
| 67.9 | 69 | 68 | 890 | 63.7 | 1998 |
| 90.0 | 79 | 80 | 2 180 | ... | |
| 60.1 | 70 | 63 | 2 074 | 44 | |


d  United Nations Educational, Scientific and Cultural Organization. (http://www.uis.unesco.org/ev.php?URL_ID=5187&URL_DO=DO_TOPIC&URL_SECTION=201)
e  The World Bank Group. (http://siteresources.worldbank.org/DATASTATISTICS/Resources/GNIPC.pdf)
f  The World Bank Group. (http://devdata.worldbank.org/wdi2005/Table2_5.htm)

*Health status: mortality*

| Country | Life expectancy at birth[a] (years) | | Healthy life expectancy (HALE) at birth[b] (years) | | Probability of dying per 1000 population between 15 and 60 years[a] (adult mortality rate) | | Probability of dying per 1000 live births under 5 years[a] (under-5 mortality rate) | Infant mortality rate[c] (per 1000 live births) | Neonatal mortality rate[d] (per 1000 live births) | Maternal mortality ratio[d] (per 100 000 live births) |
|---|---|---|---|---|---|---|---|---|---|---|
| | Males | Females | Males | Females | Males | Females | Both sexes | Both sexes | Both sexes | Females |
| | 2004 | 2004 | 2002 | 2002 | 2004 | 2004 | 2004 | 2004 | 2000 | 2000 |
| 1 Algeria | 69 | 72 | 60 | 62 | 153 | 124 | 40 | 35 | 20 | 140 |
| 2 Angola | 38 | 42 | 32 | 35 | 591 | 504 | 260 | 154 | 54 | 1 700 |
| 3 Benin | 52 | 53 | 43 | 45 | 388 | 350 | 152 | 90 | 38 | 850 |
| 4 Botswana | 40 | 40 | 36 | 35 | 786 | 770 | 116 | 75 | 40 | 100 |
| 5 Burkina Faso | 47 | 48 | 35 | 36 | 472 | 410 | 192 | 97 | 36 | 1 000 |
| 6 Burundi | 42 | 47 | 33 | 37 | 593 | 457 | 190 | 114 | 41 | 1 000 |
| 7 Cameroon | 50 | 51 | 41 | 42 | 444 | 432 | 149 | 87 | 40 | 730 |
| 8 Cape Verde | 67 | 71 | 59 | 63 | 209 | 139 | 36 | 27 | 10 | 150 |
| 9 Central African Republic | 40 | 41 | 37 | 38 | 667 | 624 | 193 | 115 | 48 | 1 100 |
| 10 Chad | 45 | 48 | 40 | 42 | 497 | 422 | 200 | 117 | 45 | 1 100 |
| 11 Comoros | 62 | 67 | 54 | 55 | 254 | 182 | 70 | 52 | 29 | 480 |
| 12 Congo | 53 | 55 | 45 | 47 | 442 | 390 | 108 | 79 | 32 | 510 |
| 13 Côte d'Ivoire | 41 | 47 | 38 | 41 | 585 | 500 | 194 | 118 | 65 | 690 |
| 14 Democratic Republic of the Congo | 42 | 47 | 35 | 39 | 576 | 446 | 205 | 129 | 47 | 990 |
| 15 Equatorial Guinea | 42 | 44 | 45 | 46 | 577 | 522 | 204 | 123 | 40 | 880 |
| 16 Eritrea | 58 | 62 | 49 | 51 | 345 | 281 | 82 | 52 | 25 | 630 |
| 17 Ethiopia | 49 | 51 | 41 | 42 | 451 | 389 | 166 | 110 | 51 | 850 |
| 18 Gabon | 55 | 59 | 50 | 53 | 411 | 344 | 91 | 59 | 31 | 420 |
| 19 Gambia | 55 | 59 | 48 | 51 | 344 | 263 | 122 | 89 | 46 | 540 |
| 20 Ghana | 56 | 58 | 49 | 50 | 349 | 319 | 112 | 68 | 27 | 540 |
| 21 Guinea | 52 | 55 | 44 | 46 | 364 | 319 | 155 | 101 | 48 | 740 |
| 22 Guinea-Bissau | 45 | 48 | 40 | 41 | 482 | 413 | 203 | 126 | 48 | 1 100 |
| 23 Kenya | 51 | 50 | 44 | 45 | 477 | 502 | 120 | 78 | 29 | 1 000 |
| 24 Lesotho | 39 | 44 | 30 | 33 | 845 | 728 | 82 | 55 | 28 | 550 |
| 25 Liberia | 39 | 44 | 34 | 37 | 596 | 477 | 235 | 157 | 66 | 760 |
| 26 Madagascar | 55 | 59 | 47 | 50 | 338 | 270 | 123 | 76 | 33 | 550 |
| 27 Malawi | 41 | 41 | 35 | 35 | 663 | 638 | 175 | 109 | 40 | 1 800 |
| 28 Mali | 44 | 47 | 37 | 38 | 490 | 414 | 219 | 121 | 55 | 1 200 |
| 29 Mauritania | 55 | 60 | 43 | 46 | 325 | 246 | 125 | 78 | 70 | 1 000 |
| 30 Mauritius | 69 | 75 | 60 | 65 | 217 | 112 | 15 | 12 | 12 | 24 |
| 31 Mozambique | 44 | 46 | 36 | 38 | 627 | 549 | 152 | 102 | 48 | 1 000 |
| 32 Namibia | 52 | 55 | 43 | 44 | 548 | 489 | 63 | 42 | 25 | 300 |
| 33 Niger | 42 | 41 | 36 | 35 | 506 | 478 | 259 | 152 | 43 | 1 600 |
| 34 Nigeria | 45 | 46 | 41 | 42 | 513 | 478 | 197 | 103 | 53 | 800 |
| 35 Rwanda | 44 | 47 | 36 | 40 | 518 | 435 | 203 | 118 | 45 | 1 400 |
| 36 Sao Tome and Principe | 57 | 60 | 54 | 55 | 301 | 236 | 118 | 75 | 38 | ... |
| 37 Senegal | 54 | 57 | 47 | 49 | 358 | 288 | 137 | 78 | 31 | 690 |
| 38 Seychelles | 67 | 78 | 57 | 65 | 232 | 83 | 14 | 12 | 9 | ... |
| 39 Sierra Leone | 37 | 40 | 27 | 30 | 579 | 497 | 283 | 165 | 56 | 2 000 |
| 40 South Africa | 47 | 49 | 43 | 45 | 667 | 598 | 67 | 54 | 21 | 230 |
| 41 Swaziland | 36 | 39 | 33 | 35 | 823 | 741 | 156 | 102 | 38 | 370 |
| 42 Togo | 52 | 56 | 44 | 46 | 401 | 327 | 140 | 79 | 40 | 570 |
| 43 Uganda | 48 | 51 | 42 | 44 | 525 | 446 | 138 | 81 | 32 | 880 |
| 44 United Republic of Tanzania | 47 | 49 | 40 | 41 | 551 | 524 | 126 | 78 | 43 | 1 500 |
| 45 Zambia | 40 | 40 | 35 | 35 | 683 | 656 | 182 | 104 | 40 | 750 |
| 46 Zimbabwe | 37 | 34 | 34 | 33 | 857 | 849 | 129 | 78 | 33 | 1 100 |
| **Region** | | | | | | | | | | |
| African Region | 47 | 49 | 40 | 42 | 519 | 465 | 167 | 100 | 43 | 910 |

... Data not available or not applicable.

[a] *World health report 2006: working together for health.* Geneva, World Health Organization, 2006. (http://www.who.int/whr/2006/annex/en)

[b] *World health report 2004: changing history.* Geneva, World Health Organization, 2004. (http://www.who.int/whr/2004/en/index.html)

[c] (i) WHO Mortality Database. World Health Organization. (http://www.who.int/healthinfo/morttables/en/index.html);
(ii) United Nations Children's Fund. State of the World's Children 2006. New York: United Nations Children's Fund, 2005.

[d] *World health report 2005: make every mother and child count.* Geneva, World Health Organization, 2005. (http://www.who.int/whr/2005/en/index.html)

[e] *UNAIDS 2004 report on global HIV/AIDS epidemic: 4th global report.* Geneva, Joint United Nations Programme on HIV/AIDS 2004.
(http://www.unaids.org/bangkok2004/GAR2004_pdf/UNAIDSGlobalReport2004_en.pdf)

[f] These are classified as deaths from tuberculosis (A15-A19, B90) according to the ICD-10. Source: *Global tuberculosis control: surveillance, planning, financing. WHO report 2006.* Geneva, World Health Organization (WHO/HTM/TB/2006.362). (http://www.who.int/tb/publications/global_report)

| Cause-specific mortality rate (per 100 000 population) | | | Age-standardized mortality rate by cause[h,i] (per 100 000 population) | | | | Years of life lost by broader causes[h,j] (%) | | | Causes of death among children under 5 years of age[j,l] (%) | | | | | | | |
| HIV/AIDS[e] | TB among HIV-negative people[f] | TB among HIV-positive people[g] | Non-communicable diseases | Cardiovascular diseases | Cancer | Injuries | Communicable diseases[k] | Non-communicable diseases | Injuries | Neonatal causes | HIV/AIDS | Diarrhoeal diseases | Measles | Malaria | Pneumonia | Injuries | Other |
| Both sexes | | | Both sexes | | | | Both sexes | | | Both sexes | | | | | | | |
| 2003 | 2004 | 2004 | 2002 | 2002 | 2002 | 2002 | 2002 | 2002 | 2002 | 2000 | 2000 | 2000 | 2000 | 2000 | 2000 | 2000 | 2000 |
|---|---|---|---|---|---|---|---|---|---|---|---|---|---|---|---|---|---|
| <10 | 2 | <1 | 598 | 314 | 103 | 85 | 50 | 30 | 20 | 48.0 | 0.0 | 11.9 | 0.9 | 0.5 | 13.7 | 5.0 | 20.0 |
| 140 | 25 | 7 | 982 | 486 | 179 | 231 | 84 | 8 | 8 | 22.2 | 2.2 | 19.1 | 4.8 | 8.3 | 24.8 | 1.4 | 17.2 |
| 73 | 14 | 2 | 852 | 432 | 154 | 116 | 82 | 10 | 8 | 25.0 | 2.2 | 17.1 | 5.3 | 27.2 | 21.1 | 2.1 | 0.0 |
| 1 863 | 37 | 58 | 653 | 338 | 124 | 72 | 93 | 4 | 3 | 40.3 | 53.8 | 1.1 | 0.1 | 0.0 | 1.4 | 3.3 | 0.0 |
| 234 | 38 | 16 | 901 | 459 | 162 | 149 | 87 | 7 | 7 | 18.3 | 4.0 | 18.8 | 3.4 | 20.3 | 23.3 | 1.5 | 10.4 |
| 355 | 59 | 33 | 843 | 439 | 146 | 301 | 81 | 7 | 12 | 23.3 | 8.0 | 18.2 | 3.0 | 8.4 | 22.8 | 1.8 | 14.6 |
| 311 | 19 | 12 | 848 | 436 | 150 | 118 | 81 | 11 | 8 | 24.8 | 7.2 | 17.3 | 4.1 | 22.8 | 21.5 | 2.2 | 0.0 |
| ... | 35 | 1 | 692 | 356 | 127 | 39 | 51 | 37 | 12 | 25.9 | 3.7 | 12.2 | 4.4 | 4.3 | 13.3 | 3.5 | 32.6 |
| 584 | 55 | 58 | 863 | 445 | 154 | 146 | 84 | 9 | 7 | 27.2 | 12.4 | 14.7 | 6.5 | 18.5 | 18.7 | 2.0 | 0.0 |
| 197 | 60 | 22 | 869 | 443 | 156 | 131 | 85 | 8 | 7 | 24.0 | 4.1 | 18.1 | 7.0 | 22.3 | 22.8 | 1.8 | 0.1 |
| ... | 7 | <1 | 736 | 381 | 128 | 83 | 70 | 18 | 12 | 37.3 | 3.7 | 13.6 | 5.9 | 19.4 | 16.3 | 3.4 | 0.5 |
| 257 | 52 | 18 | 762 | 393 | 134 | 147 | 79 | 11 | 11 | 30.9 | 9.3 | 11.2 | 6.6 | 25.7 | 13.6 | 2.6 | 0.0 |
| 267 | 67 | 37 | 873 | 436 | 160 | 179 | 78 | 11 | 10 | 34.9 | 5.6 | 14.8 | 2.5 | 20.5 | 19.6 | 2.2 | 0.0 |
| 184 | 57 | 21 | 909 | 465 | 161 | 273 | 82 | 7 | 11 | 25.7 | 3.7 | 18.1 | 4.7 | 16.9 | 23.1 | 1.6 | 6.3 |
| ... | 30 | 27 | 864 | 438 | 155 | 144 | 79 | 12 | 9 | 27.5 | 7.4 | 13.6 | 7.4 | 24.0 | 17.3 | 2.5 | 0.3 |
| 155 | 52 | 9 | 762 | 398 | 133 | 92 | 81 | 11 | 8 | 27.4 | 6.2 | 15.6 | 2.5 | 13.6 | 18.6 | 3.0 | 13.0 |
| 163 | 60 | 19 | 859 | 435 | 147 | 104 | 82 | 12 | 6 | 30.2 | 3.8 | 17.3 | 4.2 | 6.1 | 22.3 | 1.7 | 14.3 |
| 224 | 33 | 22 | 813 | 410 | 158 | 103 | 72 | 18 | 9 | 35.1 | 10.1 | 8.8 | 4.4 | 28.3 | 10.7 | 2.5 | 0.0 |
| 42 | 38 | 2 | 805 | 413 | 144 | 109 | 75 | 15 | 10 | 36.6 | 1.3 | 12.2 | 2.5 | 29.4 | 15.5 | 2.6 | 0.0 |
| 141 | 40 | 10 | 786 | 404 | 138 | 97 | 74 | 16 | 10 | 28.5 | 5.7 | 12.2 | 2.9 | 33.0 | 14.6 | 3.0 | 0.0 |
| 100 | 44 | 12 | 853 | 432 | 156 | 147 | 80 | 11 | 9 | 28.8 | 2.3 | 16.5 | 5.5 | 24.5 | 20.9 | 1.4 | 0.0 |
| ... | 33 | 9 | 883 | 449 | 159 | 138 | 86 | 8 | 6 | 24.1 | 2.6 | 18.6 | 3.4 | 21.0 | 23.4 | 1.4 | 5.5 |
| 458 | 90 | 43 | 782 | 401 | 139 | 95 | 81 | 11 | 8 | 24.2 | 14.6 | 16.5 | 3.2 | 13.6 | 19.9 | 2.7 | 5.3 |
| 1 611 | 41 | 58 | 785 | 404 | 139 | 88 | 90 | 7 | 3 | 32.8 | 56.2 | 3.9 | 0.1 | 0.0 | 4.7 | 2.2 | 0.0 |
| 223 | 46 | 27 | 955 | 485 | 169 | 270 | 83 | 7 | 10 | 29.1 | 3.6 | 17.3 | 6.0 | 18.9 | 23.0 | 1.7 | 0.3 |
| 43 | 37 | 6 | 837 | 430 | 147 | 112 | 79 | 12 | 9 | 25.6 | 1.3 | 16.9 | 5.0 | 20.1 | 20.7 | 2.4 | 8.0 |
| 681 | 48 | 49 | 835 | 430 | 150 | 105 | 89 | 6 | 5 | 21.7 | 14.0 | 18.1 | 0.3 | 14.1 | 22.6 | 1.7 | 7.6 |
| 94 | 62 | 11 | 909 | 456 | 166 | 145 | 86 | 8 | 6 | 25.9 | 1.6 | 18.3 | 6.1 | 16.9 | 23.9 | 1.4 | 5.9 |
| 17 | 57 | 3 | 884 | 451 | 158 | 138 | 79 | 12 | 9 | 39.4 | 0.3 | 16.2 | 1.7 | 12.2 | 22.3 | 1.9 | 5.9 |
| ... | 11 | <1 | 701 | 434 | 79 | 42 | 11 | 75 | 13 | 66.0 | 0.0 | 1.2 | 0.0 | 0.0 | 3.9 | 5.2 | 23.6 |
| 577 | 62 | 67 | 720 | 371 | 124 | 66 | 91 | 7 | 2 | 29.0 | 12.9 | 16.5 | 0.3 | 18.9 | 21.2 | 1.0 | 0.1 |
| 806 | 44 | 41 | 754 | 385 | 146 | 93 | 83 | 10 | 6 | 38.5 | 53.0 | 2.5 | 0.1 | 0.0 | 3.0 | 3.0 | 0.0 |
| 37 | 31 | 3 | 916 | 456 | 169 | 163 | 87 | 7 | 6 | 16.7 | 0.6 | 19.8 | 7.3 | 14.3 | 25.1 | 1.4 | 14.8 |
| 246 | 56 | 27 | 889 | 452 | 157 | 132 | 83 | 10 | 7 | 26.1 | 5.0 | 15.7 | 6.3 | 24.1 | 20.1 | 1.9 | 0.8 |
| 251 | 69 | 33 | 831 | 425 | 150 | 126 | 85 | 8 | 7 | 21.7 | 5.0 | 18.5 | 1.6 | 4.6 | 23.2 | 1.8 | 23.7 |
| ... | 28 | <1 | 764 | 396 | 133 | 87 | 67 | 21 | 12 | 32.1 | 3.7 | 16.0 | 4.8 | 0.6 | 21.2 | 3.5 | 18.1 |
| 31 | 49 | 3 | 832 | 426 | 146 | 125 | 76 | 13 | 11 | 22.8 | 1.0 | 17.1 | 8.1 | 27.6 | 20.7 | 2.6 | 0.2 |
| ... | 6 | <1 | 657 | 336 | 131 | 69 | 16 | 64 | 21 | 27.2 | 0.0 | 0.0 | 0.0 | 0.0 | 10.1 | 12.3 | 50.3 |
| ... | 92 | 13 | 1 017 | 515 | 181 | 250 | 86 | 6 | 8 | 21.9 | 1.3 | 19.7 | 5.3 | 12.4 | 25.5 | 1.2 | 12.7 |
| 789 | 56 | 78 | 808 | 410 | 154 | 120 | 77 | 15 | 8 | 35.1 | 57.1 | 0.8 | 0.0 | 0.0 | 0.9 | 5.0 | 1.1 |
| 1 643 | 93 | 176 | 732 | 364 | 162 | 72 | 91 | 5 | 4 | 26.8 | 47.0 | 9.6 | 0.2 | 0.2 | 11.8 | 3.8 | 0.5 |
| 171 | 77 | 21 | 831 | 427 | 147 | 117 | 79 | 12 | 9 | 29.0 | 5.8 | 13.8 | 6.6 | 25.3 | 17.1 | 2.5 | 0.0 |
| 290 | 71 | 22 | 824 | 422 | 146 | 154 | 84 | 8 | 8 | 23.6 | 7.7 | 17.2 | 3.0 | 23.1 | 21.1 | 2.2 | 2.1 |
| 433 | 47 | 31 | 847 | 435 | 151 | 115 | 85 | 8 | 6 | 26.9 | 9.3 | 16.8 | 1.3 | 22.7 | 21.1 | 2.0 | 0.0 |
| 788 | 70 | 68 | 700 | 359 | 122 | 58 | 92 | 6 | 2 | 22.9 | 16.1 | 17.5 | 1.2 | 19.4 | 21.8 | 1.0 | 0.1 |
| 1 322 | 62 | 89 | 685 | 347 | 122 | 103 | 90 | 7 | 4 | 28.1 | 40.6 | 12.1 | 2.9 | 0.2 | 14.7 | 1.2 | 0.3 |
| 313 | 53 | 28 | 800 | 404 | 144 | 133 | 59 | 10 | 8 | 26.2 | 6.8 | 16.6 | 4.3 | 17.5 | 21.1 | 1.9 | 5.6 |


g These deaths are classified under "HIV disease resulting in tuberculosis (B20.0)" according to the ICD-10. They are already counted in the number of deaths from HIV/AIDS (B20-B24). Source: *Global tuberculosis control: surveillance, planning, financing. WHO report 2006*. Geneva, World Health Organization (WHO/HTM/TB/2006.362). (http://www.who.int/tb/publications/global_report)

h Mortality and burden of disease estimates for WHO Member States in 2002. World Health Organization, December 2004. (http://www.who.int/entity/healthinfo/statistics/bodgbddeathdalyestimates.xls)

i Rates are age-standardized to the WHO world standard population. Source: Ahmad OB, Boschi-Pinto C, Lopez AD, Murray CJL, Lozano R, Inoue M. Age standardization of rates: a new WHO standard. GPE Discussion Paper Series: No.31. EIP/GPE/EBD. World Health Organization. 2001. (http://www3.who.int/whosis/discussion_papers)

j Sum of individual proportions may not add up to 100% due to rounding.

k "Communicable diseases" include maternal causes, conditions arising in the perinatal period and nutritional deficiencies.

l Neonatal causes include diarrhoea during the neonatal period. Sources: (i) Bryce J, Boschi-Pinto C, Shibuya K, Black RE; WHO Child Health Epidemiology Reference Group. WHO estimates of the causes of death in children. *Lancet*, 2005;365:1147-52; (ii) WHO mortality profiles. (http://www.who.int/whostatistics/mortality)

| Country | HIV prevalence among adults[a] (15-49) (%) | TB prevalence[b] (per 100 000 population) | TB incidence[b] (per 100 000 population) | Number of confirmed polio cases[c] |
|---|---|---|---|---|
| | Both sexes 2003 | Both sexes 2004 | Both sexes 2004 | Both sexes 2005 |
| 1 Algeria | 0.1 | 54 | 54 | 0 |
| 2 Angola | 3.9 | 310 | 259 | 10 |
| 3 Benin | 1.9 | 142 | 87 | 0 |
| 4 Botswana | 37.3 | 553 | 670 | 0 |
| 5 Burkina Faso | 4.2 | 365 | 191 | 0 |
| 6 Burundi | 6 | 564 | 343 | 0 |
| 7 Cameroon | 6.9 | 227 | 179 | 1 |
| 8 Cape Verde | ... | 314 | 172 | 0 |
| 9 Central African Republic | 13.5 | 549 | 322 | 0 |
| 10 Chad | 4.8 | 566 | 279 | 2 |
| 11 Comoros | ... | 95 | 46 | 0 |
| 12 Congo | 4.9 | 464 | 377 | 0 |
| 13 Côte d'Ivoire | 7 | 651 | 393 | 0 |
| 14 Democratic Republic of the Congo | 4.2 | 551 | 366 | 0 |
| 15 Equatorial Guinea | ... | 322 | 239 | 0 |
| 16 Eritrea | 2.7 | 437 | 271 | 1 |
| 17 Ethiopia | 4.4 | 533 | 353 | 22 |
| 18 Gabon | 8.1 | 339 | 280 | 0 |
| 19 Gambia | 1.2 | 329 | 233 | 0 |
| 20 Ghana | 3.1 | 376 | 206 | 0 |
| 21 Guinea | 3.2 | 410 | 240 | 0 |
| 22 Guinea-Bissau | ... | 306 | 199 | 0 |
| 23 Kenya | 6.7 | 888 | 619 | 0 |
| 24 Lesotho | 28.9 | 544 | 696 | 0 |
| 25 Liberia | 5.9 | 447 | 310 | 0 |

... Data not available or not applicable.

[a] *UNAIDS 2004 report on global HIV/AIDS epidemic: 4th global report.* Geneva, Joint United Nations Programme on HIV/AIDS 2004. (http://www.unaids.org/bangkok2004/GAR2004_pdf/UNAIDSGlobalReport2004_en.pdf)

[b] All forms of TB, including TB in people with HIV infection. Source: Global tuberculosis control: surveillance, planning, financing. WHO report 2006. Geneva, World Health Organization (WHO/HTM/TB/2006.362). (http://www.who.int/tb/publications/global_report)

[c] World Health Organization, Polio Eradication Initiative. Data as of 25 April 2006. (http://www.who.int/immunization_monitoring/en/diseases/poliomyelitis/case_count.cfm)

| | Country | HIV prevalence among adults[a] (15-49) (%) | TB prevalence[b] (per 100 000 population) | TB incidence[b] (per 100 000 population) | Number of confirmed polio cases[c] |
|---|---|---|---|---|---|
| | | Both sexes 2003 | Both sexes 2004 | Both sexes 2004 | Both sexes 2005 |
| 26 | Madagascar | 1.7 | 351 | 218 | 4 |
| 27 | Malawi | 14.2 | 501 | 413 | 0 |
| 28 | Mali | 1.9 | 578 | 281 | 3 |
| 29 | Mauritania | 0.6 | 502 | 287 | 0 |
| 30 | Mauritius | ... | 135 | 64 | 0 |
| 31 | Mozambique | 12.2 | 635 | 460 | 0 |
| 32 | Namibia | 21.3 | 586 | 717 | 0 |
| 33 | Niger | 1.2 | 288 | 157 | 10 |
| 34 | Nigeria | 5.4 | 531 | 290 | 801 |
| 35 | Rwanda | 5.1 | 660 | 371 | 0 |
| 36 | Sao Tome and Principe | ... | 253 | 107 | 0 |
| 37 | Senegal | 0.8 | 451 | 245 | 0 |
| 38 | Seychelles | ... | 83 | 34 | 0 |
| 39 | Sierra Leone | ... | 847 | 443 | 0 |
| 40 | South Africa | 21.5 | 670 | 718 | 0 |
| 41 | Swaziland | 38.8 | 1120 | 1226 | 0 |
| 42 | Togo | 4.1 | 718 | 355 | 0 |
| 43 | Uganda | 4.1 | 646 | 402 | 0 |
| 44 | United Republic of Tanzania | 8.8 | 479 | 347 | 0 |
| 45 | Zambia | 16.5 | 707 | 680 | 0 |
| 46 | Zimbabwe | 24.6 | 673 | 674 | 0 |
| | * Imported cases of malaria | (update 2004) | | | |
| | | 7.1 | 518 | 356 | 854 |

| Country | Year | Probability of dying per 1000 live births under 5 years[a] (under-5 mortality rate) | | | | | | | | | Children under 5 years stunted for age[a] (%) | | | | | |
| | | Place of residence | | | Wealth quintile | | | Educational level of mother[b] | | | Place of residence | | | Wealth quintile | | |
| | | Rural | Urban | Rural–urban ratio | Lowest | Highest | Lowest–highest ratio | Lowest | Highest | Lowest–highest ratio | Rural | Urban | Rural–urban ratio | Lowest | Highest | Lowest–highest ratio |
|---|---|---|---|---|---|---|---|---|---|---|---|---|---|---|---|---|
| 1 Benin | 2001 | 175.5 | 133.6 | 1.3 | 198.2 | 93.1 | 2.1 | 174.5 | 80.8 | 2.2 | 33.4 | 24.2 | 1.4 | 35.4 | 18.2 | 1.9 |
| 2 Botswana | 1988 | 55.2 | 55.3 | 1.0 | ... | ... | ... | 62.0 | 46.3 | 1.3 | ... | ... | ... | ... | ... | ... |
| 3 Burkina Faso | 2003 | 201.5 | 136.4 | 1.5 | 206.0 | 144.0 | 1.4 | 198.4 | 108.0 | 1.8 | 41.4 | 19.8 | 2.1 | 45.7 | 20.6 | 2.2 |
| 4 Burundi | 1987 | 184.2 | 163.7 | 1.1 | ... | ... | ... | 191.2 | 80.7 | 2.4 | 48.6 | 27.1 | 1.8 | ... | ... | ... |
| 5 Cameroon | 2004 | 168.8 | 119.3 | 1.4 | 189.0 | 88.0 | 2.1 | 185.7 | 93.3 | 2.0 | 38.2 | 23.1 | 1.7 | 40.9 | 12.3 | 3.3 |
| 6 Central African Republic | 1994-95 | 178.4 | 128.6 | 1.4 | 192.9 | 98.3 | 2.0 | 175.2 | 83.1 | 2.1 | 37.2 | 28.6 | 1.3 | 42.3 | 25.0 | 1.7 |
| 7 Chad | 2004 | 208.0 | 179.0 | 1.2 | 176.0 | 187.0 | 0.9 | 200.0 | 143.0 | 1.4 | 43.0 | 32.3 | 1.3 | 50.7 | 31.7 | 1.6 |
| 8 Comoros | 1996 | 122.6 | 80.7 | 1.5 | 128.9 | 86.6 | 1.5 | 120.6 | 74.5 | 1.6 | 35.0 | 29.9 | 1.2 | 44.8 | 23.3 | 1.9 |
| 9 Côte d'Ivoire | 1998-99 | 196.8 | 125.2 | 1.6 | ... | ... | ... | 192.7 | 79.4 | 2.4 | 28.6 | 18.3 | 1.6 | ... | ... | ... |
| 10 Eritrea | 2002 | 117.1 | 86.1 | 1.4 | 100.0 | 65.0 | 1.5 | 120.6 | 58.5 | 2.1 | 42.6 | 27.8 | 1.5 | 44.8 | 17.6 | 2.5 |
| 11 Ethiopia | 2000 | 192.5 | 148.6 | 1.3 | 159.2 | 147.1 | 1.1 | 197.4 | 89.2 | 2.2 | 52.3 | 41.6 | 1.3 | 52.9 | 43.2 | 1.2 |
| 12 Gabon | 2000 | 99.9 | 88.4 | 1.1 | 93.1 | 55.4 | 1.7 | 112.0 | 87.1 | 1.3 | 29.0 | 17.4 | 1.7 | 32.8 | 11.5 | 2.9 |
| 13 Ghana | 2003 | 118.3 | 92.7 | 1.3 | 128.0 | 88.0 | 1.5 | 124.9 | 84.5 | 1.5 | 34.0 | 19.9 | 1.7 | 41.8 | 13.2 | 3.2 |
| 14 Guinea | 1999 | 210.6 | 148.7 | 1.4 | 229.9 | 133.0 | 1.7 | 203.8 | 104.2 | 2.0 | 29.4 | 18.2 | 1.6 | 32.4 | 15.7 | 2.1 |
| 15 Kenya | 2003 | 116.9 | 93.5 | 1.3 | 149.0 | 91.0 | 1.6 | 126.5 | 62.9 | 2.0 | 32.0 | 23.8 | 1.3 | 38.1 | 19.2 | 2.0 |
| 16 Liberia | 1986 | 239.7 | 217.8 | 1.1 | ... | ... | ... | 242.1 | 176.1 | 1.4 | ... | ... | ... | ... | ... | ... |
| 17 Madagascar | 2003-04 | 120.0 | 73.3 | 1.6 | 141.8 | 49.4 | 2.9 | 148.6 | 65.4 | 2.3 | 48.9 | 40.9 | 1.2 | 50.5 | 38.2 | 1.3 |
| 18 Malawi | 2000 | 210.3 | 147.9 | 1.4 | 230.8 | 149.0 | 1.5 | 214.5 | 118.0 | 1.8 | 51.3 | 34.2 | 1.5 | 57.8 | 33.5 | 1.7 |
| 19 Mali | 2001 | 253.2 | 184.6 | 1.4 | 247.8 | 148.1 | 1.7 | 246.9 | 89.6 | 2.8 | 42.1 | 23.2 | 1.8 | 44.8 | 19.7 | 2.3 |
| 20 Mauritania | 2000-01 | 96.2 | 110.7 | 0.9 | 98.1 | 78.5 | 1.2 | 110.5 | 85.5 | 1.3 | 37.9 | 30.2 | 1.3 | 38.7 | 23.4 | 1.7 |
| 21 Mozambique | 2003 | 192.0 | 143.2 | 1.3 | 196.0 | 108.0 | 1.8 | 200.5 | 85.7 | 2.3 | 45.7 | 28.5 | 1.6 | 49.3 | 20.0 | 2.5 |
| 22 Namibia | 2000 | 66.1 | 49.5 | 1.3 | 55.4 | 31.4 | 1.8 | 83.6 | 47.1 | 1.8 | 23.0 | 21.7 | 1.1 | 26.7 | 15.3 | 1.7 |
| 23 Niger | 1998 | 327.4 | 178.1 | 1.8 | 281.8 | 183.7 | 1.5 | 314.0 | 129.6 | 2.4 | 43.0 | 31.2 | 1.4 | 41.9 | 32.3 | 1.3 |
| 24 Nigeria | 2003 | 242.7 | 152.9 | 1.6 | 257.0 | 79.0 | 3.3 | 269.4 | 107.2 | 2.5 | 42.9 | 28.9 | 1.5 | 48.8 | 17.9 | 2.7 |
| 25 Rwanda | 2000 | 216.2 | 141.3 | 1.5 | 246.4 | 154.1 | 1.6 | 232.7 | 116.7 | 2.0 | 44.9 | 27.8 | 1.6 | 49.4 | 26.9 | 1.8 |
| 26 Senegal | 1999 | 171.2 | 92.1 | 1.9 | ... | ... | ... | 159.9 | 80.1 | 2.0 | ... | ... | ... | ... | ... | ... |
| 27 South Africa | 1998 | 71.2 | 43.2 | 1.6 | 87.4 | 21.9 | 4.0 | 83.8 | 45.6 | 1.8 | ... | ... | ... | ... | ... | ... |
| 28 Sudan | 1990 | 144.0 | 117.0 | 1.2 | ... | ... | ... | 151.9 | 84.3 | 1.8 | ... | ... | ... | ... | ... | ... |
| 29 Togo | 1998 | 157.4 | 101.3 | 1.6 | 167.7 | 97.0 | 1.7 | 159.1 | 82.5 | 1.9 | 23.9 | 14.8 | 1.6 | 29.0 | 11.0 | 2.6 |
| 30 Uganda | 2000-01 | 163.8 | 100.5 | 1.6 | 191.8 | 106.4 | 1.8 | 186.9 | 93.0 | 2.0 | 39.9 | 26.5 | 1.5 | 43.3 | 25.1 | 1.7 |
| 31 United Republic of Tanzania | 1999 | 165.9 | 141.6 | 1.2 | 160.0 | 135.2 | 1.2 | 165.4 | 62.6 | 2.6 | 46.5 | 24.5 | 1.9 | 49.5 | 23.4 | 2.1 |
| 32 Zambia | 2001-02 | 182.3 | 140.0 | 1.3 | 191.7 | 92.4 | 2.1 | 197.8 | 121.1 | 1.6 | 51.1 | 37.1 | 1.4 | 54.1 | 31.6 | 1.7 |
| 33 Zimbabwe | 1999 | 99.7 | 69.0 | 1.4 | 99.5 | 62.2 | 1.6 | 118.8 | 78.7 | 1.5 | 29.2 | 20.6 | 1.4 | 32.7 | 18.6 | 1.8 |

Statistics by gender are presented elsewhere in this report.

... Data not available or not applicable.

[a] Source: Demographic and Health Surveys. (http://www.measuredhs.com)

[b] Lowest and highest mother's educational levels are "no education" and "secondary or higher", respectively.

[c] Data correspond to births in 3 years preceding survey, not 5 years.

| Births attended by skilled health personnel[a] (%) | | | | | | | | | | | | Measles immunization coverage among 1-year-olds[a] (%) | | | | | | | | |
| Educational level of mother[b] | | | Place of residence | | | Wealth quintile | | | Educational level of mother[b] | | | Place of residence | | | Wealth quintile | | | Educational level of mother[b] | | |
| Lowest | Highest | Lowest–highest ratio | Rural | Urban | Urban–rural ratio | Highest | Lowest | Highest-lowest ratio | Lowest | Highest | Highest-lowest ratio | Urban | Rural | Urban–rural ratio | Highest | Lowest | Highest-lowest ratio | Highest | Lowest | Highest-lowest ratio |
|---|---|---|---|---|---|---|---|---|---|---|---|---|---|---|---|---|---|---|---|---|
| 33.0 | 17.1 | 1.9 | 68.4 | 82.9 | 1.2 | 99.3 | 49.6 | 2.0 | 67.6 | 98.6 | 1.5 | 75.3 | 64.1 | 1.2 | 83.1 | 56.9 | 1.5 | 88.6 | 63.4 | 1.4 |
| ... | ... | ... | 71.7 | 93.5 | 1.3 | ... | ... | ... | 53.6 | 96.6 | 1.8 | 65.4 | 69.9 | 0.9 | ... | ... | ... | 63.0 | 67.8 | 0.9 |
| 40.8 | 12.4 | 3.3 | 30.5 | 87.7 | 2.9 | 90.8 | 38.8 | 2.3 | 32.7 | 94.7 | 2.9 | 73.1 | 53.3 | 1.4 | 71.3 | 48.3 | 1.5 | 80.4 | 54.3 | 1.5 |
| 49.0 | 24.6 | 2.0 | 16.8 | 85.2 | 5.1 | ... | ... | ... | 15.6 | 75.7 | 4.9 | 51.1 | 47.8 | 1.1 | ... | ... | ... | 56.3 | 45.2 | 1.2 |
| 40.1 | 21.0 | 1.9 | 44.2 | 84.2 | 1.9 | 94.5 | 29.3 | 3.2 | 22.9 | 91.7 | 4.0 | 72.5 | 58.3 | 1.2 | 83.2 | 52.1 | 1.6 | 79.3 | 46.1 | 1.7 |
| 37.2 | 24.1 | 1.5c | 23.7 | 77.7 | 3.3 | 81.7 | 14.3 | 5.7 | 29.4 | 84.8 | 2.9c | 68.4 | 40.5 | 1.7 | 79.8 | 31.3 | 2.5 | 79.2 | 38.6 | 2.1 |
| 44.3 | 22.1 | 2.0 | 6.4 | 45.6 | 7.1 | 55.4 | 3.6 | 15.4 | 9.3 | 66.7 | 7.2 | 37.5 | 19.2 | 2.0 | 38.1 | 8.2 | 4.6 | 53.7 | 18.2 | 3.0 |
| 38.2 | 25.0 | 1.5c | 43.1 | 78.9 | 1.8 | 84.8 | 26.2 | 3.2 | 40.8 | 82.9 | 2.0c | 63.0 | 63.5 | 1.0 | 86.0 | 51.1 | 1.7 | 75.5 | 58.7 | 1.3 |
| 28.3 | 14.2 | 2.0 | 32.1 | 79.1 | 2.5 | ... | ... | ... | 37.9 | 83.6 | 2.2 | 82.0 | 58.8 | 1.4 | ... | ... | ... | 94.6 | 57.8 | 1.6 |
| 44.6 | 16.2 | 2.8 | 10.4 | 64.7 | 6.2 | 81.0 | 6.7 | 12.1 | 12.0 | 87.9 | 7.3 | 93.8 | 78.5 | 1.2 | 96.4 | 83.8 | 1.2 | 95.6 | 77.1 | 1.2 |
| 52.8 | 32.5 | 1.6 | 2.3 | 34.5 | 15.0 | 25.3 | 0.9 | 28.1 | 2.5 | 45.0 | 18.0 | 63.1 | 22.3 | 2.8 | 52.2 | 18.2 | 2.9 | 61.7 | 22.1 | 2.8 |
| 22.5 | 16.5 | 1.4 | 69.4 | 92.9 | 1.3 | 97.1 | 67.2 | 1.4 | 83.9 | 92.9 | 1.1 | 61.1 | 37.1 | 1.6 | 71.3 | 34.1 | 2.1 | 63.9 | 42.3 | 1.5 |
| 38.0 | 23.7 | 1.6 | 30.9 | 79.7 | 2.6 | 90.4 | 20.6 | 4.4 | 29.7 | 67.9 | 2.3 | 85.8 | 81.8 | 1.0 | 88.8 | 75.0 | 1.2 | 89.3 | 78.2 | 1.1 |
| 27.9 | 13.3 | 2.1 | 21.3 | 75.6 | 3.5 | 81.5 | 12.1 | 6.7 | 29.1 | 83.5 | 2.9 | 66.9 | 46.7 | 1.4 | 73.0 | 33.1 | 2.2 | 82.3 | 48.4 | 1.7 |
| 36.4 | 19.0 | 1.9 | 34.5 | 72.0 | 2.1 | 75.4 | 17.0 | 4.4 | 15.8 | 72.0 | 4.6 | 85.9 | 69.7 | 1.2 | 88.0 | 54.8 | 1.6 | 84.9 | 51.1 | 1.7 |
| ... | ... | ... | 44.9 | 76.7 | 1.7 | ... | ... | ... | 49.3 | 86.6 | 1.8 | 30.2 | 28.0 | 1.1 | ... | ... | ... | 42.7 | 24.9 | 1.7 |
| 49.1 | 38.0 | 1.3 | 39.6 | 70.6 | 1.8 | 93.9 | 29.9 | 3.1 | 21.9 | 80.5 | 3.7 | 73.9 | 55.9 | 1.3 | 84.0 | 38.4 | 2.2 | 85.2 | 36.1 | 2.4 |
| 54.2 | 27.1 | 2.0 | 51.9 | 81.6 | 1.6 | 83.0 | 43.0 | 1.9 | 45.0 | 87.7 | 1.9 | 90.6 | 82.0 | 1.1 | 90.4 | 79.8 | 1.1 | 93.4 | 79.2 | 1.2 |
| 40.1 | 13.6 | 2.9 | 26.6 | 80.8 | 3.0 | 81.9 | 8.1 | 10.1 | 34.4 | 90.8 | 2.6 | 70.8 | 41.3 | 1.7 | 76.5 | 39.7 | 1.9 | 78.7 | 44.9 | 1.8 |
| 37.1 | 21.4 | 1.7 | 28.9 | 85.8 | 3.0 | 92.8 | 14.7 | 6.3 | 40.4 | 91.6 | 2.3 | 74.3 | 53.0 | 1.4 | 86.2 | 42.0 | 2.1 | 79.8 | 55.4 | 1.4 |
| 47.7 | 14.5 | 3.3 | 34.1 | 80.7 | 2.4 | 88.6 | 24.8 | 3.6 | 31.4 | 94.8 | 3.0 | 90.8 | 70.8 | 1.3 | 96.4 | 60.8 | 1.6 | 99.1 | 65.6 | 1.5 |
| 28.5 | 17.9 | 1.6 | 66.3 | 93.1 | 1.4 | 97.1 | 55.4 | 1.8 | 46.8 | 89.1 | 1.9 | 84.3 | 78.4 | 1.1 | 85.7 | 76.2 | 1.1 | 83.3 | 69.5 | 1.2 |
| 42.3 | 23.6 | 1.8c | 8.1 | 68.7 | 8.5 | 62.8 | 4.2 | 15.0 | 13.8 | 68.5 | 5.0c | 67.1 | 27.8 | 2.4 | 65.8 | 23.0 | 2.9 | 73.9 | 31.8 | 2.3 |
| 50.5 | 20.0 | 2.5 | 27.1 | 58.8 | 2.2 | 84.5 | 13.0 | 6.5 | 13.8 | 75.0 | 5.4 | 52.1 | 28.5 | 1.8 | 70.7 | 15.9 | 4.4 | 66.5 | 15.6 | 4.3 |
| 47.9 | 26.1 | 1.8 | 19.9 | 65.7 | 3.3 | 59.6 | 17.3 | 3.4 | 13.9 | 68.9 | 5.0 | 89.9 | 86.3 | 1.0 | 88.8 | 83.8 | 1.1 | 93.2 | 82.2 | 1.1 |
| ... | ... | ... | 75.7 | 95.6 | 1.3 | ... | ... | ... | 78.5 | 97.1 | 1.2 | 78.7 | 58.1 | 1.4 | ... | ... | ... | 90.9 | 54.0 | 1.7 |
| ... | ... | ... | 75.5 | 93.4 | 1.2 | 98.1 | 67.8 | 1.4 | 59.7 | 91.4 | 1.5 | 85.1 | 79.3 | 1.1 | 84.5 | 73.5 | 1.1 | 85.6 | 64.0 | 1.3 |
| ... | ... | ... | 59.3 | 85.9 | 1.4 | ... | ... | ... | 52.6 | 95.5 | 1.8 | 69.9 | 56.3 | 1.2 | ... | ... | ... | 84.8 | 50.3 | 1.7 |
| 25.5 | 12.0 | 2.1c | 39.8 | 86.4 | 2.2 | 91.2 | 25.1 | 3.6 | 36.7 | 86.8 | 2.4c | 58.0 | 38.2 | 1.5 | 63.2 | 34.5 | 1.8 | 63.7 | 36.5 | 1.7 |
| 45.5 | 28.9 | 1.6 | 33.1 | 80.4 | 2.4 | 77.3 | 19.7 | 3.9 | 21.5 | 75.8 | 3.5 | 68.4 | 55.3 | 1.2 | 64.5 | 49.1 | 1.3 | 69.4 | 54.1 | 1.3 |
| 46.7 | 16.6 | 2.8 | 34.7 | 83.3 | 2.4 | 82.8 | 28.9 | 2.9 | 25.3 | 81.5 | 3.2 | 90.3 | 75.3 | 1.2 | 89.0 | 63.4 | 1.4 | 98.1 | 63.3 | 1.5 |
| 53.8 | 36.1 | 1.5 | 27.6 | 79.0 | 2.9 | 91.1 | 19.7 | 4.6 | 17.3 | 77.8 | 4.5 | 85.5 | 83.9 | 1.0 | 88.4 | 81.2 | 1.1 | 87.2 | 79.8 | 1.1 |
| 35.3 | 22.5 | 1.6 | 64.2 | 89.4 | 1.4 | 93.5 | 56.7 | 1.6 | 42.8 | 85.6 | 2.0 | 86.2 | 75.7 | 1.1 | 85.8 | 80.2 | 1.1 | 85.2 | 69.4 | 1.2 |

| | Country | Children under-5 stunted for age[a] | | Children under-5 underweight for age[a] | | Children under-5 over-weight for age[a] | | Newborns with low birth weight[b] | Adults (≥15 years old) who are obese[c] | | |
|---|---|---|---|---|---|---|---|---|---|---|---|
| | | (%) | Year | (%) | Year | (%) | Year | (%) | (%) | | Year |
| | | Both sexes | | Both sexes | | Both sexes | | Both sexes 2000–02 | Males | Females | |
| 1 | Algeria | 19.1 | 2002 | 10.4 | 2002 | 10.1 | 2000 | 7 | ... | ... | |
| 2 | Angola | 45.2 | 2001 | 30.5 | 2001 | ... | | 12 | ... | ... | |
| 3 | Benin | 30.7 | 2001 | 22.9 | 2001 | 1.8 | 2001 | 16 | ... | 6.1 | 2001[m] |
| 4 | Botswana | 23.1 | 2000 | 12.5 | 2000 | 6.9 | 2000 | 10 | ... | ... | |
| 5 | Burkina Faso | 38.8 | 2003 | 37.7 | 2003 | 2.9 | 2003 | 19 | ... | 2.4 | 2003[m] |
| 6 | Burundi | 56.8 | 2000 | 45.1 | 2000 | 0.7 | 2000 | 16 | ... | ... | |
| 7 | Cameroon | 31.7 | 2004 | 18.1 | 2004 | 5.2 | 2004 | 11 | ... | 4.2 | 2004[m] |
| 8 | Cape Verde | ... | | ... | | ... | | 13 | ... | ... | |
| 9 | Central African Republic | ... | | ... | | ... | | 14 | ... | ... | |
| 10 | Chad | 29.1 | 2000 | 28.0 | 2000 | 1.5 | 2000 | 17 | ... | ... | |
| 11 | Comoros | 42.3 | 2000 | 25.4 | 2000 | 13.6 | 2000 | 25 | ... | ... | |
| 12 | Congo | ... | | ... | | ... | | ... | ... | ... | |
| 13 | Côte d'Ivoire | 25.1 | 1998-99 | 21.2 | 1998-99 | 2.5 | 1998-99 | 17 | ... | 5.0 | 1998-99[m] |
| 14 | Democratic Republic of the Congo | 38.1 | 2001 | 31.0 | 2001 | 3.9 | 2001 | 12 | ... | ... | |
| 15 | Equatorial Guinea | ... | | ... | | | | 13 | ... | ... | |
| 16 | Eritrea | 37.6 | 2002 | 39.6 | 2002 | 0.7 | 2002 | 21 | ... | 1.6 | 2002[m] |
| 17 | Ethiopia | 51.5 | 2000 | 47.2 | 2000 | 1.2 | 2000 | 15 | ... | 0.3 | 2000[m] |
| 18 | Gabon | 20.7 | 2000-01 | 11.9 | 2000-01 | 3.7 | 2000-01 | 14 | ... | ... | |
| 19 | Gambia | 19.2 | 2000 | 17.2 | 2000 | 1.5 | 2000 | 17 | ... | ... | |
| 20 | Ghana | 29.9 | 2003 | 22.1 | 2003 | 2.9 | 2003 | 11 | ... | 8.1 | 2003[m] |
| 21 | Guinea | 26.1 | 1999 | 23.2 | 1999 | 2.7 | 1999 | 12 | ... | ... | |
| 22 | Guinea-Bissau | 30.5 | 2000 | 25.0 | 2000 | 3.3 | 2000 | 22 | ... | ... | |
| 23 | Kenya | 30.3 | 2003 | 19.9 | 2003 | 3.7 | 2003 | 11 | ... | 6.3 | 2003[m] |
| 24 | Lesotho | 46.1 | 2000 | 18.0 | 2000 | 12.1 | 2000 | 14 | ... | 16.2 | 2004[m] |
| 25 | Liberia | 39.5 | 1999-00 | 26.5 | 1999-00 | 2.3 | 1999-00 | ... | ... | ... | |
| 26 | Madagascar | 47.7 | 2003-04 | 41.9 | 2003-04 | 2.0 | 2003-04 | 14 | ... | 0.9 | 2003[m] |
| 27 | Malawi | 49.0 | 2000 | 25.4 | 2000 | 4.3 | 2000 | 16 | ... | 2.1 | 2000[m] |
| 28 | Mali | 38.2 | 2001 | 33.2 | 2001 | 1.5 | 2001 | 23 | ... | 3.7 | 2001[m] |
| 29 | Mauritania | 34.5 | 2000-01 | 31.8 | 2000-01 | ... | | ... | ... | 16.7 | 2000-01[m] |
| 30 | Mauritius | ... | | ... | | ... | | 13 | 8.0 | 20.0 | 1998[l] |
| 31 | Mozambique | 41.0 | 2003 | 23.7 | 2003 | 3.0 | 2003 | 14 | ... | 3.8 | 2003[m] |
| 32 | Namibia | 23.6 | 2000 | 24.0 | 2000 | 2.2 | 2000 | 14 | ... | ... | |
| 33 | Niger | 39.7 | 2000 | 40.1 | 2000 | 0.8 | 2000 | 17 | ... | ... | |
| 34 | Nigeria | 38.3 | 2003 | 28.7 | 2003 | 3.6 | 2003 | 14 | ... | 5.8 | 2003[m] |
| 35 | Rwanda | 42.6 | 2000 | 24.3 | 2000 | 4.0 | 2000 | 9 | ... | ... | |
| 36 | Sao Tome and Principe | 28.9 | 2000 | 12.9 | 2000 | ... | | ... | ... | ... | |
| 37 | Senegal | 25.4 | 2000 | 22.7 | 2000 | 2.2 | 2000 | 18 | ... | ... | |
| 38 | Seychelles | ... | | ... | | ... | | ... | ... | ... | |
| 39 | Sierra Leone | 33.8 | 2000 | 27.2 | 2000 | ... | | ... | ... | ... | |
| 40 | South Africa | 24.9 | 1999 | 11.5 | 1999 | 6.2 | 1999 | 15 | 9.4 | 30.1 | 1998 |
| 41 | Swaziland | 30.2 | 2000 | 10.3 | 2000 | ... | | 9 | ... | ... | |
| 42 | Togo | 21.7 | 1998 | 25.1 | 1998 | 1.5 | 1998 | 15 | ... | ... | |
| 43 | Uganda | 39.1 | 2000-01 | 22.9 | 2000-01 | 2.6 | 2000-01 | 12 | ... | ... | |
| 44 | United Republic of Tanzania | 43.8 | 1999 | 29.4 | 1999 | 1.7 | 1999 | 13 | ... | 4.4 | 2004-05[m] |
| 45 | Zambia | 46.8 | 2001-02 | 28.1 | 2001-02 | 3.0 | 2001-02 | 12 | ... | 3.0 | 2001-02[m] |
| 46 | Zimbabwe | 26.5 | 1999 | 13.0 | 1999 | 7.0 | 1999 | 11 | ... | 7.5 | 1999[m] |

| | Region | | | | | | | | | | |
|---|---|---|---|---|---|---|---|---|---|---|---|
| | African Region | ... | | ... | | ... | | 14 | ... | ... | |

... Data not available or not applicable.

[a] Global Database on Child Growth and Malnutrition. World Health Organization.
(http://www.who.int/nutgrowthdb/database/en/)

[b] United Nations Children's Fund and World Health Organization. Low Birthweight: Country, regional and global estimates. UNICEF, New York, 2004.
(http://www.who.int/reproductive-health/publications/low_birthweight/low_birthweight_estimates.pdf)

[c] WHO Global Database on Body Mass Index (BMI). World Health Organization. (http//www.who.int/bmi). Comparisons between countries may be limited due to differences in definitions, sample characteristics, or survey years.

[d] World Health Organization and United Nations Children's Fund. Joint Monitoring Programme for Water Supply and Sanitation. Online database.
(http://www.wssinfo.org/en/wecome.html)

[e] Programme on Household Energy and Health, Department for Public Health and Environment. World Health Organization. (http://www.who.int/indoorair/en/)

[f] In adolescents, data relate to daily or occasional tobacco use, while in adults they relate to daily or occasional tobacco smoking. Comparisons between countries may be limited due to differences in definitions, sample characteristics, or survey years.

[g] Global NCD InfoBase/Online Tool. World Health Organization. (http://www.who.int/ncd_surveillance/infobase/en)

| Access to improved water sources[d] (%) | | Access to improved sanitation[d] (%) | | Population using solid fuels[e] (%) | | Prevalence of current tobacco use (%)[f] | | | | | Condom use by young people (aged 15–24) at higher risk sex[i] (%) | | |
| | | | | | | Adolescents (13-15)[g] | | Adults (≥15)[h] | | | | | |
| Urban 2002 | Rural 2002 | Urban 2002 | Rural 2002 | Urban 2003 | Rural 2003 | Both sexes | Year | Males | Females | Year | Males | Females | Year |
|---|---|---|---|---|---|---|---|---|---|---|---|---|---|
| 92 | 80 | 99 | 82 | ... | ... | ... | | ... | ... | | ... | ... | |
| 70 | 40 | 56 | 16 | ... | ... | ... | | ... | ... | | ... | ... | |
| 79 | 60 | 58 | 12 | 88 | 99 | 14.5 | 2003 | ... | ... | | 34 | 19 | 2001 |
| 100 | 90 | 57 | 25 | ... | ... | 11.3 | 2001 | ... | ... | | 88 | 75 | 2000 |
| 82 | 44 | 45 | 5 | 91 | 100 | ... | | 24.2 | 11.1 | 2003[l] | 67 | 54 | 2003 |
| 90 | 78 | 47 | 35 | 98 | 100 | ... | | ... | ... | | ... | ... | |
| 84 | 41 | 63 | 33 | 62 | 98 | ... | | ... | ... | | 57 | 46 | 2004 |
| 86 | 73 | 61 | 19 | ... | ... | ... | | ... | ... | | ... | ... | |
| 93 | 61 | 47 | 12 | ... | ... | ... | | ... | ... | | ... | ... | |
| 40 | 32 | 30 | 0 | 95 | 98 | | | 18.3 | 3.7 | 2003[l] | 25 | 17 | 2004 |
| 90 | 96 | 38 | 15 | 46 | 90[k] | ... | | 27.5 | 17.0 | 2003[k,l] | ... | ... | |
| 72 | 17 | 14 | 2 | 84 | 98[k] | ... | | 16.5 | 1.7 | 2003[k,l] | ... | ... | |
| 98 | 74 | 61 | 23 | 63 | 95[k] | ... | | 20.7 | 3.2 | 2003[k,l] | ... | ... | |
| 83 | 29 | 43 | 23 | ... | ... | ... | | ... | ... | | ... | ... | |
| 45 | 42 | 60 | 46 | ... | ... | ... | | ... | ... | | ... | ... | |
| 72 | 54 | 34 | 3 | 31 | 97 | 6.6 | 2006 | ... | | | ... | ... | |
| 81 | 11 | 19 | 4 | 78 | 100 | ... | | 7.3 | 0.6 | 2003[l] | 30 | 17 | 2000 |
| 95 | 47 | 37 | 30 | 14 | 81 | ... | | ... | ... | | 48 | 33 | 2000 |
| 95 | 77 | 72 | 46 | ... | ... | ... | | ... | ... | | ... | ... | |
| 93 | 68 | 74 | 46 | 75 | 96 | 11.7 | 2006 | 9.9 | 1.3 | 2003[l] | 52 | 33 | 2003 |
| 78 | 38 | 25 | 6 | ... | ... | ... | | ... | ... | | ... | ... | |
| 79 | 49 | 57 | 23 | ... | ... | ... | | ... | ... | | ... | ... | |
| 89 | 46 | 56 | 43 | 17 | 94 | 12.7 | 2001 | 27.2 | 1.9 | 2003[l] | 47 | 25 | 2003 |
| 88 | 74 | 61 | 32 | ... | ... | 20.3 | 2002 | ... | ... | | 53 | 53 | 2004 |
| 72 | 52 | 49 | 7 | ... | ... | ... | | ... | ... | | ... | ... | |
| 75 | 34 | 49 | 27 | ... | ... | ... | | ... | ... | | 12 | 5 | 2003 |
| 96 | 62 | 66 | 42 | 90 | 99 | ... | | 25.3 | 5.8 | 2003[l] | 47 | 35 | 2004 |
| 76 | 35 | 59 | 38 | 99 | 100 | ... | | 24.7 | 3.0 | 2003[l] | 30 | 14 | 2001 |
| 63 | 45 | 64 | 9 | 35 | 84 | 24.7 | 2001 | 29.6 | 4.7 | 2003[l] | ... | ... | |
| 100 | 100 | 100 | 99 | 0 | 2 | 13.2 | 2003 | 42.7 | 2.8 | 2003[l] | ... | ... | |
| 76 | 24 | 51 | 14 | ... | ... | ... | | ... | ... | | 33 | 29 | 2003 |
| 98 | 72 | 66 | 14 | 24 | 84 | 25.8 | 2004 | 28.3 | 12.4 | 2003[l] | 69 | 48 | 2000 |
| 80 | 36 | 43 | 4 | 95 | 98 | 18.4 | 2001 | ... | ... | | ... | ... | |
| 72 | 49 | 48 | 30 | ... | ... | ... | | ... | 0.0 | 2003[m,n] | 46 | 24 | 2003 |
| 92 | 69 | 56 | 38 | 98 | 100 | ... | | ... | ... | | 41 | 28 | 2004 |
| 89 | 73 | 32 | 20 | ... | ... | ... | | ... | ... | | ... | ... | |
| 90 | 54 | 70 | 34 | 24 | 80 | 16.6 | 2002 | 24.1 | 1.9 | 2003[l] | ... | ... | |
| 100 | 75 | ... | 100 | ... | ... | 28.9 | 2002 | ... | ... | | ... | ... | |
| 75 | 46 | 53 | 30 | ... | ... | ... | | ... | ... | | ... | ... | |
| 98 | 73 | 86 | 44 | 7 | 40 | 23.6 | 2002 | 37.0 | 11.2 | 2003[l] | ... | ... | |
| 87 | 42 | 78 | 44 | 23 | 82 | 11.5 | 2001 | 15.1 | 3.2 | 2003[l] | ... | ... | |
| 80 | 36 | 71 | 15 | ... | ... | 16.1 | 2002 | ... | ... | | ... | ... | |
| 87 | 52 | 53 | 39 | 85 | 99 | ... | | 25.2 | 3.3 | 2001[m] | 55 | 53 | 2004 |
| 92 | 62 | 54 | 41 | ... | ... | ... | | ... | ... | | 46 | 34 | 2004 |
| 90 | 36 | 68 | 32 | 68 | 99 | ... | | 23.3 | 5.7 | 2003[l] | 42 | 33 | 2001 |
| 100 | 74 | 69 | 51 | 26 | 94 | ... | | 26.2 | 3.1 | 2003[l] | ... | ... | |
| 84 | 45 | 58 | 28 | ... | ... | ... | | ... | ... | | ... | ... | |

[h] (i) Global NCD InfoBase/Online Tool. World Health Organization. (http://www.who.int/ncd_surveillance/infobase/en); (ii) Ustun TB, Chatterji S, Mechbal A, Murray CJL, WHS Collaborating Groups. The World Health Surveys in Health Systems Performance Assessment: Debates, Methods and Empiricism (eds. Murray CJL and Evans D), World Health Organization, Geneva, 2003; (iii) Results from the World Health Survey. World Health Organization. (http://www.who.int/healthinfo/survey/en/)

[i] Multiple Indicator Cluster Survey (http://childinfo.org) and Demographic and Health Surveys (http://www.measuredhs.com).

[j] Self-reported data.

[k] Sample is not necessarily nationally representative.

[l] Lower age limit above 15.

[m] Upper age limit at 50.

[n] Cigarettes are the only smoked tobacco product under consideration.

| # | Country | Immunization coverage among 1-year-olds[a] | | | Antenatal care coverage[b] | | | Births attended by skilled health personnel[c] | | Contraceptive prevalence[d] | |
|---|---------|---------|------|------|--------------|---------------|------|---------|------|---------|------|
| | | Measles | DTP3 | HepB3 | At least 1 visit | At least 4 visits | | | | | |
| | | (%) 2004 | (%) 2004 | (%) 2004 | (%) | (%) | Year | (%) | Year | (%) | Year |
| 1 | Algeria | 81 | 86 | 81 | 79 | ... | 2000 | 92 | 2000 | 64.0 | 2000 |
| 2 | Angola | 64 | 59 | ... | ... | ... | | 47 | 2000 | 6.2 | 2001 |
| 3 | Benin | 85 | 83 | 89 | 88 | 61 | 2001 | 66 | 2001 | 18.6 | 2001 |
| 4 | Botswana | 90 | 97 | 79 | 99 | 97 | 2001 | 94 | 2000 | 40.4 | 2000 |
| 5 | Burkina Faso | 78 | 88 | ... | 72 | 18 | 2003 | 57[k] | 2003 | 13.8 | 2003 |
| 6 | Burundi | 75 | 74 | 83 | 93 | 79 | 2001 | 25 | 2000 | 15.7 | 2000 |
| 7 | Cameroon | 64 | 73 | ... | 77 | 52 | 1998 | 62 | 2004 | 26.0 | 2004 |
| 8 | Cape Verde | 69 | 75 | 68 | ... | 99 | 2001 | 89[k] | 1998 | 52.9 | 1998 |
| 9 | Central African Republic | 35 | 40 | ... | ... | ... | | 44 | 2000 | 27.9 | 2000 |
| 10 | Chad | 56 | 50 | ... | 51 | 13 | 1997 | 14 | 2004 | 7.9 | 2000 |
| 11 | Comoros | 73 | 76 | 77 | ... | ... | | 62 | 2000 | 25.7 | 2000 |
| 12 | Congo | 65 | 67 | ... | ... | ... | | ... | | ... | |
| 13 | Côte d'Ivoire | 49 | 50 | 50 | 84 | 35 | 1998-99 | 63 | 2000 | 15.0 | 1998-99 |
| 14 | Democratic Republic of the Congo | 64 | 64 | ... | ... | ... | | 61 | 2001 | 31.4 | 2001 |
| 15 | Equatorial Guinea | 51 | 33 | ... | ... | 37 | 2001 | 65 | 2000 | ... | |
| 16 | Eritrea | 84 | 83 | 83 | ... | 49 | 2001 | 28 | 2002 | 8.0 | 2002 |
| 17 | Ethiopia | 71 | 80 | ... | 27 | 10 | 2000 | 6 | 2000 | 8.1 | 2000 |
| 18 | Gabon | 55 | 38 | ... | 94 | 63 | 2000 | 86 | 2000 | 32.7 | 2000 |
| 19 | Gambia | 90 | 92 | 90 | 92 | ... | 2000 | 55 | 2000 | 9.6 | 2000 |
| 20 | Ghana | 83 | 80 | 80 | 90 | 69 | 2003 | 47 | 2003 | 25.2 | 2003 |
| 21 | Guinea | 73 | 69 | ... | 74 | 48 | 1999 | 35 | 1999 | 6.2 | 1999 |
| 22 | Guinea-Bissau | 80 | 80 | ... | 89 | 62 | 2001 | 35 | 2000 | 7.6 | 2000 |
| 23 | Kenya | 73 | 73 | 73 | 88 | 52 | 2003 | 42 | 2003 | 39.3 | 2003 |
| 24 | Lesotho | 70 | 78 | 67 | 91 | 88 | 2001 | 55 | 2004 | 30.4 | 2000 |
| 25 | Liberia | 42 | 31 | ... | ... | 84 | 2001 | 51 | 2000 | ... | |
| 26 | Madagascar | 59 | 61 | 61 | 91 | 38 | 1997 | 51 | 2003-04 | 27.1 | 2003-04 |
| 27 | Malawi | 80 | 89 | 89 | 94 | 55 | 2000 | 61 | 2002 | 30.6 | 2000 |
| 28 | Mali | 75 | 76 | 73 | 53 | 30 | 2001 | 41 | 2001 | 8.1 | 2001 |
| 29 | Mauritania | 64 | 70 | ... | 63 | 16 | 2000-01 | 57[k] | 2001 | 8.0 | 2000-01 |
| 30 | Mauritius | 98 | 98 | 98 | ... | ... | | 99 | 1998 | ... | |
| 31 | Mozambique | 77 | 72 | 72 | 71 | 41 | 1997 | 48 | 2003 | 16.5 | 2003 |
| 32 | Namibia | 70 | 81 | ... | 85 | 69 | 2000 | 76 | 2000 | 43.9 | 2000 |
| 33 | Niger | 74 | 62 | ... | 39 | 11 | 1998 | 16 | 2000 | 14.0 | 2000 |
| 34 | Nigeria | 35 | 25 | ... | 61 | 47 | 2003 | 35 | 2003 | 12.6 | 2003 |
| 35 | Rwanda | 84 | 89 | 89 | 93 | 10 | 2001 | 31 | 2000 | 13.2 | 2000 |
| 36 | Sao Tome and Principe | 91 | 99 | 99 | 91 | ... | 2000 | 79 | 2000 | 29.3 | 2000 |
| 37 | Senegal | 57 | 87 | 54 | 82 | 64 | 1999 | 58 | 2000 | 10.5 | 1999 |
| 38 | Seychelles | 99 | 99 | 99 | ... | ... | | ... | | ... | |
| 39 | Sierra Leone | 64 | 61 | ... | 82 | 68 | 2001 | 42 | 2000 | 4.3 | 2000 |
| 40 | South Africa | 81 | 93 | 92 | 89 | 72 | 1998 | 84 | 1998 | 56.3 | 1998 |
| 41 | Swaziland | 70 | 83 | 78 | ... | ... | | 70 | 2000 | 27.7 | 2000 |
| 42 | Togo | 70 | 71 | ... | 78 | 46 | 1998 | 49 | 2000 | 25.7 | 2000 |
| 43 | Uganda | 91 | 87 | 87 | 92 | 40 | 2000-01 | 39 | 2000 | 22.8 | 2000-01 |
| 44 | United Republic of Tanzania | 94 | 95 | 95 | 96 | 69 | 1999 | 46 | 2004-05 | 25.4 | 1999 |
| 45 | Zambia | 84 | 80 | ... | 94 | 71 | 2001-02 | 43 | 2001-02 | 34.2 | 2001-02 |
| 46 | Zimbabwe | 80 | 85 | 85 | 82 | 64 | 1999 | 73 | 1999 | 53.5 | 1999 |
| | **Region** | | | | | | | | | | |
| | African Region | 66 | 66 | 35 | ... | ... | | ... | | ... | |

... Data not available or not applicable.

[a] WHO/UNICEF estimates of national coverage for year 2004 (as of September 2005). (http://www.who.int/immunization_monitoring/routine/immunization_coverage/en/index4.html)

[b] *World health report 2005: make every mother and child count.* Geneva, World Health Organization, 2005. (http://www.who.int/whr/2005/en/index.html)

[c] WHO Database on Skilled Attendant at Delivery. World Health Organization. (http://www.who.int//reproductive-health/global_monitoring/data.html)

[d] World Contraceptive Use 2005 database. Population Division, Department of Economic and Social Affairs, United Nations.

[e] *World malaria report 2005.* Geneva, World Health Organization and United Nations Children's Fund, 2005. Values for Cameroon and Chad have been updated.

[f] *Progress on global access to HIV antiretroviral therapy. A report on "3 by 5" and beyond.* Geneva, World Health Organization and Joint United Nations Programme on HIV/AIDS, March 2006. Data for high-income countries have been added to the original list which consisted of 152 low- and middle-income countries. Regional values relate to low- and middle-income countries only. (http://www.who.int/hiv/fullreport_en_highres.pdf)

| Children under-5 sleeping under insecticide-treated nets[e] | | Antiretroviral therapy coverage[f] | TB detection rate under DOTS[g] | TB treatment success under DOTS[h] | Children under-5 with ARI symptoms taken to facility[i] | | Children under-5 with diarrhoea receiving ORT[i] | | Children under-5 with fever who received treatment with any antimalarial[e] | | Children 6–59 months who received vitamin A supplementation[j] | Births by Caesarean section[b] | |
|---|---|---|---|---|---|---|---|---|---|---|---|---|---|
| (%) | Year | (%) Dec 2005 | (%) 2004 | (%) 2003 cohort | (%) | Year | (%) | Year | (%) | Year | (%) 2002 | (%) | Year |
| … | | 39 | 105 | 90 | … | | … | | … | | … | 6 | 2000 |
| 2.3 | 2001 | 6 | 94 | 68 | … | | … | | 63.0 | 2001 | 87.5 | … | |
| 7.4 | 2001 | 33 | 82 | 81 | 35.1 | 2001 | 39.3 | 2001 | 60.4 | 2001 | 84.6 | 4 | 2001 |
| … | | 85 | 67 | 77 | … | | … | | … | | … | … | |
| 1.6 | 2003 | 24 | 18 | 66 | 35.9 | 2003 | 49.0 | 2003 | 49.6 | 2003 | 97.0 | 1 | 2003 |
| 1.3 | 2000 | 14 | 29 | 79 | … | | … | | 31.3 | 2000 | 89.2 | … | |
| 0.9 | 2004 | 36 | 91 | … | 36.6 | 2000 | 47.7 | 2004 | 53.1 | 2004 | 86.1 | 3 | 1998 |
| … | | >75 | … | … | … | | … | | … | | … | 6 | 1998 |
| 1.5 | 2000 | … | 4 | 59 | … | | … | | 68.8 | 2000 | … | 2 | 1994-95 |
| 0.6 | 2000 | 3 | 16 | 78 | 11.8 | 2004 | 27.8 | 2004 | 55.8 | 2004 | 85.3 | 1 | 1996-97 |
| 9.3 | 2000 | 43 | 39 | … | … | | … | | 62.7 | 2000 | … | 5 | 1996 |
| … | | … | 65 | 69 | … | | … | | … | | 85.6 | … | |
| 1.1 | 2000 | 80 | 38 | 72 | … | | … | | 57.5 | 2000 | … | 3 | 1998-99 |
| 0.7 | 2001 | 4 | 70 | 83 | … | | … | | 45.4 | 2001 | 61.7 | … | |
| 0.7 | 2000 | 0 | 82 | 51 | … | | … | | 48.6 | 2000 | … | … | |
| 4.2 | 2002 | 5 | 14 | 85 | 43.6 | 2002 | 38.2 | 2002 | 3.6 | 2002 | 51.1 | 2 | 1995 |
| … | | 7 | 36 | 70 | 15.8 | 2000 | 34.9 | 2000 | 3.0 | 2000 | … | 1 | 2000 |
| … | | 23 | 81 | 34 | 47.7 | 2000 | 62.7 | 2000 | … | | 86.6 | 6 | 2000 |
| 14.7 | 2000 | 9 | 66 | 75 | … | | … | | 55.2 | 2000 | 93.0 | … | |
| 3.5 | 2003 | 7 | 37 | 66 | 44.0 | 2003 | 39.6 | 2003 | 62.8 | 2003 | 98.6 | 4 | 2003 |
| … | | 9 | 52 | 75 | 38.4 | 1999 | … | | … | | 94.5 | 2 | 1999 |
| 7.4 | 2000 | 1 | 75 | 80 | … | | … | | 58.4 | 2000 | 79.7 | … | |
| 4.6 | 2003 | 24 | 46 | 80 | 49.1 | 2003 | 34.2 | 2003 | 26.5 | 2003 | 91.4 | 4 | 2003 |
| … | | 14 | 86 | 70 | 54.4 | 2004 | 32.1 | 2004 | … | | … | … | |
| … | | 3 | 58 | 73 | … | | … | | … | | 40.0 | … | |
| 0.2 | 2000 | 0 | 74 | 71 | 47.9 | 2003-04 | 34.9 | 2004 | 41.1 | 2004 | 95.0 | 1 | 1997 |
| 35.5 | 2004 | 20 | 40 | 73 | 26.7 | 2000 | 35.4 | 2000 | 31.6 | 2004 | 85.8 | 3 | 2000 |
| … | | 31 | 19 | 65 | 35.6 | 2001 | 53.5 | 2001 | 37.6 | 2003 | 68.3 | 1 | 2001 |
| 2.1 | 2003-04 | 40 | 43 | 58 | 40.7 | 2000-01 | … | | 33.4 | 2003-04 | 89.0 | 3 | 2000-01 |
| … | | … | 33 | 87 | … | | … | | … | | … | … | |
| … | | 9 | 46 | 76 | 55.4 | 2003 | 46.7 | 2003 | … | | … | 3 | 1997 |
| … | | 71 | 88 | 63 | 53.1 | 2000 | 15.3 | 2000 | 14.4 | 2000 | 96.4 | 7 | 1992 |
| 1.0 | 2000 | 5 | 46 | 70 | … | | … | | 48.1 | 2000 | 76.6 | 1 | 1998 |
| 1.2 | 2003 | 6 | 21 | 59 | 32.8 | 2003 | 20.4 | 2003 | 33.8 | 2003 | 79.0 | 2 | 2003 |
| 5.0 | 2000 | 39 | 29 | 67 | 15.5 | 2000 | 17.3 | 2000 | 12.6 | 2000 | 36.2 | 2 | 2000 |
| 22.8 | 2000 | … | … | … | … | | … | | 61.2 | 2000 | … | … | |
| 1.7 | 2000 | 47 | 52 | 70 | … | | 48.3 | 1999 | 36.2 | 2000 | 82.7 | 2 | 1997 |
| … | | … | 106 | 100 | … | | … | | … | | … | … | |
| 1.5 | 2000 | 2 | 36 | 83 | … | | … | | 60.7 | 2000 | 87.2 | 2 | 1997 |
| … | | 21 | 83 | 67 | 73.9 | 1998 | … | | … | | … | 16 | 1998 |
| 0.1 | 2000 | 31 | 38 | 42 | … | | … | | 25.5 | 2000 | … | … | |
| 2.0 | 2000 | 27 | 17 | 63 | … | | … | | 60.0 | 2000 | 95.0 | 2 | 1998 |
| 0.2 | 2000-01 | 51 | 43 | 68 | 66.5 | 2000-01 | 27.7 | 2000-01 | … | | 46.0 | 3 | 2000-01 |
| 2.1 | 1999 | 7 | 47 | 81 | 45.8 | 2003 | 36.3 | 2003 | 53.4 | 1999 | 94.2 | 3 | 1999 |
| 6.5 | 2001-02 | 26 | 54 | 75 | 69.1 | 2001-02 | 40.9 | 2000-02 | 51.9 | 2001-02 | 79.8 | 2 | 2001-02 |
| … | | 8 | 42 | 66 | 49.0 | 1999 | 51.0 | 1999 | … | | 78.2 | 7 | 1999 |
| … | | 17 | 48 | 72 | … | | … | | … | | … | … | |

[g] The number of new smear-positive cases notified to WHO divided by the estimated number of new smear-positive cases. Source: *Global tuberculosis control: surveillance, planning, financing. WHO report 2006.* Geneva, World Health Organization (WHO/HTM/TB/2006.362).

[h] The percentage of new smear-positive patients registered for treatment under DOTS during 2003 who were cured (with laboratory confirmation) or completed their course of treatment. Source: *Global tuberculosis control: surveillance, planning, financing.*

[i] Demographic and Health Surveys. (http://www.measuredhs.com)

[j] UNICEF Global Database on Vitamin A Supplementation Coverage. The United Nations Children's Fund. (http://www.childinfo.org/eddb/vita_a/framedb.htm)

[k] Data do not exactly relate to "skilled health personnel" as defined in the document: Making pregnancy safer: the critical role of the skilled attendant: a joint statement by WHO, ICM and FIGO. Geneva, World Health Organization, 2004. Further information can be found on http://www.who.int/whosis.

| Country | Human resources for health[a] | | | | | | | | | | | |
| | Physicians | | | Nurses | | | Midwives | | | Dentists | | |
| | Number | Density per 1000 | Year | Number | Density per 1000 | Year | Number | Density per 1000 | Year | Number | Density per 1000 | Year |
|---|---|---|---|---|---|---|---|---|---|---|---|---|
| 1 Algeria | 35 368 | 1.13 | 2002 | 68 950 | 2.21 | 2002 | 799 | 0.03 | 2002 | 9 553 | 0.31 | 2002 |
| 2 Angola | 881 | 0.08 | 1997 | 13 135 | 1.15 | 1997 | 492 | 0.04 | 1997 | 2 | 0.00 | 1997 |
| 3 Benin | 311 | 0.04 | 2004 | 5 789 | 0.84 | 2004 | ... | ... | | 12 | 0.00 | 2004 |
| 4 Botswana | 715 | 0.40 | 2004 | 4 753 | 2.65 | 2004 | ... | ... | | 38 | 0.02 | 2004 |
| 5 Burkina Faso | 789 | 0.06 | 2004 | 5 518 | 0.41 | 2004 | 1 732 | 0.13 | 2004 | 58 | 0.00 | 2004 |
| 6 Burundi | 200 | 0.03 | 2004 | 1 348 | 0.19 | 2004 | ... | ... | | 14 | 0.00 | 2004 |
| 7 Cameroon | 3 124 | 0.19 | 2004 | 26 042 | 1.60 | 2004 | ... | ... | | 147 | 0.01 | 2004 |
| 8 Cape Verde | 231 | 0.49 | 2004 | 410 | 0.87 | 2004 | ... | ... | | 11 | 0.02 | 2004 |
| 9 Central African Republic | 331 | 0.08 | 2004 | 1 188 | 0.30 | 2004 | 519 | 0.13 | 2004 | 13 | 0.00 | 2004 |
| 10 Chad | 345 | 0.04 | 2004 | 2 387 | 0.27 | 2004 | 112 | 0.01 | 2004 | 15 | 0.00 | 2004 |
| 11 Comoros | 115 | 0.15 | 2004 | 588 | 0.74 | 2004 | ... | ... | | 29 | 0.04 | 2004 |
| 12 Congo | 756 | 0.20 | 2004 | 3 672 | 0.96 | 2004 | ... | ... | | 12 | 0.00 | 2004 |
| 13 Côte d'Ivoire | 2 081 | 0.12 | 2004 | 10 180 | 0.60 | 2004 | ... | ... | | 339 | 0.02 | 2004 |
| 14 Democratic Republic of the Congo | 5 827 | 0.11 | 2004 | 28 789 | 0.53 | 2004 | ... | ... | | 159 | 0.00 | 2004 |
| 15 Equatorial Guinea | 153 | 0.30 | 2004 | 228 | 0.45 | 2004 | 43 | 0.08 | 2004 | 15 | 0.03 | 2004 |
| 16 Eritrea | 215 | 0.05 | 2004 | 2 505 | 0.58 | 2004 | ... | ... | | 16 | 0.00 | 2004 |
| 17 Ethiopia | 1 936 | 0.03 | 2003 | 14 893 | 0.21 | 2003 | 651 | 0.01 | 2003 | 93 | 0.00 | 2003 |
| 18 Gabon | 395 | 0.29 | 2004 | 6 974 | 5.16 | 2004 | ... | ... | | 66 | 0.05 | 2004 |
| 19 Gambia | 156 | 0.11 | 2003 | 1 719 | 1.21 | 2003 | 162 | 0.11 | 2003 | 43 | 0.03 | 2003 |
| 20 Ghana | 3 240 | 0.15 | 2004 | 19 707 | 0.92 | 2004 | ... | ... | | 393 | 0.02 | 2004 |
| 21 Guinea | 987 | 0.11 | 2004 | 4 757 | 0.55 | 2004 | 64 | 0.01 | 2004 | 60 | 0.01 | 2004 |
| 22 Guinea-Bissau | 188 | 0.12 | 2004 | 1 037 | 0.67 | 2004 | 35 | 0.02 | 2004 | 22 | 0.01 | 2004 |
| 23 Kenya | 4 506 | 0.14 | 2004 | 37 113 | 1.14 | 2004 | ... | ... | | 1 340 | 0.04 | 2004 |
| 24 Lesotho | 89 | 0.05 | 2003 | 1 123 | 0.62 | 2003 | ... | ... | | 16 | 0.01 | 2003 |
| 25 Liberia | 103 | 0.03 | 2004 | 613 | 0.18 | 2004 | 422 | 0.12 | 2004 | 13 | 0.00 | 2004 |
| 26 Madagascar | 5 201 | 0.29 | 2004 | 5 661 | 0.32 | 2004 | ... | ... | | 410 | 0.02 | 2004 |
| 27 Malawi | 266 | 0.02 | 2004 | 7 264 | 0.59 | 2004 | ... | ... | | ... | ... | |
| 28 Mali | 1 053 | 0.08 | 2004 | 6 538 | 0.49 | 2004 | 573 | 0.04 | 2004 | 84 | 0.01 | 2004 |
| 29 Mauritania | 313 | 0.11 | 2004 | 1 893 | 0.64 | 2004 | ... | ... | | 64 | 0.02 | 2004 |
| 30 Mauritius | 1 303 | 1.06 | 2004 | 4 550 | 3.69 | 2004 | 54 | 0.04 | 2004 | 233 | 0.19 | 2004 |
| 31 Mozambique | 514 | 0.03 | 2004 | 3 954 | 0.21 | 2004 | 2 229 | 0.12 | 2004 | 159 | 0.01 | 2004 |
| 32 Namibia | 598 | 0.30 | 2004 | 6 145 | 3.06 | 2004 | ... | ... | | 113 | 0.06 | 2004 |
| 33 Niger | 377 | 0.03 | 2004 | 2 716 | 0.22 | 2004 | 21 | 0.00 | 2004 | 15 | 0.00 | 2004 |
| 34 Nigeria | 34 923 | 0.28 | 2003 | 210 306 | 1.70 | 2003 | ... | ... | | 2 482 | 0.02 | 2003 |
| 35 Rwanda | 401 | 0.05 | 2004 | 3 593 | 0.42 | 2004 | 54 | 0.01 | 2004 | 21 | 0.00 | 2004 |
| 36 Sao Tome and Principe | 81 | 0.49 | 2004 | 256 | 1.55 | 2004 | 52 | 0.32 | 2004 | 11 | 0.07 | 2004 |
| 37 Senegal | 594 | 0.06 | 2004 | 3 287 | 0.32 | 2004 | ... | ... | | 97 | 0.01 | 2004 |
| 38 Seychelles | 121 | 1.51 | 2004 | 634 | 7.93 | 2004 | ... | ... | | 94 | 1.17 | 2004 |
| 39 Sierra Leone | 168 | 0.03 | 2004 | 1 841 | 0.36 | 2004 | ... | ... | | 5 | 0.00 | 2004 |
| 40 South Africa | 34 829 | 0.77 | 2004 | 184 459 | 4.08 | 2004 | ... | ... | | 5 995 | 0.13 | 2004 |
| 41 Swaziland | 171 | 0.16 | 2004 | 6 828 | 6.30 | 2004 | ... | ... | | 32 | 0.03 | 2004 |
| 42 Togo | 225 | 0.04 | 2004 | 2 141 | 0.43 | 2004 | 5 | 0.00 | 2004 | 19 | 0.00 | 2004 |
| 43 Uganda | 2 209 | 0.08 | 2004 | 16 221 | 0.61 | 2004 | 3 104 | 0.12 | 2004 | 363 | 0.01 | 2004 |
| 44 United Republic of Tanzania | 822 | 0.02 | 2002 | 13 292 | 0.37 | 2002 | ... | ... | | 267 | 0.01 | 2002 |
| 45 Zambia | 1 264 | 0.12 | 2004 | 19 014 | 1.74 | 2004 | 2 996 | 0.27 | 2004 | 491 | 0.04 | 2004 |
| 46 Zimbabwe | 2 086 | 0.16 | 2004 | 9 357 | 0.72 | 2004 | ... | ... | | 310 | 0.02 | 2004 |

... Data not available or not applicable.

[a] *World health report 2006: working together for health.* Geneva, World Health Organization, 2006. (http://www.who.int/whr/2006/annex/en)

| Pharmacists | | | Public and environmental health workers | | | Community health workers | | | Lab technicians | | | Other health workers | | | Health management and support workers | | |
|---|---|---|---|---|---|---|---|---|---|---|---|---|---|---|---|---|---|
| Number | Density per 1000 | Year | Number | Density per 1000 | Year | Number | Density per 1000 | Year | Number | Density per 1000 | Year | Number | Density per 1000 | Year | Number | Density per 1000 | Year |
| 6 333 | 0.20 | 2002 | 2 534 | 0.08 | 2002 | 1 062 | 0.03 | 2002 | 8 838 | 0.28 | 2002 | 5 088 | 0.16 | 2002 | 60 882 | 1.95 | 2002 |
| 24 | 0.00 | 1997 | ... | ... | | ... | ... | | ... | ... | | ... | ... | | ... | ... | |
| 11 | 0.00 | 2004 | 178 | 0.03 | 2004 | 88 | 0.01 | 2004 | 477 | 0.07 | 2004 | 128 | 0.02 | 2004 | 3 281 | 0.47 | 2004 |
| 333 | 0.19 | 2004 | 172 | 0.10 | 2004 | ... | ... | | 277 | 0.15 | 2004 | ... | ... | | 829 | 0.46 | 2004 |
| 343 | 0.03 | 2004 | 46 | 0.00 | 2004 | 1 291 | 0.10 | 2004 | 424 | 0.03 | 2004 | 975 | 0.07 | 2004 | 325 | 0.02 | 2004 |
| 76 | 0.01 | 2004 | ... | ... | | 657 | 0.09 | 2004 | 147 | 0.02 | 2004 | 1 186 | 0.17 | 2004 | 2 087 | 0.30 | 2004 |
| 700 | 0.04 | 2004 | 28 | 0.00 | 2004 | ... | ... | | 1 793 | 0.11 | 2004 | 16 | 0.00 | 2004 | 5 902 | 0.36 | 2004 |
| 43 | 0.09 | 2004 | 9 | 0.02 | 2004 | 65 | 0.14 | 2004 | 78 | 0.16 | 2004 | 42 | 0.09 | 2004 | 74 | 0.16 | 2004 |
| 17 | 0.00 | 2004 | 55 | 0.01 | 2004 | 211 | 0.05 | 2004 | 48 | 0.01 | 2004 | 367 | 0.09 | 2004 | 167 | 0.04 | 2004 |
| 37 | 0.00 | 2004 | 230 | 0.03 | 2004 | 268 | 0.03 | 2004 | 317 | 0.04 | 2004 | 153 | 0.02 | 2004 | 1 502 | 0.17 | 2004 |
| 41 | 0.05 | 2004 | 17 | 0.02 | 2004 | 41 | 0.05 | 2004 | 63 | 0.08 | 2004 | 9 | 0.01 | 2004 | 272 | 0.34 | 2004 |
| 99 | 0.03 | 2004 | 9 | 0.00 | 2004 | 124 | 0.03 | 2004 | 554 | 0.15 | 2004 | 957 | 0.25 | 2004 | 987 | 0.26 | 2004 |
| 1 015 | 0.06 | 2004 | 155 | 0.01 | 2004 | ... | ... | | 1 165 | 0.07 | 2004 | 172 | 0.01 | 2004 | 2 107 | 0.12 | 2004 |
| 1 200 | 0.02 | 2004 | ... | ... | | ... | ... | | 512 | 0.01 | 2004 | 1 042 | 0.02 | 2004 | 15 013 | 0.28 | 2004 |
| 130 | 0.26 | 2004 | 18 | 0.04 | 2004 | 1 275 | 2.51 | 2004 | 75 | 0.15 | 2004 | ... | ... | | 74 | 0.15 | 2004 |
| 107 | 0.02 | 2004 | 88 | 0.02 | 2004 | ... | ... | | 248 | 0.06 | 2004 | 56 | 0.01 | 2004 | 765 | 0.18 | 2004 |
| 1 343 | 0.02 | 2003 | 1 347 | 0.02 | 2003 | 18 652 | 0.26 | 2003 | 2 703 | 0.04 | 2003 | 7 354 | 0.10 | 2003 | ... | ... | |
| 63 | 0.05 | 2004 | 150 | 0.11 | 2004 | ... | ... | | 276 | 0.20 | 2004 | 1 | 0.00 | 2004 | 144 | 0.11 | 2004 |
| 48 | 0.03 | 2003 | 33 | 0.02 | 2003 | 968 | 0.68 | 2003 | 99 | 0.07 | 2003 | 3 | 0.00 | 2003 | 391 | 0.27 | 2003 |
| 1 388 | 0.06 | 2004 | ... | ... | | ... | ... | | 899 | 0.04 | 2004 | 7 132 | 0.33 | 2004 | 19 151 | 0.90 | 2004 |
| 530 | 0.06 | 2004 | 135 | 0.02 | 2004 | 93 | 0.01 | 2004 | 268 | 0.03 | 2004 | 17 | 0.00 | 2004 | 511 | 0.06 | 2004 |
| 40 | 0.03 | 2004 | 13 | 0.01 | 2004 | 4 486 | 2.92 | 2004 | 230 | 0.15 | 2004 | 61 | 0.04 | 2004 | 38 | 0.02 | 2004 |
| 3 094 | 0.10 | 2004 | 6 496 | 0.20 | 2004 | ... | ... | | 7 000 | 0.22 | 2004 | 5 610 | 0.17 | 2004 | 1 797 | 0.06 | 2004 |
| 62 | 0.03 | 2003 | 55 | 0.03 | 2003 | ... | ... | | 146 | 0.08 | 2003 | 23 | 0.01 | 2003 | 18 | 0.01 | 2003 |
| 35 | 0.01 | 2004 | 150 | 0.04 | 2004 | 142 | 0.04 | 2004 | 218 | 0.06 | 2004 | 540 | 0.15 | 2004 | 518 | 0.15 | 2004 |
| 175 | 0.01 | 2004 | 130 | 0.01 | 2004 | 385 | 0.02 | 2004 | 172 | 0.01 | 2004 | 530 | 0.03 | 2004 | 6 036 | 0.34 | 2004 |
| ... | ... | | 26 | 0.00 | 2004 | ... | ... | | 46 | 0.00 | 2004 | 707 | 0.06 | 2004 | ... | ... | |
| 351 | 0.03 | 2004 | 231 | 0.02 | 2004 | 1 295 | 0.10 | 2004 | 264 | 0.02 | 2004 | 377 | 0.03 | 2004 | 652 | 0.05 | 2004 |
| 81 | 0.03 | 2004 | ... | ... | | 429 | 0.14 | 2004 | 106 | 0.04 | 2004 | 48 | 0.02 | 2004 | 1 056 | 0.35 | 2004 |
| 1 428 | 1.16 | 2004 | 238 | 0.19 | 2004 | 236 | 0.19 | 2004 | 324 | 0.26 | 2004 | 134 | 0.11 | 2004 | 2 038 | 1.65 | 2004 |
| 618 | 0.03 | 2004 | 564 | 0.03 | 2004 | ... | ... | | 941 | 0.05 | 2004 | 1 633 | 0.09 | 2004 | 9 517 | 0.50 | 2004 |
| 288 | 0.14 | 2004 | 240 | 0.12 | 2004 | ... | ... | | 481 | 0.24 | 2004 | 597 | 0.30 | 2004 | 7 782 | 3.87 | 2004 |
| 20 | 0.00 | 2004 | 268 | 0.02 | 2004 | ... | ... | | 294 | 0.02 | 2004 | 213 | 0.02 | 2004 | 513 | 0.04 | 2004 |
| 6 344 | 0.05 | 2004 | ... | ... | | 115 761 | 0.91 | 2004 | 690 | 0.01 | 2004 | 1 220 | 0.01 | 2004 | ... | ... | |
| 278 | 0.03 | 2004 | 101 | 0.01 | 2004 | 12 000 | 1.41 | 2004 | 39 | 0.00 | 2004 | 521 | 0.06 | 2004 | 1 419 | 0.17 | 2004 |
| 24 | 0.15 | 2004 | 19 | 0.12 | 2004 | 374 | 2.27 | 2004 | 51 | 0.31 | 2004 | 291 | 1.76 | 2004 | 288 | 1.75 | 2004 |
| 85 | 0.01 | 2004 | 705 | 0.07 | 2004 | ... | ... | | 66 | 0.01 | 2004 | 704 | 0.07 | 2004 | 564 | 0.05 | 2004 |
| 61 | 0.76 | 2004 | 77 | 0.96 | 2004 | ... | ... | | 59 | 0.74 | 2004 | 35 | 0.44 | 2004 | ... | ... | |
| 340 | 0.07 | 2004 | 130 | 0.03 | 2004 | 1 227 | 0.24 | 2004 | ... | ... | | ... | ... | | 4 | 0.00 | 2004 |
| 12 521 | 0.28 | 2004 | 2 529 | 0.06 | 2004 | 9 160 | 0.20 | 2004 | 1 968 | 0.04 | 2004 | 40 526 | 0.90 | 2004 | 28 005 | 0.62 | 2004 |
| 70 | 0.06 | 2004 | 110 | 0.10 | 2004 | 4 700 | 4.34 | 2004 | 78 | 0.07 | 2004 | 551 | 0.51 | 2004 | 374 | 0.35 | 2004 |
| 134 | 0.03 | 2004 | 289 | 0.06 | 2004 | 475 | 0.09 | 2004 | 528 | 0.11 | 2004 | 397 | 0.08 | 2004 | 1 335 | 0.27 | 2004 |
| 688 | 0.03 | 2004 | 1 042 | 0.04 | 2004 | ... | ... | | 1 702 | 0.06 | 2004 | 3 617 | 0.14 | 2004 | 6 499 | 0.24 | 2004 |
| 365 | 0.01 | 2002 | 1 831 | 0.05 | 2002 | ... | ... | | 1 520 | 0.04 | 2002 | 29 722 | 0.82 | 2002 | 689 | 0.02 | 2002 |
| 1 039 | 0.10 | 2004 | 1 027 | 0.09 | 2004 | ... | ... | | 1 415 | 0.13 | 2004 | 3 330 | 0.30 | 2004 | 10 853 | 0.99 | 2004 |
| 883 | 0.07 | 2004 | 1 803 | 0.14 | 2004 | ... | ... | | 917 | 0.07 | 2004 | 743 | 0.06 | 2004 | 581 | 0.04 | 2004 |

Figures computed to assure comparability;[a] they are not necessarily the official statistics of Member States, which may use alternative methods

| Member State | Total expenditure on health as % of gross domestic product | | | | | General government expenditure on health as % of total expenditure on health[b] | | | | | Private expenditure on health as % of total expenditure on health[b] | | | | | General government expenditure on health as % of total government expenditure | | | | |
|---|---|---|---|---|---|---|---|---|---|---|---|---|---|---|---|---|---|---|---|---|
| | 1999 | 2000 | 2001 | 2002 | 2003 | 1999 | 2000 | 2001 | 2002 | 2003 | 1999 | 2000 | 2001 | 2002 | 2003 | 1999 | 2000 | 2001 | 2002 | 2003 |
| 1 Algeria | 3.7 | 3.5 | 3.8 | 4.2 | 4.1 | 71.9 | 73.3 | 77.4 | 78.9 | 80.8 | 28.1 | 26.7 | 22.6 | 21.1 | 19.2 | 9 | 9 | 9.5 | 9.6 | 10 |
| 2 Angola | 3.2 | 2.5 | 3.3 | 2.4 | 2.8 | 45.3 | 82.2 | 84.6 | 80.9 | 84.2 | 54.7 | 17.8 | 15.4 | 19.1 | 15.8 | 2.4 | 3.4 | 5.5 | 4.1 | 5.3 |
| 3 Benin | 4.8 | 4.7 | 5 | 4.7 | 4.4 | 43.8 | 44.5 | 46.9 | 43.5 | 43.1 | 56.2 | 55.5 | 53.1 | 56.5 | 56.9 | 11.1 | 10 | 9.8 | 8 | 9.8 |
| 4 Botswana | 5.2 | 5.4 | 4.8 | 5.1 | 5.6 | 54.3 | 57.2 | 50.4 | 54 | 58.2 | 45.7 | 42.8 | 49.6 | 46 | 41.8 | 6.7 | 7.4 | 6 | 6.4 | 7.5 |
| 5 Burkina Faso | 5.4 | 5.2 | 5 | 5.4 | 5.6 | 44 | 42.4 | 39.5 | 44.2 | 46.8 | 56 | 57.6 | 60.5 | 55.8 | 53.2 | 10 | 9.4 | 10.5 | 12.8 | 12.7 |
| 6 Burundi | 3 | 3.1 | 3.1 | 3.1 | 3.1 | 19.9 | 17.9 | 21.6 | 21 | 23.3 | 80.1 | 82.1 | 78.4 | 79 | 76.7 | 2.8 | 2 | 2.2 | 2 | 2 |
| 7 Cameroon | 4.9 | 4.4 | 4.5 | 4.6 | 4.2 | 24.4 | 28 | 27.6 | 27.6 | 28.9 | 75.6 | 72 | 72.4 | 72.4 | 71.1 | 7.2 | 9.6 | 8 | 8.4 | 8 |
| 8 Cape Verde | 4.5 | 4.6 | 5 | 5 | 4.6 | 73.9 | 73.5 | 75.8 | 75.1 | 73.2 | 26.1 | 26.5 | 24.2 | 24.9 | 26.8 | 9 | 9.6 | 12.4 | 11.1 | 11.1 |
| 9 Central African Republic | 3.6 | 4 | 3.9 | 4 | 4 | 38 | 41.1 | 38.6 | 41.2 | 38.6 | 62 | 58.9 | 61.4 | 58.8 | 61.4 | 6.7 | 10 | 11.5 | 11.2 | 12.4 |
| 10 Chad | 6.1 | 6.7 | 6.8 | 6.3 | 6.5 | 33.6 | 42 | 40.9 | 35.5 | 39.9 | 66.4 | 58 | 59.1 | 64.5 | 60.1 | 11.9 | 13.1 | 13.8 | 9.4 | 10.5 |
| 11 Comoros | 3.2 | 2.7 | 2.3 | 2.9 | 2.7 | 60.8 | 54.9 | 47.7 | 58 | 54.1 | 39.2 | 45.1 | 52.3 | 42 | 45.9 | 10.5 | 9.5 | 5 | 6.4 | 6.4 |
| 12 Congo | 2.4 | 1.8 | 2 | 1.9 | 2 | 63.8 | 66.5 | 67 | 66.9 | 64.2 | 36.2 | 33.5 | 33 | 33.1 | 35.8 | 4.9 | 4.8 | 4.2 | 3.7 | 4.3 |
| 13 Côte d'Ivoire[c] | 5.1 | 4.7 | 3.9 | 3.8 | 3.6 | 17.4 | 19.8 | 18.3 | 31.6 | 27.6 | 82.6 | 80.2 | 81.7 | 68.4 | 72.4 | 4.5 | 5.2 | 4.3 | 6.2 | 5 |
| 14 Democratic Republic of Congo | 3.2 | 3.7 | 3.1 | 3.3 | 4 | 7.7 | 5.3 | 6.8 | 13.1 | 18.3 | 92.3 | 94.7 | 93.2 | 86.9 | 81.7 | 2.6 | 2.6 | 4.7 | 4.2 | 5.4 |
| 15 Equatorial Guinea | 2.8 | 2 | 1.7 | 1.8 | 1.5 | 60.8 | 67.6 | 70.2 | 72.2 | 67.5 | 39.2 | 32.4 | 29.8 | 27.8 | 32.5 | 9.9 | 11 | 10.1 | 8.8 | 7 |
| 16 Eritrea | 3.8 | 4.5 | 4.6 | 4.5 | 4.4 | 70.3 | 66.9 | 59.2 | 50.9 | 45.5 | 29.7 | 33.1 | 40.8 | 49.1 | 54.5 | 2.9 | 4.4 | 4.6 | 3.9 | 4 |
| 17 Ethiopia | 5.4 | 5.7 | 5.8 | 6 | 5.9 | 53 | 54.6 | 53.2 | 56.9 | 58.4 | 47 | 45.4 | 46.8 | 43.1 | 41.6 | 8.9 | 9.3 | 10.5 | 9.9 | 9.6 |
| 18 Gabon | 4.5 | 4.2 | 4.2 | 4.4 | 4.4 | 68.4 | 73.1 | 73 | 69.8 | 66.6 | 31.6 | 26.9 | 27 | 30.2 | 33.4 | 10.9 | 13.9 | 9.9 | 10.7 | 12.8 |
| 19 Gambia | 7 | 7.9 | 7.8 | 7.5 | 8.1 | 32.3 | 40.5 | 40.1 | 40.9 | 40 | 67.7 | 59.5 | 59.9 | 59.1 | 60 | 10 | 14.4 | 9.4 | 12 | 13.9 |
| 20 Ghana | 5.5 | 5.4 | 4.8 | 4.7 | 4.5 | 35.3 | 35.3 | 28.8 | 30.5 | 31.8 | 64.7 | 64.7 | 71.2 | 69.5 | 68.2 | 7.8 | 6.8 | 4.2 | 5.4 | 5 |
| 21 Guinea | 4.7 | 4.8 | 4.8 | 5.2 | 5.4 | 13.4 | 13.5 | 18.3 | 14.7 | 16.6 | 86.6 | 86.5 | 81.7 | 85.3 | 83.4 | 3.9 | 3.9 | 4.7 | 4.2 | 4.9 |
| 22 Guinea-Bissau | 4.8 | 4.1 | 4.3 | 6.2 | 5.6 | 29.7 | 23.7 | 21.3 | 40.8 | 45.8 | 70.3 | 76.3 | 78.7 | 59.2 | 54.2 | 4.6 | 2.2 | 2.1 | 6.6 | 6.9 |
| 23 Kenya | 4.6 | 4.3 | 4.2 | 4.5 | 4.3 | 41.1 | 46.5 | 42.8 | 44 | 38.7 | 58.9 | 53.5 | 57.2 | 56 | 61.3 | 4.1 | 11.1 | 8 | 9.2 | 7.2 |
| 24 Lesotho | 5.4 | 5.8 | 5.6 | 6.5 | 5.2 | 80.9 | 82.6 | 82 | 83.1 | 79.7 | 19.1 | 17.4 | 18 | 16.9 | 20.3 | 9.1 | 9.7 | 10.1 | 10.9 | 9.5 |
| 25 Liberia | 6.3 | 4.8 | 4.1 | 3.9 | 4.7 | 67.7 | 57.7 | 50.3 | 47.7 | 56.7 | 32.3 | 42.3 | 49.7 | 52.3 | 43.3 | 18.1 | 13 | 12.4 | 10.5 | 17.6 |
| 26 Madagascar | 2.2 | 2.1 | 1.9 | 2.8 | 2.7 | 53.7 | 53 | 64.7 | 63 | 63.4 | 46.3 | 47 | 35.3 | 37 | 36.6 | 6.9 | 6.5 | 7 | 11.4 | 9.3 |
| 27 Malawi | 9.8 | 8.6 | 10.5 | 9.4 | 9.3 | 36.9 | 30.2 | 45.2 | 34 | 35.2 | 63.1 | 69.8 | 54.8 | 66 | 64.8 | 12.2 | 7.5 | 11.7 | 9.1 | 9.1 |
| 28 Mali | 4 | 4.7 | 4.3 | 4.5 | 4.8 | 42.9 | 49.5 | 50.1 | 52.6 | 57.4 | 57.1 | 50.5 | 49.9 | 47.4 | 42.6 | 6.6 | 8.5 | 8.2 | 9 | 9.2 |
| 29 Mauritania | 2.7 | 2.5 | 2.9 | 3.9 | 4.2 | 64.2 | 63.3 | 67.9 | 74.2 | 76.8 | 35.8 | 36.7 | 32.1 | 25.8 | 23.2 | 8.6 | 6.5 | 6.8 | 9.2 | 14.3 |
| 30 Mauritius | 3.1 | 3.3 | 3.5 | 3.6 | 3.7 | 62 | 58.7 | 60.5 | 60.7 | 60.8 | 38 | 41.3 | 39.5 | 39.3 | 39.2 | 7.2 | 6.6 | 9 | 9.4 | 9.2 |
| 31 Mozambique | 4.7 | 5.5 | 4.8 | 5.1 | 4.7 | 63 | 67.8 | 66.2 | 67.6 | 61.7 | 37 | 32.2 | 33.8 | 32.4 | 38.3 | 12.1 | 12.9 | 10.7 | 11.5 | 10.9 |
| 32 Namibia | 7 | 7 | 6.4 | 5.9 | 6.4 | 73.3 | 68.9 | 69.4 | 68.6 | 70 | 26.7 | 31.1 | 30.6 | 31.4 | 30 | 13.1 | 12.3 | 11.1 | 11 | 12.4 |
| 33 Niger | 4.5 | 4.4 | 4.3 | 4.3 | 4.7 | 49.7 | 52.4 | 53.1 | 52.8 | 53 | 50.3 | 47.6 | 46.9 | 47.2 | 47 | 12.5 | 12.3 | 12 | 11.5 | 12.4 |
| 34 Nigeria | 5.4 | 4.3 | 5.3 | 5 | 5 | 29.1 | 33.5 | 31.4 | 25.6 | 25.5 | 70.9 | 66.5 | 68.6 | 74.4 | 74.5 | 5.4 | 4.2 | 3.2 | 3.1 | 3.2 |
| 35 Rwanda | 4.6 | 4.3 | 4.1 | 4.2 | 3.7 | 47.7 | 34.6 | 38.8 | 47 | 43.5 | 52.3 | 65.4 | 61.2 | 53 | 56.5 | 9.9 | 8 | 7.7 | 10.2 | 7.2 |
| 36 Sao Tome and Principe | 10 | 8.6 | 10.5 | 9 | 8.6 | 87.3 | 85.9 | 85.8 | 85 | 83.9 | 12.7 | 14.1 | 14.2 | 15 | 16.1 | 12.5 | 11.2 | 10.9 | 11.3 | 11.1 |
| 37 Senegal | 4.5 | 4.4 | 4.7 | 5 | 5.1 | 36.2 | 36.4 | 38.5 | 39.8 | 41.8 | 63.8 | 63.6 | 61.5 | 60.2 | 58.2 | 7.8 | 8.1 | 8 | 9.5 | 9.3 |
| 38 Seychelles | 5.3 | 5.2 | 5.1 | 5.1 | 5.9 | 74.8 | 75 | 74.7 | 74.9 | 73.2 | 25.2 | 25 | 25.3 | 25.1 | 26.8 | 6.9 | 6.8 | 8.1 | 7 | 10.2 |
| 39 Sierra Leone | 3.1 | 3.8 | 3.4 | 3.5 | 3.5 | 46.1 | 55.5 | 53.7 | 63.6 | 58.3 | 53.9 | 44.5 | 46.3 | 36.4 | 41.7 | 6.9 | 7.6 | 6.4 | 7.9 | 7.9 |
| 40 South Africa | 8.7 | 8.1 | 8.4 | 8.4 | 8.4 | 41.1 | 42.4 | 41.2 | 40.6 | 38.6 | 58.9 | 57.6 | 58.8 | 59.4 | 61.4 | 10.7 | 10.9 | 11.2 | 11.6 | 10.2 |
| 41 Swaziland | 6.4 | 6.1 | 6 | 5.9 | 5.8 | 59 | 58.6 | 57.8 | 59.3 | 57.3 | 41 | 41.4 | 42.2 | 40.7 | 42.7 | 11.8 | 11.6 | 11.3 | 10.9 | 10.9 |
| 42 Togo[d] | 5.4 | 4.6 | 5.4 | 4.9 | 5.6 | 40 | 29 | 25.2 | 18.7 | 24.8 | 60 | 71 | 74.8 | 81.3 | 75.2 | 12.4 | 7.5 | 8.6 | 6.9 | 9.3 |
| 43 Uganda | 6.3 | 6.6 | 7.3 | 7.6 | 7.3 | 30.6 | 26.8 | 27.3 | 31.1 | 30.4 | 69.4 | 73.2 | 72.7 | 68.9 | 69.6 | 9.4 | 9 | 9.6 | 10.8 | 10.7 |
| 44 United Republic of Tanzania | 4.3 | 4.4 | 4.5 | 4.5 | 4.3 | 43.4 | 48.1 | 48.5 | 51.6 | 55.4 | 56.6 | 51.9 | 51.5 | 48.4 | 44.6 | 12.4 | 12.6 | 12.8 | 12.8 | 12.7 |
| 45 Zambia | 5.7 | 5.5 | 5.8 | 6 | 5.4 | 48.8 | 50.6 | 56.5 | 56.7 | 51.4 | 51.2 | 49.4 | 43.5 | 43.3 | 48.6 | 9.5 | 9.1 | 10.2 | 10.6 | 11.8 |
| 46 Zimbabwe | 8.1 | 7.8 | 9.1 | 8.4 | 7.9 | 48.9 | 48.3 | 38.6 | 37.7 | 35.9 | 51.1 | 51.7 | 61.4 | 62.3 | 64.1 | 10 | 7.4 | 9.3 | 9.8 | 9.2 |

Equatorial Guinea, Gabon, Guinea Bissau, Liberia and Sao Tome and Principe: estimates for these countries should be read with caution as these are derived from limited sources (mostly macro data that are publicly accessible).

Burkina Faso, Guinea, Mauritius and Rwanda: new NHA reports, surveys, and/or country consultations provided new bases for the estimates.

[a] See explanatory notes for sources and methods.
[b] In some cases the sum of the ratios of general government and private expenditures on health may not add to 100 because of rounding.
[c] The series was adjusted for the removal of social security expenditure on health, which could not be confirmed due to incomplete information.
[d] Togo data on health research and development and training were adjusted to harmonize with the standard methodology used for World Health Reports.

n/a Used when the information accessed indicates that a cell should have an entry but no estimates could be made.
0 Used when no evidence of the schemes to which the cell relates exist. Some estimates yielding a ratio below 0.04% are shown as '0'.

| External resources for health as % of total expenditure on health | | | | | Social security expenditure on health as % of general government expenditure on health | | | | | Out-of-pocket expenditure as % of private expenditure on health | | | | | Private prepaid plans as % of private expenditure on health | | | | |
|---|---|---|---|---|---|---|---|---|---|---|---|---|---|---|---|---|---|---|---|
| 1999 | 2000 | 2001 | 2002 | 2003 | 1999 | 2000 | 2001 | 2002 | 2003 | 1999 | 2000 | 2001 | 2002 | 2003 | 1999 | 2000 | 2001 | 2002 | 2003 |
| 0.1 | 0.1 | 0.1 | 0 | 0 | 40.8 | 35.5 | 33.3 | 29.1 | 28.4 | 97 | 96.7 | 96 | 95.7 | 95.3 | 2.9 | 3.1 | 3.8 | 4.1 | 4.4 |
| 5.7 | 17.5 | 16.7 | 8.3 | 6.7 | 0 | 0 | 0 | 0 | 0 | 100 | 100 | 100 | 100 | 100 | 0 | 0 | 0 | 0 | 0 |
| 14.6 | 16.8 | 12.2 | 8.5 | 11.5 | n/a | n/a | n/a | n/a | n/a | 91 | 91 | 90.6 | 90.3 | 90.3 | 8.4 | 8.4 | 8.7 | 9 | 9 |
| 2.2 | 1.8 | 2.9 | 3.4 | 2.9 | n/a | n/a | n/a | n/a | n/a | 30.3 | 31.3 | 31.5 | 29.7 | 28.8 | 22.7 | 20.6 | 20 | 19.6 | 21.8 |
| 10.2 | 9.9 | 10.1 | 7 | 7.4 | 0.3 | 0.8 | 1.2 | 0.7 | 1 | 98.1 | 98.1 | 98.1 | 98.1 | 98.1 | 0.9 | 0.9 | 0.9 | 0.9 | 0.9 |
| 10.7 | 8 | 10.6 | 10.3 | 14.1 | n/a | n/a | n/a | n/a | n/a | 100 | 100 | 100 | 100 | 100 | n/a | n/a | n/a | n/a | n/a |
| 5.2 | 6 | 6.9 | 2.3 | 3.2 | 0.1 | 0.1 | 0.1 | 0.1 | 0.1 | 94.2 | 93.3 | 93.4 | 93.6 | 98.3 | n/a | n/a | n/a | n/a | n/a |
| 8.4 | 13.5 | 15.1 | 15.2 | 10 | 36.9 | 36.1 | 35.1 | 33.6 | 35.5 | 99.7 | 99.6 | 99.5 | 99.8 | 99.7 | 0.3 | 0.4 | 0.5 | 0.2 | 0.3 |
| 20 | 20 | 15.4 | 13.4 | 2.9 | n/a | n/a | n/a | n/a | n/a | 95.1 | 95.5 | 95.5 | 95.5 | 95.3 | n/a | n/a | n/a | n/a | n/a |
| 29.1 | 36.6 | 33.8 | 17 | 11.8 | n/a | n/a | n/a | n/a | n/a | 96.7 | 96.5 | 96.6 | 96.5 | 96.3 | 0.3 | 0.4 | 0.4 | 0.4 | 0.4 |
| 47.6 | 35.9 | 26.2 | 43 | 40.5 | 0 | 0 | 0 | 0 | 0 | 100 | 100 | 100 | 100 | 100 | 0 | 0 | 0 | 0 | 0 |
| 2.8 | 2.4 | 2.5 | 2.4 | 2.2 | 0 | 0 | 0 | 0 | 0 | 100 | 100 | 100 | 100 | 100 | n/a | n/a | n/a | n/a | n/a |
| 2.7 | 2.9 | 3.5 | 3.7 | 3.4 | n/a | n/a | n/a | n/a | n/a | 94 | 93.4 | 92.1 | 90.3 | 90.5 | 6 | 6.6 | 7.9 | 9.7 | 9.5 |
| 6 | 4.9 | 6.6 | 12.7 | 15.1 | 0 | 0 | 0 | 0 | 0 | 100 | 100 | 100 | 100 | 100 | n/a | n/a | n/a | n/a | n/a |
| 9.2 | 7.7 | 5.9 | 3.6 | 5.5 | 0 | 0 | 0 | 0 | 0 | 91.8 | 83.9 | 81.3 | 80.5 | 80.5 | 0 | 0 | 0 | 0 | 0 |
| 20.2 | 30.6 | 24.1 | 22.5 | 19.6 | 0 | 0 | 0 | 0 | 0 | 100 | 100 | 100 | 100 | 100 | 0 | 0 | 0 | 0 | 0 |
| 22.6 | 19.3 | 23.4 | 21.7 | 26 | 0.4 | 0.4 | 0.4 | 0.4 | 0.4 | 79.7 | 79.1 | 79.8 | 79.3 | 78.7 | 0.4 | 0.5 | 0.5 | 0.5 | 0.5 |
| 2.4 | 1 | 1.6 | 0.7 | 0.7 | 1.7 | 1.6 | 1.7 | 1.7 | 1.7 | 100 | 100 | 100 | 100 | 100 | n/a | n/a | n/a | n/a | n/a |
| 29.8 | 35.8 | 30.8 | 18.5 | 21.8 | 0 | 0 | 0 | 0 | 0 | 68.1 | 69.3 | 69.6 | 69.2 | 67 | n/a | n/a | n/a | n/a | n/a |
| 6.4 | 12.8 | 20.7 | 14.4 | 15.8 | n/a | n/a | n/a | n/a | n/a | 100 | 100 | 100 | 100 | 100 | 0 | 0 | 0 | 0 | 0 |
| 5.5 | 5.8 | 10.5 | 6.3 | 7.3 | 1.8 | 1.8 | 1.5 | 1.7 | 1.5 | 99.4 | 99.4 | 99.4 | 99.5 | 99.4 | 0 | 0 | 0 | 0 | 0 |
| 22.4 | 16 | 15.8 | 35.5 | 26.8 | 1.2 | 2.1 | 3 | 1.5 | 2.2 | 85.1 | 83.7 | 85.2 | 84.1 | 80.2 | 0 | 0 | 0 | 0 | 0 |
| 13.3 | 13.2 | 17.2 | 16.4 | 15.3 | 16.7 | 11.7 | 14.8 | 9.2 | 10 | 79.3 | 80.1 | 80.5 | 80 | 82.6 | 7.4 | 7.1 | 6.8 | 6.9 | 6 |
| 3.6 | 10.8 | 16.2 | 6.4 | 8.2 | 0 | 0 | 0 | 0 | 0 | 20 | 20 | 19.4 | 18.6 | 18.2 | n/a | n/a | n/a | n/a | n/a |
| 55.7 | 43.6 | 31.2 | 25.5 | 32.3 | 0 | 0 | 0 | 0 | 0 | 98.5 | 98.5 | 98.5 | 98.5 | 98.5 | 0 | 0 | 0 | 0 | 0 |
| 40.5 | 43.3 | 39.1 | 31.6 | 22 | n/a | n/a | n/a | n/a | n/a | 89.7 | 90.5 | 87.1 | 91.6 | 91.7 | 10.3 | 9.5 | 12.9 | 8.4 | 8.3 |
| 26.1 | 18.5 | 31 | 23 | 25.1 | 0 | 0 | 0 | 0 | 0 | 42.3 | 41.7 | 42 | 42.5 | 42.7 | 1.7 | 1.6 | 1.7 | 1.6 | 1.6 |
| 18.8 | 24.1 | 20.8 | 3.4 | 13.7 | 24 | 21.8 | 22.9 | 27.7 | 26 | 89.3 | 88.6 | 89.1 | 89.2 | 89.3 | 0 | 0 | 0 | 0 | 0 |
| 5.5 | 5.7 | 4.9 | 2.5 | 4.7 | 0 | 0 | 0 | 0 | 0 | 100 | 100 | 100 | 100 | 100 | 0 | 0 | 0 | 0 | 0 |
| 1.2 | 1.1 | 1.6 | 1.4 | 1 | 6.5 | 7.8 | 8.3 | 8.3 | 8.7 | 100 | 100 | 100 | 100 | 100 | n/a | n/a | n/a | n/a | n/a |
| 39.6 | 42.9 | 47.6 | 38.3 | 40.8 | 0 | 0 | 0 | 0 | 0 | 38.5 | 39 | 34.3 | 32 | 38.8 | 0.6 | 0.6 | 0.6 | 0.6 | 0.5 |
| 2.4 | 3.8 | 4 | 4.3 | 5.3 | 1.2 | 1.8 | 2 | 2 | 1.9 | 21.3 | 18.2 | 20.1 | 20.4 | 19.2 | 74.7 | 77.3 | 75.1 | 74.9 | 76 |
| 28.6 | 46.6 | 23.1 | 22.7 | 32.8 | 2.6 | 2.8 | 2.6 | 2.4 | 2.2 | 88.9 | 88 | 88.2 | 88.8 | 89.2 | 6.4 | 7.4 | 7.3 | 7 | 7.2 |
| 13.8 | 16.2 | 5.6 | 6.1 | 5.3 | 0 | 0 | 0 | 0 | 0 | 94.8 | 92.7 | 91.4 | 90.4 | 91.2 | 3.4 | 5.1 | 6.5 | 6.7 | 6.7 |
| 43 | 48.9 | 38.2 | 46.9 | 54.5 | 5.1 | 6.8 | 8.3 | 9 | 9.8 | 41.4 | 35.6 | 39.2 | 43.8 | 41.7 | 3.8 | 5.6 | 6.5 | 7.5 | 7.1 |
| 59.9 | 62.5 | 62.9 | 74.9 | 56 | 0 | 0 | 0 | 0 | 0 | 100 | 100 | 100 | 100 | 100 | 0 | 0 | 0 | 0 | 0 |
| 12.6 | 14 | 19.2 | 10.3 | 15.4 | 19 | 19.2 | 18.8 | 16.6 | 15.8 | 96.7 | 96.6 | 96.5 | 95.4 | 95.3 | 2.1 | 2.2 | 2.2 | 3.3 | 3.4 |
| 1.3 | 0.6 | 0.4 | 0.5 | 2 | 5.3 | 5.2 | 5.1 | 4.8 | 3.3 | 62.5 | 61.8 | 62.5 | 62.5 | 62.5 | 0 | 0 | 0 | 0 | 0 |
| 8.8 | 11.8 | 14.8 | 5.8 | 15.5 | 0 | 0 | 0 | 0 | 0 | 100 | 100 | 100 | 100 | 100 | 0 | 0 | 0 | 0 | 0 |
| 0.1 | 0.4 | 0.4 | 0.4 | 0.5 | 3.5 | 3.3 | 3.1 | 3.8 | 4.6 | 17.1 | 18.9 | 17.8 | 16.8 | 17.1 | 77.4 | 75.6 | 76.7 | 77.7 | 77.7 |
| 10.3 | 5.5 | 5.2 | 5.1 | 5.5 | 0 | 0 | 0 | 0 | 0 | 40.9 | 42.4 | 41.8 | 41.7 | 42.4 | 18.6 | 18.9 | 20 | 20 | 19.6 |
| 4.9 | 7.1 | 4.8 | 11.4 | 2.3 | 8.1 | 13.4 | 11.6 | 14.4 | 14.6 | 87 | 86.6 | 87.8 | 87.7 | 88 | 5.1 | 5.4 | 4.3 | 4.3 | 4.1 |
| 27.6 | 28.3 | 27.4 | 29.1 | 28.5 | 0 | 0 | 0 | 0 | 0 | 61.5 | 56.7 | 51.8 | 51 | 52.8 | 0.2 | 0.1 | 0.2 | 0.2 | 0.2 |
| 29.3 | 32.1 | 34.1 | 29.6 | 21.9 | 0 | 0 | 5 | 3.2 | 2.6 | 83.5 | 83.6 | 83.8 | 83.5 | 81.1 | 4.5 | 4.5 | 4.5 | 4.7 | 5.4 |
| 8.9 | 18.2 | 13.7 | 18.3 | 44.7 | 0 | 0 | 0 | 0 | 0 | 82 | 81.1 | 74.9 | 72.7 | 68.2 | n/a | n/a | n/a | n/a | n/a |
| 15.7 | 11.7 | 5.6 | 1.4 | 6.8 | 0 | 0 | 0 | 0 | 0 | 44.9 | 46.7 | 50.7 | 51.7 | 56.7 | 39.6 | 31.1 | 29 | 25.9 | 21 |

**Figures computed to assure comparability;[a] they are not necessarily the official statistics of Member States, which may use alternative methods**

| Member State | Per capita total expenditure on health at average exchange rate (US$) | | | | | Per capita total expenditure on health at international dollar rate | | | | | Per capita government expenditure on health at average exchange rate (US$) | | | | | Per capita government expenditure on health at international dollar rate | | | | |
|---|---|---|---|---|---|---|---|---|---|---|---|---|---|---|---|---|---|---|---|---|
| | 1999 | 2000 | 2001 | 2002 | 2003 | 1999 | 2000 | 2001 | 2002 | 2003 | 1999 | 2000 | 2001 | 2002 | 2003 | 1999 | 2000 | 2001 | 2002 | 2003 |
| 1 Algeria | 61 | 63 | 68 | 75 | 89 | 137 | 132 | 149 | 174 | 186 | 43 | 46 | 53 | 60 | 71 | 99 | 97 | 115 | 137 | 150 |
| 2 Angola | 15 | 16 | 21 | 18 | 26 | 43 | 34 | 48 | 41 | 49 | 7 | 13 | 18 | 15 | 22 | 20 | 28 | 41 | 33 | 41 |
| 3 Benin | 16 | 15 | 16 | 16 | 20 | 34 | 34 | 38 | 37 | 36 | 7 | 7 | 7 | 7 | 9 | 15 | 15 | 18 | 16 | 16 |
| 4 Botswana | 138 | 152 | 132 | 144 | 232 | 259 | 294 | 284 | 312 | 375 | 75 | 87 | 67 | 78 | 135 | 141 | 168 | 143 | 169 | 218 |
| 5 Burkina Faso | 15 | 12 | 12 | 15 | 19 | 55 | 54 | 55 | 62 | 68 | 6 | 5 | 5 | 6 | 9 | 24 | 23 | 22 | 27 | 32 |
| 6 Burundi | 4 | 3 | 3 | 3 | 3 | 14 | 14 | 15 | 15 | 15 | 1 | 1 | 1 | 1 | 1 | 3 | 3 | 3 | 3 | 4 |
| 7 Cameroon | 31 | 29 | 29 | 32 | 37 | 62 | 58 | 62 | 66 | 64 | 8 | 8 | 8 | 9 | 11 | 15 | 16 | 17 | 18 | 19 |
| 8 Cape Verde | 61 | 55 | 61 | 66 | 78 | 148 | 163 | 186 | 193 | 185 | 45 | 41 | 46 | 50 | 57 | 110 | 119 | 141 | 145 | 135 |
| 9 Central African Republic | 10 | 10 | 10 | 11 | 12 | 44 | 50 | 49 | 51 | 47 | 4 | 4 | 4 | 4 | 5 | 17 | 20 | 19 | 21 | 18 |
| 10 Chad | 11 | 11 | 12 | 12 | 16 | 37 | 40 | 43 | 44 | 51 | 4 | 4 | 5 | 4 | 7 | 12 | 17 | 18 | 16 | 20 |
| 11 Comoros | 11 | 8 | 7 | 10 | 11 | 30 | 25 | 21 | 27 | 25 | 6 | 4 | 3 | 6 | 6 | 18 | 14 | 10 | 16 | 14 |
| 12 Congo | 17 | 17 | 16 | 16 | 19 | 25 | 20 | 23 | 22 | 23 | 11 | 11 | 10 | 11 | 12 | 16 | 13 | 15 | 15 | 15 |
| 13 Côte d'Ivoire | 39 | 30 | 24 | 25 | 28 | 87 | 79 | 65 | 62 | 57 | 7 | 6 | 4 | 8 | 8 | 15 | 16 | 12 | 20 | 16 |
| 14 Democratic Republic of Congo | 8 | 10 | 4 | 3 | 4 | 12 | 13 | 10 | 11 | 14 | 1 | 1 | <1 | <1 | 1 | 1 | 1 | 1 | 1 | 3 |
| 15 Equatorial Guinea | 46 | 54 | 67 | 85 | 96 | 125 | 106 | 152 | 193 | 179 | 28 | 37 | 47 | 61 | 65 | 76 | 72 | 107 | 139 | 121 |
| 16 Eritrea | 8 | 8 | 8 | 7 | 8 | 47 | 48 | 53 | 51 | 50 | 6 | 5 | 5 | 4 | 4 | 33 | 32 | 31 | 26 | 23 |
| 17 Ethiopia | 5 | 5 | 5 | 5 | 5 | 17 | 19 | 21 | 21 | 20 | 3 | 3 | 3 | 3 | 3 | 9 | 10 | 11 | 12 | 12 |
| 18 Gabon | 165 | 164 | 148 | 158 | 196 | 250 | 229 | 235 | 244 | 255 | 113 | 120 | 108 | 111 | 130 | 171 | 167 | 171 | 171 | 170 |
| 19 Gambia | 24 | 25 | 23 | 20 | 21 | 76 | 88 | 92 | 84 | 96 | 8 | 10 | 9 | 8 | 8 | 24 | 36 | 37 | 34 | 38 |
| 20 Ghana | 22 | 13 | 12 | 14 | 16 | 100 | 102 | 94 | 95 | 98 | 8 | 5 | 4 | 4 | 5 | 35 | 36 | 27 | 29 | 31 |
| 21 Guinea | 20 | 18 | 17 | 19 | 22 | 74 | 76 | 81 | 90 | 95 | 3 | 2 | 3 | 3 | 4 | 10 | 10 | 15 | 13 | 16 |
| 22 Guinea-Bissau | 8 | 6 | 6 | 9 | 9 | 45 | 38 | 38 | 49 | 45 | 2 | 2 | 1 | 4 | 4 | 13 | 9 | 8 | 20 | 21 |
| 23 Kenya | 16 | 18 | 18 | 19 | 20 | 60 | 61 | 62 | 66 | 65 | 7 | 8 | 8 | 8 | 8 | 25 | 28 | 27 | 29 | 25 |
| 24 Lesotho | 28 | 28 | 24 | 25 | 31 | 91 | 100 | 103 | 125 | 106 | 23 | 23 | 20 | 21 | 25 | 74 | 83 | 84 | 104 | 84 |
| 25 Liberia | 10 | 8 | 7 | 7 | 6 | 26 | 23 | 21 | 20 | 17 | 6 | 5 | 3 | 3 | 4 | 18 | 13 | 10 | 10 | 10 |
| 26 Madagascar[b] | 5 | 5 | 5 | 7 | 8 | 20 | 20 | 19 | 24 | 24 | 3 | 3 | 3 | 5 | 5 | 11 | 10 | 12 | 15 | 15 |
| 27 Malawi | 16 | 13 | 15 | 15 | 13 | 47 | 41 | 48 | 44 | 46 | 6 | 4 | 7 | 5 | 5 | 17 | 12 | 22 | 15 | 16 |
| 28 Mali | 11 | 11 | 11 | 12 | 16 | 27 | 32 | 32 | 35 | 39 | 5 | 5 | 5 | 6 | 9 | 11 | 16 | 16 | 18 | 22 |
| 29 Mauritania | 10 | 9 | 10 | 14 | 17 | 32 | 32 | 38 | 53 | 59 | 7 | 6 | 7 | 10 | 13 | 21 | 20 | 26 | 39 | 46 |
| 30 Mauritius | 113 | 127 | 132 | 143 | 172 | 281 | 331 | 373 | 398 | 430 | 70 | 74 | 80 | 87 | 105 | 174 | 194 | 226 | 242 | 261 |
| 31 Mozambique | 11 | 12 | 10 | 11 | 12 | 34 | 40 | 39 | 45 | 45 | 7 | 8 | 6 | 7 | 7 | 21 | 27 | 26 | 30 | 28 |
| 32 Namibia | 127 | 126 | 107 | 95 | 145 | 328 | 340 | 323 | 318 | 359 | 93 | 87 | 75 | 65 | 101 | 240 | 235 | 224 | 218 | 252 |
| 33 Niger | 8 | 6 | 6 | 7 | 9 | 27 | 25 | 26 | 27 | 30 | 4 | 3 | 3 | 4 | 5 | 14 | 13 | 14 | 15 | 16 |
| 34 Nigeria | 17 | 18 | 19 | 19 | 22 | 48 | 39 | 50 | 49 | 51 | 5 | 6 | 6 | 5 | 6 | 14 | 13 | 16 | 12 | 13 |
| 35 Rwanda | 11 | 10 | 8 | 9 | 7 | 33 | 32 | 31 | 35 | 32 | 5 | 3 | 3 | 4 | 3 | 16 | 11 | 12 | 17 | 14 |
| 36 Sao Tome and Principe | 34 | 29 | 35 | 31 | 34 | 94 | 84 | 107 | 95 | 93 | 30 | 25 | 30 | 26 | 29 | 82 | 72 | 92 | 81 | 78 |
| 37 Senegal | 21 | 18 | 20 | 23 | 29 | 44 | 45 | 51 | 55 | 58 | 8 | 7 | 8 | 9 | 12 | 16 | 16 | 19 | 22 | 24 |
| 38 Seychelles | 431 | 405 | 403 | 456 | 522 | 548 | 555 | 535 | 554 | 599 | 322 | 304 | 301 | 342 | 382 | 410 | 417 | 400 | 415 | 439 |
| 39 Sierra Leone | 5 | 5 | 6 | 7 | 7 | 19 | 24 | 25 | 32 | 34 | 2 | 3 | 3 | 4 | 4 | 9 | 13 | 13 | 21 | 20 |
| 40 South Africa | 257 | 236 | 216 | 198 | 295 | 595 | 579 | 626 | 649 | 669 | 105 | 100 | 89 | 80 | 114 | 244 | 245 | 258 | 263 | 258 |
| 41 Swaziland | 87 | 83 | 73 | 68 | 107 | 305 | 302 | 308 | 315 | 324 | 51 | 48 | 42 | 40 | 61 | 180 | 177 | 178 | 187 | 185 |
| 42 Togo | 16 | 11 | 13 | 13 | 16 | 59 | 49 | 58 | 54 | 62 | 7 | 3 | 3 | 2 | 4 | 24 | 14 | 15 | 10 | 15 |
| 43 Uganda | 16 | 16 | 17 | 18 | 18 | 55 | 60 | 70 | 75 | 75 | 5 | 4 | 5 | 5 | 5 | 17 | 16 | 19 | 23 | 23 |
| 44 United Republic of Tanzania | 11 | 12 | 12 | 12 | 12 | 23 | 25 | 27 | 28 | 29 | 5 | 6 | 6 | 6 | 7 | 10 | 12 | 13 | 15 | 16 |
| 45 Zambia | 17 | 17 | 19 | 20 | 21 | 45 | 46 | 51 | 53 | 51 | 8 | 9 | 11 | 11 | 11 | 22 | 23 | 29 | 30 | 26 |
| 46 Zimbabwe | 36 | 44 | 65 | 132 | 40 | 185 | 168 | 184 | 161 | 132 | 17 | 21 | 25 | 50 | 14 | 91 | 81 | 71 | 61 | 47 |

[a] See explanatory notes for sources and methods.
[b] The currency now called Ariary is worth one fifth of the Francs previously used.

# Explanatory notes

The following provides the definition of the health statistics categories included in this statistical annex, as well as the rationale for including them and the estimation methods used to produce them.

## 1. Life expectancy at birth

Rationale for use: life expectancy at birth reflects the overall mortality level of a population. It summarizes the mortality pattern that prevails across all age groups — children and adolescents, adults and the elderly.

Definition: average number of years that a newborn is expected to live if current mortality rates continue to apply.

Methods of estimation: WHO has developed a model life table based on about 1800 life tables from vital registration judged to be of good quality. For countries with vital registration, the level of completeness of recorded mortality data in the population is assessed and mortality rates are adjusted accordingly. Where vital registration data for 2003 were available, these were used directly to construct the life table. For countries where the information system provided a time series of annual life tables, parameters from the life table were projected using a weighted regression model, giving more weight to recent years. Projected values of the two life table parameters were then applied to the modified logit life table model, where the most recent national data provided an age pattern, to predict the full life table for 2003. In case of inadequate sources of age-specific mortality rates, the life table is derived from estimated under-5 mortality rates and adult mortality rates that are applied to a global standard (defined as the average of all the 1800 life tables using a modified logit model.)

## 2. Healthy life expectancy (HALE)

Rationale for use: substantial resources are devoted to reducing the incidence, duration and severity of major diseases that cause morbidity but not mortality and to reducing their impact on people's lives. It is important to capture both fatal and non-fatal health outcomes in a summary measure of average levels of population health. Healthy life expectancy (HALE) at birth adds up expectation of life for different health states, adjusted for severity distribution making it sensitive to changes over time or differences between countries in the severity distribution of health states.

Definition: average number of years that a person can expect to live in "full health" by taking into account years lived in less than full health due to disease and/or injury.

Methods of estimation: since comparable health state prevalence data are not available for all countries, a four-stage strategy is used. Data from the WHOGBD study are used to estimate severity-adjusted prevalence by age and sex for all countries. Data from the WHOMCSS and WHS are used to make independent estimates of severity-adjusted prevalence by age and sex for survey countries. Prevalence for all countries is calculated based on GBD, MCSS and WHS estimates. Life tables constructed by WHO are used with Sullivan's method to compute HALE for countries.

## 3. Probability of dying (per 1000) between ages 15 and 60 years (adult mortality rate)

Rationale for use: disease burden from noncommunicable diseases among adults — the most economically productive age span — is rapidly increasing in developing countries due to ageing and health transitions. Therefore, the level of adult mortality is becoming an important indicator for the comprehensive assessment of the mortality pattern in a population.

Definition: probability that a 15-year-old person will die before reaching his/her 60th birthday.

## 4. Life table (see life expectancy at birth).

Data sources: civil or sample registration: Mortality by age and sex are used to calculate age specific rates. Census: Mortality by age and sex tabulated from questions on recent deaths that occurred in the household during a given period preceding the census (usually 12 months). Census or surveys: Direct or indirect methods provide adult mortality rates based on information on survival of parents or siblings.

Methods of estimation: empirical data from different sources are consolidated to obtain estimates of the level and trend in adult mortality by fitting a curve to the observed mortality points. However, to obtain the best possible estimates, judgement needs to be made on data quality and how representative it is of the population. Recent statistics based on data availability in most countries are point estimates dated by at least 3–4 years which need to be projected forward in order to obtain estimates of adult mortality for the current year. When no adequate source of age-specific mortality exists, the life table is derived as described in the life expectancy indicator.

## 5. Probability of dying (per 1000) under age five years (under-five mortality rate)

### Probability of dying (per 1000) under age one year (infant morality rate)

Rationale for use: under-five mortality rate and infant mortality rate are leading indicators of the level of child health and overall development in countries. They are also MDG indicators.

Definition: under-five mortality rate is the probability of a child born in a specific year or period dying before reaching the age of five, if subject to age-specific mortality rates of that period. Infant mortality rate is the probability of a child born in a specific year or period dying before reaching the age of one, if subject to age-specific mortality rates of that period.

Methods of estimation: empirical data from different sources are consolidated to obtain estimates of the level and trend in under-five mortality by fitting a curve to the observed mortality points. However, to obtain the best possible estimates, judgement needs to be made on data quality and how representative it is of the population. Recent statistics based on data availability in most countries are point estimates dated by at least 3–4 years which need to be projected forward in order to obtain estimates of under-five mortality for the current year. Those are then converted to their corresponding infant mortality rates through model life table systems: the one developed by WHO for countries with adequate vital registration data; Coale-Demeny model life tables for the other countries. It should be noted that the infant mortality from surveys are exposed to recall bias, hence their estimates are derived from under-five mortality, which leads to a supplementary step to estimate infant mortality rates.

### 6. Neonatal mortality rate (per 1000 live births)

Rationale for use: neonatal deaths account for a large proportion of child deaths. Mortality during neonatal period is considered a useful indicator of both maternal and newborn health and care.

Definition: number of deaths during the first 28 completed days of life per 1000 live births in a given year or period. Neonatal deaths may be subdivided into early neonatal deaths, occurring during the first seven days of life, and late neonatal deaths, occurring after the seventh day but before the 28 completed days of life.

### 7. Maternal mortality ratio (per 100 000 live births)

Rationale for use: complications during pregnancy and childbirth are leading causes of death and disability among women of reproductive age in developing countries. Maternal mortality ratio (MMR) represents the risk associated with each pregnancy, i.e. the obstetric risk. It is also an MDG indicator for monitoring goal 5 of improving maternal health.

Definition: number of maternal deaths per 100 000 live births during a specified time period, usually one year.

Methods of estimation: measuring maternal mortality accurately is difficult except where comprehensive registration of deaths and their causes exist. Elsewhere, censuses or surveys can be used to measure levels of maternal mortality. Data derived from health services records are problematic where not all births take place in health facilities because of biases whose dimensions and direction cannot be determined. Reproductive-age mortality studies (RAMOS) use triangulation of different sources of data on deaths of women of reproductive age including record review and/or verbal autopsy to accurately identify maternal deaths. Based on multiple sources of information, RAMOS are considered the best way to estimate levels of maternal mortality. Estimates derived from household surveys are usually based on information retrospectively collected about the deaths of sisters of the respondents and could refer back up to an average 12 years and they are subject to wide confidence intervals. For countries without any reliable data on maternal mortality, statistical models are applied. Global and regional estimates of maternal mortality are developed every five years, using a regression model.

### 8. Estimated rate of adults (15 years and older) dying of HIV/AIDS (per 1000)

### Estimated rate of children below 15 years of age dying of HIV/AIDS (per 1000)

Rationale for use: adult and children below 15 mortality rate are leading indicators of the level of impact of HIV/AIDS epidemic and impact of interventions specially scale up of treatment and prevention to mother to child transmission in countries.

Definition: estimated mortality due to HIV/AIDS is the number of adults and children that have died in a specific year based in the modeling of HIV surveillance data using standard and appropriate tools.

Methods of estimation: empirical data from different HIV surveillance sources are consolidated to obtain estimates of the level and trend in adults and children mortality by using standard methods and tools for HIV estimates appropriate to the level of HIV epidemic. However, to obtain the best possible estimates, judgement needs to be made on data quality and how representative it is of the population. UNAIDS/WHO produce country specific estimates every two years.

### 9. Tuberculosis mortality

Rationale for use: prevalence and mortality are direct indicators of the burden of tuberculosis (TB), indicating the number of people suffering from the disease at a given point in time, and the number dying each year. Furthermore, prevalence and mortality respond quickly to improvements in control, as timely and effective treatment reduce the average duration of disease (thus decreasing prevalence) and the likelihood of dying from the disease (thus reducing disease-specific mortality).

Definition: estimated number of deaths due to TB in given time period. Expressed in this database as deaths per 100 000 population per year. Includes deaths from all forms of TB, and deaths from TB in people with HIV.

Methods of estimation: estimates of TB incidence, prevalence and mortality are based on a consultative and analytical process in WHO and are published annually. The methods used to estimate TB mortality rates are described in detail elsewhere. Country-specific estimates of TB mortality are, in most instances, derived from estimates of incidence, combined with assumptions about the case fatality rate. The case fatality rate is assumed to vary according to whether the disease is smear-positive or not; whether the individual receives treatment in a DOTS programme or non-DOTS programmes, or is not treated at all; and whether the individual is infected with HIV.

### 10. Age-standardized death rates per 100 000 by cause

Rationale for use: the numbers of deaths per 100 000 population are influenced by the age distribution of the population. Two populations with the same age-specific mortality rates for a cause of death will have different overall death rates if the age distributions of their populations are different. Age-standardized mortality rates adjust for differences in population age distribution by applying the observed age-specific mortality rates for each population to a standard population.

Definition: the age-standardized mortality rate is a weighted average of the age-specific mortality rates per 100 000 persons, where the weights are the proportions of persons in the corresponding age groups of the WHO standard population.

### 11. Years of life lost (percentage of total)

Rationale for use: years of life are lost (YLL) take into account the age at which deaths occur by giving greater weight to deaths at younger age and lower weight to deaths at older age. The years of life lost (percentage of total) indicator measures the YLL due to a cause as a proportion of the total YLL lost in the population due to premature mortality.

Definition: YLL are calculated from the number of deaths multiplied by a standard life expectancy at the age at which death occurs. The standard life expectancy used for YLL at each age is the same for deaths in all regions of the world and is the same as that used for the calculation of disability-adjusted-life-years (DALY). Additionally 3% time discounting and non-uniform age weights which give less weight to years lived at young and older ages were used as for the DALY. With non-uniform age weights and 3% discounting, a death in infancy corresponds to 33 YLL, and deaths at ages 5 to 20 to around 36 YLL.

### 12. The disability-adjusted-life-year or DALY

DALY is a health gap measure that extends the concept of potential years of life lost due to premature death (PYLL) to include equivalent years of "healthy" life lost by virtue of being in states of poor health or disability (1). DALYs for a disease or health condition are calculated as the sum of the years of life lost due to premature mortality (YLL) in the population and the years lost due to disability (YLD) for incident cases of the health condition.

Methods of estimation: life tables specifying all-cause mortality rates by age and sex for 192 WHO Member States were developed for 2002 from available death registration data, sample registration systems (India, China) and data on child and adult mortality from censuses and surveys. Cause of death distributions were estimated from death registration data for 107 countries, together with data from population-based epidemiological studies, disease registers and notifications systems for selected specific causes of death. Causes of death for populations without useable death registration data were estimated using cause-of-death models together with data from population-based epidemiological studies, disease registers and notifications systems for 21 specific causes of death.

## 13. Causes of death among children under five years of age (percentage)

Rationale for use: MDG4 consists in the reduction of under-five mortality by two-thirds in 2015, from its level in 1990. Child survival efforts can be effective only if they are based on reasonably accurate information about the causes of childhood deaths. Cause-of-death information is needed to prioritize interventions and plan for their delivery, to determine the effectiveness of disease-specific interventions, and to assess trends in disease burden in relation to national and international goals.

Definition: the cause(s) of death (CoD) as entered on the medical certificate of cause of death in countries with civil (vital) registration system. The underlying CoD is being analysed. In countries with incomplete or no civil registration, causes of death are those reported as such in epidemiological studies that use verbal autopsy algorithms to establish CoD.

Methods of estimation: CoD data from civil registration systems were evaluated for their completeness. Complete and nationally-representative data were then grouped by ICD codes into the cause categories and their proportions to total under-five deaths were then computed. For countries with incomplete data or no data, the distribution of deaths by cause was estimated in two steps. In the first step, a statistical model was used to assign deaths to one of three broad categories of causes: communicable diseases; noncommunicable diseases; or injuries and external causes.

In a second step, cause specific under five mortality estimates from Child Health Epidemiology Reference Group (CHERG), WHO Technical Programmes, and the Joint United Nations Programme on HIV/AIDS (UNAIDS) were taken into account in assigning the distribution of deaths to specific causes. A variety of methods, including proportional mortality and natural history models, were used by CHERG and WHO to develop country-level cause-specific mortality estimates. All CHERG working groups developed comparable and standardized procedures to generate estimates from the databases.

## 14. HIV prevalence among the population aged 15–49 years

Rationale for use: HIV and AIDS has become a major public health problem in many countries and monitoring the course of the epidemic and impact of interventions is crucial. Both the Millenium Development Goals (MDG) and the United Nations General Assembly Special Session on HIV and AIDS (UNGAS) have set goals of reducing HIV prevalence.

Definition: percent of people with HIV infection among all people aged 15–49 years.

Methods of estimation: HIV prevalence data from HIV sentinel surveillance systems, which may include national population surveys with HIV testing, are used to estimate HIV prevalence using standardized tools and methods of estimation developed by UNAIDS and WHO in collaboration with the UNAIDS Reference Group on Estimation, Modelling and Projections. Tools for estimating the level of HIV infection are different for generalized epidemics, and concentrated or low level epidemic.

## 15. Incidence of tuberculosis

Rationale for use: incidence (cases arising in a given time period) gives an indication of the burden of tuberculosis (TB) in a population, and of the size of the task faced by a national TB control programme. Incidence can change as the result of changes in transmission (the rate at which people become infected with *M. tuberculosis*, the bacterium which causes TB), or changes in the rate at which people infected with *M. tuberculosis* develop TB disease (e.g. as a result of changes in nutritional status or of HIV infection). Because TB can develop in people who became infected many years previously, the effect of TB control on incidence is less immediate than the effect on prevalence or mortality. Millennium Development Goal 6, Target 8 is "have halted by 2015 and begun to reverse the incidence of" TB. WHO estimates that in 2004 the per capita incidence of TB was stable or falling in 5 out of 6 WHO regions, but growing globally at 0.6% per year. The exception was the African Region, where incidence is apparently still increasing, but less rapidly each year. Implementation of the Stop TB Strategy, following the Global Plan to Stop TB 2006–2015, is expected to reverse the rise in incidence globally by 2015.

Definition: estimated number of TB cases arising in a given time period (expressed as per capita rate). All forms of TB are included, as are cases in people with HIV.

Methods of estimation: estimates of TB incidence, prevalence and mortality are based on a consultative and analytical process in WHO and are published annually. Estimates of incidence for each country are derived using one or more of four approaches, depending on the available data:

1. incidence = case notifications / proportion of cases detected

2. incidence = prevalence / duration of condition

3. incidence = annual risk of TB infection x Stýblo coefficient

4. incidence = deaths / proportion of incident cases that die.

## 16. Prevalence of tuberculosis

Rationale for use: prevalence and mortality are direct indicators of the burden of tuberculosis (TB), indicating the number of people suffering from the disease at a given point in time, and the number dying each year. Furthermore, prevalence and mortality respond quickly to improvements in control, as timely and effective treatment reduce the average duration of disease (thus decreasing prevalence) and the likelihood of dying from the disease (thus reducing disease-specific mortality). Millennium Development Goal 6 is "to combat HIV/AIDS, malaria and other diseases" [including TB]. This goal is linked to Target 8 – "to have halted by 2015 and begun to reverse the incidence of malaria and other major diseases" – and indicator 24 – "prevalence and mortality rates associated with TB". The Stop TB Partnership has endorsed the related targets of reducing per capita TB prevalence and mortality by 50% relative to 1990, by the year 2015. There are few good data with which to establish TB prevalence and mortality, particularly for the baseline year of 1990. However, current best estimates suggest that implementation of the Global Plan to Stop TB 2006–2015 will halve 1990 prevalence and mortality rates globally and in most regions by 2015, though not in Africa and eastern Europe.

Definition: the number of cases of TB (all forms) in a population at a given point in time (sometimes referred to as "point prevalence") expressed in this database as number of cases per 100 000 population.

Methods of estimation: estimates of TB incidence, prevalence and mortality are based on a consultative and analytical process in WHO and are published annually. The methods used to estimate TB prevalence and mortality rates are described in detail elsewhere. Country-specific estimates of prevalence are, in most instances, derived from estimates of incidence [please link to incidence page of compendium], combined with assumptions about the duration of disease. The duration of disease is assumed to vary according to whether the disease is smear-positive or not; whether the individual receives treatment in a DOTS programme, non-DOTS programmes, or is not treated at all; and whether the individual is infected with HIV.

### 17. Number of poliomyelitis cases

Rationale for use: the 1988 World Health Assembly (WHA) called for the global eradication of poliomyelitis. The number of poliomyelitis cases is used to monitor progress towards this goal and to inform eradication strategies. Countries implement strategies supplementing routine immunization e.g. national immunization days and sub-national campaigns – or more targeted mop-up activities, depending on the levels of poliomyelitis cases.

Definition: suspected polio cases (acute-flaccid paralysis – AFP, other paralytic diseases, and contacts with polio cases) that are confirmed by laboratory examination or are consistent with polio infection.

Methods of estimation: estimates of polio cases are based exclusively on unadjusted surveillance data.

### 18. One-year-olds immunized with:

**one dose of measles (%)**

**three doses of diphtheria, tetanus toxoid and pertussis (DTP3) (%)**

**three doses of hepatitis B (HepB3 )(%)**

Rationale for use: immunization coverage estimates are used to monitor immunization services, to guide disease eradication and elimination efforts, and are a good indicator of health systems performance.

Definition: measles immunization coverage is the percentage of one-year-olds who have received at least one dose of measles containing vaccine in a given year. For countries recommending the first dose of measles among children older than 12 months of age, the indicator is calculated as the proportion of children less than 24 months of age receiving one dose of measles containing vaccine. DTP3 immunization coverage is the percentage of one-year-olds who have received three doses of the combined diphtheria and tetanus toxoid and pertussis vaccine in a given year. HepB3 immunization coverage is the percentage of one-year-olds who have received three doses of Hepatitis B3 vaccine in a given year.

Methods of estimation: WHO and UNICEF rely on reports from countries, household surveys and other sources such as research studies. Both organizations have developed common review process and estimation methodologies. Draft estimates are made, reviewed by country and external experts and then finalized.

### 19. Antenatal care coverage (%)

Rationale for use: antenatal care coverage is an indicator of access and utilization of health care during pregnancy.

Definition: percentage of women who utilized antenatal care provided by skilled health personnel for reasons related to pregnancy at least once during pregnancy as a percentage of live births in a given time period.

Methods of estimation: empirical data from household surveys are used. At global level, facility data are not used.

### 20. Births attended by skilled health personnel (%)

Rationale for use: all women should have access to skilled care during pregnancy and at delivery to ensure detection and management of complications. Moreover, because it is difficult to measure accurately maternal mortality and model-based maternal mortality ratio (MMR) estimates cannot be used for monitoring short -term trends. The proportion of births attended by skilled health personnel is used as a proxy indicator for this purpose.

Definition: percentage of live births attended by skilled health personnel in a given period of time.

Methods of estimation: empirical data from household surveys are used. At global level, facility data are not used.

### 21. Contraceptive prevalence (%)

Rationale for use: contraceptive prevalence is an indicator of health, population, development and women's empowerment. It also serves as a proxy measure of access to reproductive health services that are essential for meeting many of the Millennium Development Goals (MDG)s, especially the child mortality, maternal health HIV/AIDS, and gender related goals.

Definition: contraceptive prevalence is the proportion of women of reproductive age who are using (or whose partner is using) a contraceptive method at a given point in time

Methods of estimation: empirical data only.

### 22. Children under five years of age sleeping under insecticide-treated nets (%)

Rationale for use: in areas of intense malaria transmission, malaria-related morbidity and mortality are concentrated in young children, and the use of insecticide-treated nets (ITN) by children under 5 years of age has been demonstrated to considerably reduce malaria disease incidence, malaria-related anaemia and all-cause under-5 mortality. Vector control through the use of ITNs constitute one of the four intervention strategies of the Roll Back Malaria Initiative. It is also listed as an MDG indicator.

Definition: percentage of children under five years of age in malaria endemic areas who slept under an ITN the previous night, ITN being defined as a mosquito net that has been treated within 12 months or is a long-lasting insecticidal net (LLIN).

Methods of estimation: empirical data only.

### 23. People with advanced HIV infection receiving antiretroviral (ARV) combination therapy (%)

Rationale for use: as the HIV epidemic matures, increasing numbers of people are reaching advanced stages of HIV infection. ARV combination therapy has been shown to reduce mortality among those infected and efforts are being made to make it more affordable even in less developed countries. This indicator assesses the progress in providing ARV combination therapy to everyone with advanced HIV infection.

Definition: percentage of people with advanced HIV infection receiving ARV therapy according to nationally approved treatment protocol (or WHO/Joint UN Programme on HIV and AIDS standards) among the estimated number of people with advanced HIV infection.

Methods of estimation: the denominator of the coverage estimate is obtained from models that also generate the HIV prevalence, incidence and mortality estimates. The number of adults with advanced HIV infection who need to start treatment is estimated as the number of AIDS cases in the current year times two. The total number of adults needing ARV therapy is calculated by adding the number of adults that need to start ARV therapy to the number of adults who are being treated in the previous year and have survived into the current year.

## 24. Tuberculosis: DOTS case detection rate

Rationale for use: the proportion of estimated new smear-positive cases which are detected (diagnosed and notified to WHO) by DOTS programmes provides an indication of how effective national tuberculosis programmes are in finding people with tuberculosis and diagnosing the disease.

Methods of estimation: estimates of incidence are based on a consultative and analytical process in WHO and are published annually. The DOTS detection rate for new smear-positive cases is calculated by dividing the number of new smear-positive cases notified to WHO by the estimated number of incident smear-positive cases for the same year.

## 25 . Tuberculosis: DOTS treatment success

Rationale for use: treatment success is an indicator of the performance of national tuberculosis control programmes. In addition to the obvious benefit to individual patients, successful treatment of infectious cases of TB is essential to prevent the spread of the infection. Detecting and successfully treating a large proportion of TB cases should have an immediate impact on TB prevalence and mortality. By reducing transmission, successfully treating the majority of cases will also affect, with some delay, the incidence of disease.

Definition: the proportion of new smear-positive TB cases registered under DOTS in a given year that successfully completed treatment, whether with bacteriologic evidence of success ("cured") or without ("treatment completed"). At the end of treatment, each patient is assigned one of the following six mutually exclusive treatment outcomes: cured; completed; died; failed; defaulted; and transferred out with outcome unknown. The proportions of cases assigned to these outcomes, plus any additional cases registered for treatment but not assigned to an outcome, add up to 100% of cases registered.

## 26. Children under five years of age with acute respiratory infection and fever (ARI) taken to facility

Rationale for use: respiratory infections are responsible for almost 20% of all under-five deaths worldwide. Under-fives with ARI that are taken to an appropriate health provider is a key indicator for both coverage of intervention and care-seeking and provides critical inputs to the monitoring of progress towards the child survival related millennium development goals (MDGs) and strategies.

Definition: proportion of children aged 0-59 months who had presumed pneumonia (ARI) in the last two weeks and were taken to an appropriate health provider.

Methods of estimation: empirical data.

## 27. Children under five years of age with diarrhoea who received ORT

Rationale for use: diarrhoeal diseases remain one of the major causes of under-five mortality, accounting for 1.8 million child deaths worldwide, despite all the progress in its management and the undeniable success of the oral rehydration therapy (ORT). Therefore, the monitoring of the coverage of this very cost-effective intervention is crucial for the monitoring of progress towards the child survival related Millennium Development Goals (MDGs) and strategies.

Definition: proportion of children aged 0–59 months of age who had diarrhoea in the last two weeks and were treated with oral rehydration salts or an appropriate household solution (ORT)

Methods of estimation: empirical data.

## 28. Children under five years of age with fever who received treatment with any antimalarial (%)

Rationale for use: prompt treatment with effective anti-malaria drugs for children with fever in malaria risk areas is a key intervention to reduce mortality. In addition to be listed as a global MDG indicator under Goal 6, malaria effective treatment is also identified by WHO, UNICEF, and the World Bank as one of the four main interventions to reduce the burden of malaria in Africa: (i) use of insecticide-treated nets (ITNs), (ii) prompt access to effective treatments in or near the home, (iii) providing antimalarial drugs to symptom-free pregnant women in stable transmission areas, and (iv) improved forecasting, prevention and response, essential to respond quickly and effectively to malaria epidemics. In areas of sub-Saharan Africa with stable levels of malaria transmission, it is essential that access to prompt treatment is ensured. This requires drug availability at household or community level and, for complicated cases, availability of transport to the nearest equipped facility. Reserve drug stocks, transport, and hospital capacity are needed to mount an appropriate response to malaria cases and prevent the onset of malaria to degenerate to a highly lethal complicated malaria picture.

Definition: percentage of population under five years of age in malaria-risk areas with fever being treated with effective antimalarial drugs:

Methods of estimation: for prevention, the indicator is calculated as the percentage of children under five years of age who received effective anti-malaria drugs upon a fever episode. The information is obtained directly from household surveys. The empiric values are directly reported without further estimation.

## 29. Children 6–59 months of age who received vitamin A supplementation

Rationale for use: vitamin A supplementation is considered a critically important intervention for child survival due to the strong evidence that exists of its impact on child mortality. Therefore, measuring the proportion of children who have received vitamin A in the last six months is crucial for monitoring coverage of interventions towards the child survival related MDGs and strategies.

Definition: proportion of children 6–59 months of age who have received a high dose vitamin A supplement in the last 6 months

Methods of estimation: empirical data.

## 30. Births by caesarean section (%)

Rationale for use: births by caesarean section is an indicator of access to and utilization of health care during childbirth.

Definition: percentage of births by caesarean section among all live births in a given time period.

Methods of estimation: empirical data from household surveys are used.

## 31. Children under five years of age

- stunted for age (%)
- underweight for age (%)
- overweight for age (%)

Rationale for use: all three indicators measure growth in young children. Child growth is internationally recognized as an important public health indicator for monitoring nutritional status and health in populations. In addition, children who suffer from growth retardation as a result of poor diets and/or recurrent infections tend to have greater risks of illness and death.

Definition: percentage of children stunted describes how many children under five years old have a height-for-age below minus two standard deviations of the National Center for Health Statistics (NCHS)/WHO reference median. Percentage of children underweight describes how many children under five years have a weight-for-age below minus two standard deviations of the NCHS/WHO reference median. Percentage of children overweight describes how many children under five years have a weight-for-height above two standard deviations of the NCHS/WHO reference median.

Methods of estimation: empirical values are used. Several countries have limited data for recent years and current estimations are made using models that make projections based on past trends.

## 32. Newborns with low birth weight (%)

Rationale for use: the low-birth-weight rate at the population level is an indicator of a public health problem that includes long-term maternal malnutrition, ill-health and poor health care. On an individual basis, low birth weight is an important predictor of newborn health and survival.

Definition: percentage of live born infants with birth weight less than 2500 g* in a given time period. Low birth weight may be subdivided into very low birth weight (less than 1500 g) and extremely low birth weight (less than 1000 g).

Methods of estimation: where reliable health service statistics with a high level of coverage exist : "Percentage of low birth weight" births. For household survey data different adjustments are made according to the type of information available (numerical birth weight data or subjective assessment of the mother).

## 33. Prevalence of adults (15 years and older) who are obese (%)

Rationale for use: the prevalence of overweight and obesity in adults has been increasing globally. Obese adults (BMI = 30.0) are at increased risk of adverse metabolic outcomes including increased blood pressure, cholesterol, triglycerides, and insulin resistance. Subsequently, an increase in BMI exponentially increases the risk of noncommunicable diseases (NCDs), such as coronary heart disease, ischaemic stroke and type-2 diabetes mellitus. Raised BMI is also associated with an increased risk of cancer.

Definition: percentage of adults classified as obese (BMI = 30.0 kg/m²) among total adult population (15 years and older).

Methods of estimation: estimates are still under development and will be published later in 2006. Only nationally representative surveys with either anthropometric data collection or self-reported weight and height (mostly in high income countries) are included in the 2006 *World health statistics*.

## 34. Population with:

- **sustainable access to an improved water source (%)**
- **access to improved sanitation (%)**

Rationale for use: access to drinking water and improved sanitation is a fundamental need and a human right vital for the dignity and health of all people. The health and economic benefits of improved water supply to households and individuals (especially children) are well documented. Both indicators are used to monitor progress towards the MDGs.

Definition: access to an improved water source is the percentage of population with access to an improved drinking water source in a given year. Access to improved sanitation is the percentage of population with access to improved sanitation in a given year.

Methods of estimation: estimates are generated through analysis of survey data and linear regression of data points. Coverage estimates are updated every two years.

## 35. Population using solid fuels (%)

Rationale for use: the use of solid fuels in households is associated with increased mortality from pneumonia and other acute lower respiratory diseases among children as well as increased mortality from chronic obstructive pulmonary disease and lung cancer (where coal is used) among adults. It is also a Millennium Development Goal indicator.

Definition: percentage of population using solid fuels.

Methods of estimation: the data from surveys and censuses are used as reported in the surveys and censuses. All countries with a Gross National Income (GNI) per capita above US$ 10 500 are assumed to have made a complete transition to cooking with non-solid fuels. For low- and middle-income countries with a GNI per capita below US$ 10 500 and for which no household solid fuel use data are available, a regression model based on GNI, percentage of rural population and location or non-location within the Eastern Mediterranean Region is used to estimate the indicator.

## 36. Prevalence of current tobacco use in adolescents (13–15 years of age)

Rationale for use: the risk of chronic diseases starts early in childhood and such behaviour continues to adulthood. Tobacco is an addictive substance and smoking often starts in adolescence, before the development of risk perception. By the time the risk to health is recognized, the addicted individuals find it difficult to stop tobacco use.

Definition: prevalence of tobacco use (including smoking, oral tobacco and snuff) on more than one occasion in the 30 days preceding the survey, among adolescent 13–15 year olds.

### 37. Prevalence of current (daily or occasional) tobacco smoking among adults (15 years and older) (%)

Rationale for use: prevalence of current tobacco smoking among adults is an important measure of the health and economic burden of tobacco, and provides a baseline for evaluating the effectiveness of tobacco control programmes over time. While a more general measure of tobacco use, including both smoked and smokeless products, would be ideal, data limitations restrict the present indicator to smoked tobacco. Occasional tobacco smoking constitutes a significant risk factor for tobacco-related disease, and is therefore included along with daily tobacco smoking.

Definition: prevalence of current tobacco smoking (including cigarettes, cigars, pipes or any other smoked tobacco products). Current smoking includes both daily and non-daily or occasional smoking.

Methods of estimation: empirical data only.

### 38. Condom use at higher risk sex among young people aged 15–24 years (percentage)

Rationale for use: consistent correct use of condoms within non-regular sexual partnerships substantially reduces the risk of sexual HIV transmission.

Definition: percentage of young people aged 15–24 years reporting the use of a condom during the last sexual intercourse with a non-regular partner among those who had sex with a non-regular partner in the last 12 months.

Methods of estimation: empirical data only. Survey respondents aged 15-24 years are asked whether they have commenced sexual activity. Those who report sexual activity and have had sexual intercourse with a non-regular partner in the last 12 months, are further asked about the number of non-regular partners and condom use the last time they had sex with a non-regular partner.

### 39. Number of:

-physicians per 1000 population

-nurses per 1000 population

-midwives per 1000 population

-dentists per 1000 population

-pharmacists per 1000 population

-public and environmental health workers per 1000 population

-community health workers per 1000 population

-laboratory health workers per 1000 population

-other health workers per 1000 population

-health management and support workers per 1000 population

Rationale for use: the availability and composition of human resources for health is an important indicator of the strength of the health system. Even though there is no consensus about the optimal level of health workers for a population, there is ample evidence that worker numbers and quality are positively associated with immunization coverage, outreach of primary care, and infant, child and maternal survival.

Definition:

**Physicians**: includes generalists and specialists.

**Nurses**: includes professional nurses, auxiliary nurses, enrolled nurses and other nurses, such as dental nurses and primary care nurses.

**Midwives**: includes professional midwives, auxiliary midwives and enrolled midwives. Traditional birth attendants, who are counted as community health workers, appear elsewhere.

**Dentists:** includes dentists, dental assistants and dental technicians.

**Pharmacists:** includes pharmacists, pharmaceutical assistants and pharmaceutical technicians.

**Laboratory health workers:** includes laboratory scientists, laboratory assistants, laboratory technicians and radiographers.

**Environment and public health workers:** includes environmental and public health officers, sanitarians, hygienists, environmental and public health technicians, district health officers, malaria technicians, meat inspectors, public health supervisors and similar professions.

**Community health workers:** includes traditional medicine practitioners, faith healers, assistant/community health education workers, community health officers, family health workers, lady health visitors, health extension package workers, community midwives, institution-based personal care workers and traditional birth attendants.

**Other health workers:** includes a large number of occupations such as dieticians and nutritionists, medical assistants, occupational therapists, operators of medical and dentistry equipment, optometrists and opticians, physiotherapists, podiatrists, prosthetic/orthetic engineers, psychologists, respiratory therapists, speech pathologists, medical trainees and interns.

**Health management and support workers:** includes general managers, statisticians, lawyers, accountants, medical secretaries, gardeners, computer technicians, ambulance staff, cleaning staff, building and engineering staff, skilled administrative staff and general support staff.

Methods of estimation: no methods of estimation have been developed.

### 40. Total expenditure on health as percentage of GDP

### 41. General government expenditure on health as percentage of total general government expenditure

### 42. Per capita total expenditure on health at international dollar rate

Rationale for use: health financing is a critical component of health systems. National health accounts (NHA) provide large set of indicators based on the expenditure information collected within a internationally recognized framework. NHA are a synthesis of the financing and spending flows recorded in the operation of a health system, from funding sources to the distribution of funds across providers and functions of health systems and benefits across geographical, demographic, socioeconomic and epidemiological dimensions.

Definition: total health expenditure as percentage of gross domestic product (GDP).

Percentage of total general government expenditure that is spent on health.

Per capita total expenditure on health at international dollar rate.

Data sources & Methods of estimation.

Only about 95 countries either have produced full NHA or report expenditure on health to OECD. Standard accounting estimation and extrapolation techniques have been used to provide time series. The principal international references used are the International Monetary Fund (IMF) Government finance statistics and International financial statistics; OECD health data and International development statistics; and the United Nations National accounts statistics. National sources include: national health accounts reports, public expenditure reports, statistical yearbooks and other periodicals, budgetary documents, national accounts reports, statistical data on official web sites, central bank reports, nongovernmental organization reports, academic studies, and reports and data provided by central statistical offices and ministries.

## 43. General government expenditure on health as percentage of total expenditure on health

## 44. General government expenditure on health as percentage of total government expenditure

## 45. External resources for health as percentage of total expenditure on health

## 46. Social security expenditure on health as percentage of general government expenditure on health

## 47. Out-of-pocket expenditure as percentage of private expenditure on health

## 48. Private prepaid plans as percentage of private expenditure on health

## 49. Per capita total expenditure on health at average exchange rate (US$)

## 50. Per capita government expenditure on health at average exchange rate (US$)

## 51. Per capita government expenditure on health at international dollar rate

Rationale for use: health financing is a critical component of health systems. National health accounts (NHA) provide large set of indicators based on the expenditure information collected within a internationally recognized framework. NHA are a synthesis of the financing and spending flows recorded in the operation of a health system, from funding sources to the distribution of funds across providers and functions of health systems and benefits across geographical, demographic, socioeconomic and epidemiological dimensions.

Definition: key indicators for which the data are available:

Level of **total expenditure on health** as % of GDP, and per capita health expenditures in US dollars and in international dollars.

Distribution of public and private sectors in financing health and their main components, such as:

- Extent of social and private health insurance

- Burden on households' through out-of-pocket spending

- Reliance on external resources in financing health

Associated terms:

**Gross domestic product** (GDP) is the value of all goods and services provided in a country by residents and non-residents. This corresponds to the total sum of expenditure (consumption and investment) of the private and government agents of the economy during the reference year.

**General government expenditure** (GGE) includes consolidated direct outlays and indirect outlays, such as subsidies and transfers, including capital, of all levels of government social security institutions, autonomous bodies, and other extrabudgetary funds.

**Total expenditure on health** (THE) is the sum of general government health expenditure and private health expenditure in a given year, calculated in national currency units in current prices. It comprises the outlays earmarked for health maintenance, restoration or enhancement of the health status of the population, paid for in cash or in kind

**General government expenditure on health** (GGHE) is the sum of outlays by government entities to purchase health care services and goods. It comprises the outlays on health by all levels of government, social security agencies, and direct expenditure by parastatals and public firms. Expenditures on health include final consumption, subsidies to producers, and transfers to households (chiefly reimbursements for medical and pharmaceutical bills). It includes both recurrent and investment expenditures (including capital transfers) made during the year. Besides domestic funds it also includes external resources (mainly as grants passing through the government or loans channelled through the national budget).

**Social security expenditure on health** (SSHE) includes outlays for purchases of health goods and services by schemes that are mandatory and controlled by government. Such social security schemes that apply only to a selected group of the population, such as public sector employees only, are also included here.

**External resources health expenditure** (ExtHE) includes all grants and loans whether passing through governments or private entities for health goods and services, in cash or in kind.

**Private health expenditure** (PvtHE) is defined as the sum of expenditures on health by the following entities:

**Prepaid plans** and risk-pooling arrangements (PrepaidHE): the outlays of private insurance schemes and private social insurance schemes (with no government control over payment rates and participating providers but with broad guidelines from government)

**Firms' expenditure on health**: the outlays by private enterprises for medical care and health enhancing benefits other than payment to social security or other pre-paid schemes.

**Non-profit institutions serving mainly households**: outlays of those entities whose status do not permit them to be a source of financial gain for the units that establish, control or finance them. This includes funding from internal and external sources.

**Household out-of-pocket spending** (OOPS): the direct outlays of households, including gratuities and in-kind payments made to health practitioners and to suppliers of pharmaceuticals, therapeutic appliances and other goods and services. This includes household direct payments to public and private providers of health care services, non-profit institutions, and non-reimbursable cost sharing, such as deductibles, copayments and fee for services.

**Exchange rate**: the annual average or year end number of units at which a currency is traded in the banking system.

**International dollars**: derived by dividing local currency units by an estimate of their Purchasing Power Parity (PPP) compared to the US dollar, i.e. the measure which minimizes the consequences of differences in price levels between countries.

Data sources & methods of estimation: about 100 countries either have produced full national health accounts or report expenditure on health to OECD. Standard accounting estimation and extrapolation techniques have been used to provide time series (1998-2004). Ministries of Health have responded to the draft updates sent for their inputs and comments.

For details on sources and methods see www.who.int/nha.

## 52. Coverage of vital registration of deaths

Rationale for use: health information is an essential component of health systems. The registration of births and deaths with causes of death, called "civil registration (vital registration)", is an important component of a country health information system.

Definition: percentage of estimated total deaths that are "counted" through civil registration system.

Methods of estimation: expected numbers of deaths by age and sex are estimated from current life tables, based on multiple sources. Reported numbers are compared with expected numbers by age and sex to obtain an estimate of coverage of the vital registration system.

## 53. Number of hospital beds per 10 000 population

Rationale for use: service delivery is an important component of health systems. To capture availability, access and distribution of health services delivery a range of indicators or a composite indicator is needed. Currently, there is no such data for the majority of countries. Inpatient beds density is one of the few available indicators on a component of level of health service delivery.

Definition: number of inpatient beds per 100 000 population.

Methods of estimation: empirical data only with possible adjustment for underreporting (e.g. missing private facilities).

# *Glossary*

Terms used in the African Regional Health Report

**Active surveillance**: a method of using outreach to identify cases that would be missed by passive case detection and reporting.

**Acute flaccid paralysis**: loss of power of voluntary movement in a muscle, with a loss of muscle tone and reflexes; can be associated with an infectious disease, usually viral in origin, that causes fever, pain and gastrointestinal symptoms; such as that caused by the poliovirus.

**Acute respiratory infection**: infection of the lungs or airways, usually caused by viruses or bacteria.

**Aflatoxins**: toxic metabolites of some fungi, which can cause disease in humans and animals eating peanut meal and other food contaminated by these fungi, and through long exposure, play a role in the etiology of acute hepatitis, and liver cancer in humans.

**Amodiaquine**: a drug used for treating malaria

**Anaemia**: insufficient concentrations of red blood cells or the haemoglobin that they contain; resulting in pallor, shortness of breath, palpitations, lethargy.

**Antenatal care**: care provided to mothers during pregnancy, which can include counselling about diet, hygiene, HIV status, birth preparedness, care and feeding of the newborn, and screening for, and treatment of, conditions such as anaemia, malnutrition, tuberculosis, malaria, hypertension and diabetes.

**Antiretrovirals**: drugs that are used for treating HIV infection; they work by preventing the virus from replicating.

**Artemether-lumefantrine**: an artemisinin combination treatment used for malaria.

**Artemisinin combination therapies (ACTs)**: drugs used for the treatment of malaria, one of the active ingredients of which is extracted from the plant *Artemesia annua* (also known as sweet wormwood or Qinghao).

**Bacteria**: a one-celled organism that usually multiplies by cell division; smaller than parasites and bigger than viruses.

**BCG vaccination (bacille Calmette–Guérin)**: a suspension of a weakened strain of *Mycobacterium tuberculosis*, which is inoculated into the skin to prevent tuberculosis.

**Blood alcohol concentration**: the amount of alcohol present in the bloodstream, usually measured in milligrams per decilitre (mg/dl).

**Body mass index**: a person's weight in kilos, divided by height in metres squared. Less than 18.5 is considered underweight, 20–25 normal, 25.0–29.9 overweight, more than 30 obese, and more than 40, very obese.

**Bronchitis**: inflammation of the airways of the lung.

**Buruli ulcer**: an ulcer of the skin with widespread necrosis of subcutaneous fat, due to infection with *Mycobacterium ulcerans*; named after the Buruli district in Uganda where it was first described.

***Campylobacter***: bacteria that can cause acute gastroenteritis in people with sudden onset of diarrhoea, muscle and joint pains, and headache.

**Cancer**: a general term for any of various types of malignant growths, most of which invade surrounding tissues, metastasize to distant sites in the body, recur after attempted removal, and cause death of the patient unless adequately treated.

**Cardiovascular diseases**: diseases of the heart and blood vessels that include strokes, hypertension, heart attacks, etc.

**Case management**: treatment of the individual patient, in contrast to population-based approaches.

**Cervical cancer**: a malignant disease of the neck of the uterus.

**Chemoprophylaxis**: prevention of a disease by the use of drugs.

**Child mortality rate**: measured by the probability (per 1000 live births) of a child born in a specific year dying before reaching 5 years of age.

**Cholera**: an acute epidemic infectious disease caused by *Vibrio cholerae*, causing profuse watery diarrhoea, dehydration and collapse.

**Choloroquine**: a drug used for treating malaria.

**Conflict resources**: natural resources such as gold, oil, timber, diamonds, that provoke and finance war.

**Contagious**: transmitted by contact

**Corruption**: the process of changing for the worse, particularly in a moral sense, as by bribing.

**Cost-effectiveness**: the amount of value for money that a particular intervention gives.

**Cysticercosis**: disease caused by the larvae of tapeworms encysting in humans.

**DALY**: Disability-adjusted life year; a unit for measuring the burden of disease —calculated as the sum of the years of life lost due to premature mortality and disability in the population.

**Demography**: the study of populations, especially with reference to birth, death and health of the people.

**DHS:** Demographic and health surveys, done by the Opinion Research Corporation (ORC Macro), are nationally-representative household surveys with large sample sizes (usually between 5000 and 30 000 households) that are used to obtain data on female population, health, and nutrition indicators.

**DHS+:** Demographic and health surveys that also collect data from men.

**DOTS**: a five-component strategy for tuberculosis control; including diagnosis by high-quality microscopy, political commitment, an assured supply of drugs, directly-observed treatment and systematic monitoring and accountability.

**Dracunculiasis**: guinea-worm disease: an infection with *Dracunculus medinensis*, a nematode similar to the filarial worms, that is acquired by humans drinking water containing cyclopoid copepods (water fleas) infected with guinea worm larvae. Human infection can be prevented by filtering drinking-water, preventing infected people from wading in the water, or vector control, by using insecticides to kill the water fleas.

**Emphysema**: an increase in the size of the distal air spaces in the lung, causing breathlessness.

**Epidemic**: an outbreak of an illness, or specific health-related behaviour in a community or a region that is clearly in excess of that normally encountered.

**Epilepsy**: a chronic disorder comprising seizures or fits due to bursts of neuronal discharge in the brain.

**Escherichia coli (E-coli)**: a species of bacteria that is normally found in the intestines, and can cause urinary tract infections and diarrhoea, particularly in children, and travellers.

**Essential medicines**: drugs that are determined by the WHO Expert Committee on the Selection and Use of Essential Medicines to be required for the basic health needs of a population.

**Famine**: severe general shortage of food usually caused by population explosion or failure of food crops.

**Fertility rate**: the number of live births in a year divided by the number of females of child-bearing age.

**Foodborne disease**: infections or toxic reactions that are spread by eating contaminated food.

**Gender equality**: a state of even balance and access to societal rights and privileges between men and women.

**Generic drugs**: drugs that not protected by trademark or sold as a specific brand; non-proprietary.

**Governance**: the exercise of political, economic and administrative authority in the management of a country's affairs at all levels: the complex mechanisms, processes, relationships and institutions through which citizens articulate their interests, exercise their rights and obligations and mediate their differences.

**Health systems**: the people, institutions and resources that serve to improve the health of the population, by helping people to avoid ill-health and treating disease.

**Health workers**: people with specific training and a recognized role in the provision of health care.

**Health-for-all**: the attainment by all the people of the world of a level of health that will permit them to lead socially and economically productive lives.

**Heart disease**: commonly used term that encompasses diseases of the muscle, blood vessels, or envelopes of the heart — including ischaemia, myocardial infarction, angina pectoris, arrhythmias, hypertension and heart failure.

**Hepatitis**: inflammation of the liver, usually caused by a viral infection, or toxic agents; including alcohol and drugs. Hepatitis A virus is spread by contact with faeces or blood, most often through the ingestion of contaminated food. Hepatitis B virus is shed through blood, semen, vaginal secretions and saliva; symptoms can develop after an incubation period that may be as long as six months; and people may remain asymptomatic carriers; a leading cause of chronic liver disease, cirrhosis, and liver cancer. An effective vaccine exists. Hepatitis C virus is spread mainly through blood transfusion and can cause cirrhosis, liver failure, and liver cancer.

**HIV/AIDS**: human immunodeficiency virus is the causative agent and acquired immunodeficiency syndrome is the disease that it causes. A fatal, incurable disease of humans that includes a constellation of relatively specific infections and cancers that result from the selective destruction of part of the human immune system by the virus.

**Hookworm**: common name for bloodsucking round worms of the family Ancylostomatidae, and the infection that it causes in humans, with anaemia as its main consequence.

**Human *Papillomavirus***: certain types of this virus cause cutaneous and genital warts in humans, including verruca vulgaris and condyloma acuminatum, other types cause cervical intraepithelial neoplasia; accounting for about 80% of cervical cancer and anogenital and laryngeal carcinomas.

**Human resources**: the people that make up the workforce.

**Humanitarian emergencies**: a situation in which the quality and/or continuation of people's lives are gravely endangered.

**Hypertension**: blood pressure consistently exceeding 160 mm Hg (systolic) and 95mm Hg (diastolic).

**Incidence**: the number of instances of illness commencing, or of persons falling ill, during a given period in a specified population; the number of new events, such as the new cases of a disease in a defined population, within a specific period of time.

**Infectious**: a disease that is caused by transmission of a specific pathogenic agent or its toxic products from an infected person, animal, or reservoir to a susceptible host.

**Infrastructure**: the permanent services and equipment such as roads, railways, bridges, factories and schools, needed for a country to be able to function properly.

**Insecticide**: any natural or manufactured substance that is used to kill insects.

**Insecticide-treated nets (ITN)**: mesh fabric that is soaked in a solution of chemicals designed to kill the insects that land on them; usually intended to be hung over sleeping people to protect them from the night-biting mosquito that carries malaria.

**Intermittent preventive treatment**: the practice of giving drugs at regular intervals to a defined population at risk in an area of endemic disease (regardless of whether the individual is already infected or not), in order to prevent the worst effects of this disease.

**Isoniazid**: a drug used to treat tuberculosis

**Ivermectin**: a drug used to decrease the complications and transmission of filarial diseases.

**Know–do gap**: the difference between current knowledge on a subject and what is actually done in practice.

**Knowledge management**: the handling of a set of principles, tools and practices that enable people to create, share, translate and apply what they know in order to improve effectiveness and create value.

**Larvicide**: a compound that is toxic to the stage of the insects at which they are immature, but capable of independent life

**Macroeconomics**: the study of economics on a large scale such as the nation as a whole, taking into account trade, national income, output and exchange rates, and financial policy.

**Malaria**: a parasitic disease caused by *Plasmodium* species, transmitted to humans by the bite of the female *Anopheles* mosquito; fever and anaemia are its main signs.

**Malnutrition**: various disorders resulting from inadequate food intake, an unbalanced diet (lack of protein or vitamins) or an inability to absorb nutrients from food.

**Market restrictions**: legislation covering the amount and type of trading that a country is allowed to legally pursue.

**Measles:** a contagious eruptive fever with coryza and catarrhal symptoms, caused by a virus, with about a two-week incubation period. An effective vaccine exists.

**Microbicide gel**: a gel that is formulated to destroy microbes, and designed to be used in the vagina or rectum to prevent the transmission of sexually transmitted infections.

**MICS:** Multiple Indicator Cluster Surveys — household surveys developed by UNICEF specifically to gather information on the status of women and children to measure progress towards the World Summit for Children goals.

**Mop-up campaign**: in immunization programmes, when a case of the disease is detected, a concerted effort is made to immunize all susceptible individuals in the immediate vicinity within a very short space of time.

**Morbidity**: the condition of being diseased, or sick; also the amount of sickness and disease caused by a particular agent or condition.

**Mortality rate**: the ratio of the number of people dying in a year to the total mid-year population in which the deaths occurred.

**Multidrug-resistant tuberculosis:** disease caused by strains of *M. tuberculosis* that are resistant to rifampicin and isoniazid, irrespective of resistance to other standard antituberculosis drugs.

**Mycobacteria**: slender, Gram-positive, acid-fast microorganisms resembling, and including, the bacillus which causes tuberculosis.

**Neonatal mortality rate**: the number of deaths in infants under 28 days of age in a given period, usually a year, per 1000 live births in that period.

**Noma (cancrum oris)**: a severe infection causing gangrene of the oral and facial tissues, usually occurring in debilitated patients or malnourished children; has a very poor prognosis.

**Noncommunicable disease**: a disease that is not transmitted to or between people, and does not have an infectious cause.

**Obesity**: the condition of being overweight to an unhealthy extent: for adults, a body-mass index equal to, or greater than 30.

**Onchocerciasis**: also known as river blindness; infection with filarial worms that live and breed in the nodules under the patient's skin, and can cause blindness. Transmitted by biting blackflies that breed on rocks in turbulent river water.

**Oral rehydration therapy (ORT)**: a water, salt and sugar mixture used for treating dehydration.

**Overweight**: a body mass index equal to or great than 25 in adults.

**Pandemic**: a widespread epidemic disease

**Parasite**: a plant or animal which lives upon or within another living organism at whose expense it obtains some advantage without compensation.

**Patent protection**: an official licence from the government granting a person or business the sole right for a certain period, to make and sell a particular article.

**Pesticides**: a compound used to destroy pests of any sort; including fungicides, herbicides, insecticides, rodenticides etc.

**Performance indicators:** (used for assessing polio surveillance) all three of which need to be reached for a region to be declared free of polio:

1. Every year, countries must report at least 1 case of acute flaccid paralysis that is not caused by polio, per 100 000 population aged <15 years.

2. Countries must collect adequate stool specimens from at least 80% of reported cases of acute flaccid paralysis.

3. All acute flaccid paralysis stool specimens must be analysed in laboratories accredited by WHO.

**Philanthropic**: practically benevolent towards mankind.

***Pneumocystis jiroveci***: the microorganism that causes pneumocystis pneumonia in debilitated patients.

**Poliomyelitis (polio)**: an acute viral disease characterized clinically by fever, sore throat, headache and vomiting, often with stiffness of the head and back, that may lead to involvement of the central nervous system with meningitis, destruction of the anterior horn cells of the spinal cord, and paralysis. An effective vaccine exists.

**Poverty**: poverty is pronounced deprivation in well-being. It is associated not only with insufficient income or consumption but also with insufficient outcomes with respect to health, nutrition, and literacy, and with deficient social relations, insecurity, and low self-esteem and powerlessness. Defined by the World Bank as having an income of less than US$ 1 per day.

**Poverty reduction**: actions — usually country's macroeconomic, structural and social policies and programmes — to promote economic growth and reduce poverty, as well as associated external financing needs. The Poverty Reduction Strategy Papers, prepared by governments through a participatory process involving civil society and development partners, including the World Bank and the International Monetary Fund (IMF) are presently the principal instruments for combating poverty in many low-income countries.

**Poverty trap**: [Often] extreme poverty that is pervasive and persistent, a situation from which many cannot escape without external assistance.

**Prevalence**: the number of cases of a disease in existence at a certain time in a designated area.

**Prevalence of contraceptive use**: the proportion of acts of sexual intercourse in which means to prevent conception and/or sexually transmitted infection are used.

**Psychosis**: any mental disorder characterized by delusion and/or prominent hallucinations to the extent that this disorder grossly interferes with the capacity to meet ordinary demands of life.

**Public–private partnerships**: arrangements between governments and industry to combine funding and skills in an effort to address specific problems.

**Rifampicin**: a drug used for treating tuberculosis.

**Roundworm**: members of the phylum Nematoda; *Ascaris* is the genus that causes the most infections in humans, and is acquired by ingesting eggs of the parasite in contaminated soil. The infection causes damage to the lungs when the larvae migrate through the body, intestinal colic due to large masses of adult worms in the intestines, these masses can also cause complications such as volvulus, intestinal obstruction or intussusception.

**Rumble strips**: a series of indented or raised elements on a road to alert drivers to reduce speed.

**Salmonella**: rod-shaped, Gram-negative bacteria that include the typhoid–paratyphoid bacilli, and that can cause violent painful diarrhoea.

**Saturated fat**: a fatty acid whose carbon chain contains no double or triple bonds between the carbon atoms. It is the main dietary cause of high levels of blood cholesterol.

**Scaling up**: growth in size, number and activities of organized initiatives, particularly to reach more people.

**Schistosomiasis**: a variety of infections caused by blood flukes, which are transmitted to humans by exposure to infested water. The three main forms of infection — urinary, intestinal or hepatosplenic — vary with the species of schistosome but result mostly from reactions to the eggs deposited in tissues.

**Schizophrenia**: a mental disorder which tends to be chronic, impairs functioning and includes psychotic symptoms involving disturbances of thought, perception, feeling and behaviour.

**Screening**: the systematic application of a test or enquiry, to identify individuals at sufficient risk of a specific disorder, who may benefit from further investigation or direct preventive action without having sought medical attention on account of any symptoms of that disorder.

**Shigella**: bacteria that are the usual cause of dysentery with painful bloody diarrhoea and fever; spread by the faecal oral route, contaminated food and objects, and by flies as mechanical vectors.

**Sickle cell disease**: a chronic haemolytic anaemia, characterized by sickle-shaped red blood cells due to homozygous inheritance of haemoglobin S.

**Skilled birth attendance**: the practice of having a specifically trained health worker (doctor, nurse or midwife) to assist during labour and delivery, irrespective of where the birth actually occurs.

**Smoke hoods**: a metal frame designed to draw smoke away from an open fire towards a chimney or other outlet as part of a passive extraction system.

**Social protection schemes**: arrangements for payment of an amount of money in the event of illness, injury or death, particularly for people too poor to be able to pay the premium for individual insurance contracts.

**STEPS**: Stepwise approach to surveillance. A simple standardized method for collecting, analysing and disseminating data for noncommunicable disease risk factors (www.who.int/ncd_surveillance/ steps/riskfactor/en).

**Stroke**: a sudden and severe attack caused by acute vascular lesions of the brain, such as haemorrhage, thrombosis or embolism, with functional consequences depending on the location and the extent of the lesion.

**Stunted:** not having gained full growth or development; used specifically to mean a child that is less than two standard deviations from the mean height for his or her age, due to chronic malnutrition.

**Sulfadoxine–pyrimethamine**: a long-acting sulfonamide used in combination with pyrimethamine to reduce the relapse rate of malaria.

**Sustainable development**: the use of natural resources to support human endeavour at a rate, and by methods that do not irreparably deplete or damage the source.

**Syphilis**: a contagious systemic disease caused by the spirochete *Treponema pallidum*, that can affect all organs; characterized by three clinical stages, and years of asymptomatic latency. Easily prevented and treated in its early stages by penicillin.

**Tapeworm**: a parasitic intestinal cestode worm; most human infections are caused by either *Taenia solium* (acquired by eating undercooked pork) or *Taenia saginata* (aquired by eating undercooked beef); only the former can cause cysticercosis in humans, while there are few symptoms that can be reliably attributed to the presence of the adult worms in the intestines.

**Tetanus**: an acute infectious disease caused by a toxin produced in the body by the bacteria *Clostridium tetani*, caused by soil contaminating wounds; resulting in muscular rigidity and spasms; when the respiratory muscles are involved, patients die from asphyxia. An effective vaccine exists.

**Trade tariffs**: the tax or duty to be paid on a particular class of imported or exported goods.

**Traditional birth attendants**: women usually with no formal training, who act as midwives; assisting women during labour and delivery.

**Trypanosomiasis**: in Africa, a fatal infection caused by *Trypanosoma brucei gambiense* or *T. brucei rhodesiense* that is transmitted by the bite of the tsetse flies; also called sleeping sickness.

**Tuberculin test**: a test for tuberculosis, consisting of the subcutaneous injection of 5 mg of tuberculin. The test has no effect in healthy people, but usually causes inflammation at the site of the injection in people that are infected.

**Tuberculosis**: an infectious disease caused by *Mycobacterium tuberculosis*, spread by inhalation, ingestion or inoculation, characterised by an initial predilection for the lungs, although tubercles may form in any organ

**Typhoid**: a disease with fever and rash due to infection with *Salmonella typhi*.

**Urbanization**: the process of making a district less rural and more town-like.

**Vaccine**: any preparation whose administration is intended for the prevention, amelioration or treatment of infectious diseases by stimulating the formation of antibodies to specific pathogens or toxins.

**Vector control**: control of the carrier, especially an animal, (usually an arthropod; mosquito, flea, fly, tick), which transfers an infective agent from one host to another.

**Vector-borne disease**: a disease that is transmitted by an animal, such as an insect, that transfers the pathogen from one organism to another, for example, from animal to humans, usually without itself contracting the disease.

**Verbal autopsy**: the recounting of events that surrounded the death of a person, usually by someone who has no formal health training, used as a means to attribute the cause of death in places where traditional postmortems are not practicable.

**Virus**: a minute infectious agent that can only replicate within living host cells

**Vital registration**: the process of collecting, by civil records, enumeration, or indirect estimation, data on the frequency of the occurrence of important events in human life including birth, death, fetal death, marriage, divorce, annulment, judicial separation, adoption, legitimation and recognition.

**Vitamin A supplements**: doses of the organic substance, usually present in minute amounts in natural foodstuffs, given to treat

or prevent a deficit that can lead to night blindness, xerophthalmia, dermatosis, susceptibility to infection and retarded growth.

**Wasted**: having lost flesh or strength, emaciated; abnormally thin from extreme loss of flesh; particularly a child who is less than 2 standard deviations from the mean weight for height.

Sources:

Chalmer's Dictionary. Larousse. 1995.

Dorland's Illustrated Medical Dictionary 24th ed. W.B. Philadelphia and London: Saunders Company, Philadelphia and London; 1965.

Last JM (editor). A dictionary of epidemiology. 2nd ed. Oxford: Oxford University Press; 1988.

Obesity: preventing and managing the global epidemic. Report of a WHO Consultation. WHO Technical Report Series 894. Geneva: World Health Organization, 2000.

World Health Organization. Health Promotion Glossary whqlibdoc.who.int/hq/1998/WHO_HPR_HEP_98.1.pdf

*World health statistics 2006.* Geneva: World Health Organization; 2006.

*World health report 2001 — mental health: new understanding, new hope.* Geneva: World Health Organization; 2001.